Parenting
Begins Before
Conception

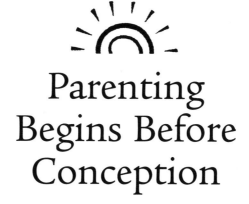

Parenting Begins Before Conception

A GUIDE TO PREPARING BODY, MIND, AND SPIRIT

FOR YOU AND YOUR FUTURE CHILD

Carista Luminare-Rosen, Ph.D.

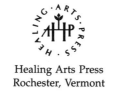

Healing Arts Press
Rochester, Vermont

Healing Arts Press
One Park Street
Rochester, Vermont 05767
www.InnerTraditions.com

Healing Arts Press is a division of Inner Traditions International

*Note to the reader: This book is intended as an informational guide. The remedies,
approaches, and techniques described herein are meant to supplement, and not to be
a substitute for, professional medical care or treatment. They should not be used to treat
a serious ailment without prior consultation with a qualified health care professional.*

Library of Congress Cataloging-in-Publication Data

Luminare-Rosen, Carista.
    Parenting Begins before Conception : a guide to preparing body, mind,
and spirit : for you and your future child / Carista Luminare-Rosen.
        p. cm.
    Includes bibliographical references and index.
    ISBN 0-89281-827-1 (alk. paper)
        1. Parenting—Religious aspects. 2. Pregnancy—Religious aspects.
    3. Reincarnation. I. Title.

BL625.8 .L86 2000
649'.1'0242—dc21
                                                                99-089235

Printed and bound in Canada

10 9 8 7 6 5 4 3 2 1

Text design and layout by Rachel Goldenberg
This book was typeset in ITC Legacy Serif

Photographs for chapters 2 and 8 courtesy of Suzanne Arms
Photographs for chapters 1, 3, 5, 6, and 9 courtesy of Photodisc
Photograph for chapter 4 courtesy of Corbis
Photograph for chapter 7 courtesy of Superstock

To my precious and beautiful daughter, Kylea Sophia,
who truly inspired this book before she was conceived, and who
blesses my every moment with her delightful and loving being.
You have gifted me with the grace and marvel of motherhood and
affirmed my inner truth that parenting begins before conception.

To all of the unborn Souls who are choosing to incarnate to express
their divine nature in human form. May you find parents who
will honor your whole being—body, mind, and spirit.

To all of the parents who are choosing to care for the personality
and soul of their child, before and after conception.

To Shekinah, who reminds me to experience the Grand Mystery of Life.

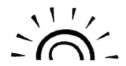

Contents

The Effects of Stress on Your Child in Utero
Nurturing Your Child's Personality Nature
Sacred Space: An Attitude for the Pregnant Mother
Creative Exercise: Optimizing Your Child's Prenatal Life

Acknowledgments

I am thankful for my beloved husband, Jared, who inspires me to be true to my Self as he always embraces me with his transformative love and bountiful wisdom.

I wish to acknowledge my mother and father, Mary Alice Borg and Donald Borg, for their lifelong love and wisdom, and for their willingness to heal and nurture our relationship, so that the challenges of the past have become a healthy, vibrant love for one another in the present.

Heartfelt gratitude to my agent, Stephanie Evans, who generously devoted her time and effort to be the literary midwife for the birth of this book. Without her to guide me through the labor and delivery, this book would still be gestating in the womb of the computer. Her compassionate wisdom and dedicated support permeate this book.

To all of my many teachers, healers, colleagues, friends, and clients who taught me the provocative power of self-healing, self-love, self-understanding, inner wisdom—and the truth of the soul and the glory of Spiritual Being.

To Laura Uplinger, my very own cosmic cheerleader, who has always shared the ideal vision of parenthood with me, and who inspires me to trust my ideal and to live it fearlessly.

To Steven Sevigny and Za Luminare for the eternal journey of our multidimensional mastery and illumination.

To Peter Gold, an effulgent fountain of inspired support, cheerfulness, and creativity.

To Shoshana Alexander, who understood my vision for this book and guided me at an auspicious moment of its unfoldment.

To Roxanne Schwabe, whose ability to creatively translate my soul purpose into brochures, newsletters, and illustrations has always been deeply appreciated.

To Kate Rabinowitz, whose generosity supported the vision of this book almost two decades ago during its preconception preparation.

To Niravi Payne, who boldly affirms the healing power of revealing the mother-father wound within each of us and of loving ourself whole.

To Angela Wu, whose profound knowledge in Chinese medicine has been a guiding light in my personal and professional life.

To Steven Katz, who taught me to respect the invaluable contribution of Western medicine as an ally for some couples preparing for parenthood.

To Thomas Verny, M.D., and David Chamberlain, Ph.D., whose pioneering work have continually inspired and empowered my soul purpose. As founders of the Association of Pre- and Perinatal Psychology and Health, they have gifted me and this world with profound and veritable research about the living reality of prebirth consciousness.

To Irene Young for her photographic "touch" and talent (and production efforts).

To Tami DeSellier for using her photographic magic to capture the front cover photo.

To John Paul, I offer profound gratitude for his extraordinary generosity and creative instinct in designing the front cover and supporting me to be true to my inner visions.

To those who gave freely of their love, inspiration, and support during critical phases of the book: Suellen Ehnebuske, Kathryn Darling, Marsha Podd, Joryel Vera, Alvita Soleil, Andrew Borg, Roberta "Sumitra" Godbe, and Mishi Silvia.

To my siblings, Douglas, Andrew, Jana, and Alexandra; I remain fascinated in discovering our souls' purpose to be related this lifetime.

To all those at Inner Traditions, who have wholeheartedly embraced the essence and form of this book. I thank Jon Graham, Rowan Jacobsen, Peri Champine, and Jeff Euber for their creative efforts and support. I am very grateful for the wisdom, warm heart, timely humor, and gracious guidance of my editor, Lee Juvan.

To the universal presence of the Divine Mother and Divine Father—and the eternal life that their union conceives. I am forever appreciative to the One Life that graces and impregnates all forms of creation.

Preface

The information and health care suggestions contained in this book are not intended to diagnose or prescribe, or to be used as a substitute for the information and care recommended by your medical or health care practitioner. I make no claims that following the suggestions in this text will provide any kind of cure. All information is for the purpose of inspiration, education, and assisting present and future parents in developing their own holistic model of preconception and prenatal health care.

This book will explore possibilities for your future child, who will be described in her many phases of development as a soul, a zygote, an embryo, a fetus, a prenate, a baby, a child, and an adult. Your child may be male or female. In honor of both sexes, and to avoid the inherent limitations of our language, I will alternate using masculine and feminine genders throughout each chapter.

Many times in this text I use the term *prospective parents*. Although the emphasis of my orientation is on those who are preparing for parenting their first child, all of the information can be applied to anyone preparing for a new human life, even those who have children already. Each child has unique needs, and it is never too early or late to begin caring for the whole health of any child—and the whole health of the parents as well.

In addition, much of the text assumes that preparing for a child involves a couple. Yet it is my experience that some children, after conception, are cared for only by the pregnant mother (whether she is single or not) before they are born. Also, given the popularity of in vitro procedures and sperm and egg donor availability, conception does not always require the sexual joining of a man and a woman. Some women are conceiving with the assistance of advanced technology—from in vitro fertilization to gamete intrafallopian transfer. Other women choose to pick up sperm at the donor center and insert it alone at home. In addition, some children are parented by two adults of the same sex.

Although in some sections I clearly specify a *female and male* partner preparing together, since a man and woman are essential for a natural human conception, the references to "prospective parents" throughout the text assume that there are two adults—most commonly a mother and father—who are choosing to be responsible for conceiving and caring for the incarnating child. However, I hope that anything I've written to be useful for couples can also be used by single parents, as well nontraditional couples, with similar benefits.

Whatever your religious choices and practices, the spiritual approaches I share in this book are meant to inspire all those who cultivate reverence for life.

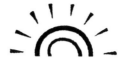

Introduction: Parenting Began Before Conception— My Personal Journey

There has been no experience more thrilling for me than giving birth to my daughter after ten years of preparation for her arrival in my life. I will never forget that slippery, wet body being laid across mine as we met each other after laboring together for a timeless day. Instantly, her brilliant and precious eyes reminded me that she was an ancient soul in a brand-new body and her innate nature was just as evolved as mine, if not more so. The human experience of giving birth to each other expanded into the profound realization that we were not only co-creating a new family as mother, father, and daughter, we were three great souls who were here to express our divine natures with each other in human form. The birth of Kylea was a human event, yet a deeply spiritual one as well.

This personal experience supported a premise I had been exploring for years. My daughter's birth was not the beginning of our relationship, it was just another natural phase of bonding that I had initiated more than a decade before as I consciously began my preparation process. It was so clear to me that the sweet being in my arms, who had many urgent primitive needs as a newborn, was also an old soul with specific reasons for choosing to be with me and my husband. Because we had been developing our psychic bond for many years through thought and feeling, I possessed the intuitive wisdom and confidence to care for her both as a newborn baby and as a magnificent spirit of light.

Just imagine if your parents had prepared for your arrival before you were even conceived or born. Can you imagine being part of a family in which your physical, emotional, mental, and spiritual needs had been consciously cared for from your first moments of life? So many of us have suffered because our parents did not understand that we were powerful souls reappearing as children, and that we depended upon our mothers and fathers to create the optimal life circumstances for us to embody our spirits in human form.

An infant arrives fresh from the spiritual realms and depends on his parents to honor and actively nurture his virtuous soul nature from the beginning of his life. But the Western human family has yet to embrace the ancient—and practical—wisdom of reincarnation and soul development. It is, however, an extraordinary time on our planet. As we come to understand the multidimensional dynamics of our sacred origin and of birth, we become able to include the revelations of the great mystical teachings in our preparation for the greatest of human tasks: readying ourselves for parenthood.

Consider that at conception, your future child is biologically enfolding ancient cosmic mysteries within herself.

Did you know that reincarnation principles can help you optimize the whole health of your child—in very practical ways—before he is conceived, and throughout his prenatal development? Are you curious to discover how angels are actually co-creating your child with you? Has anyone ever suggested to you that you can learn to bond with your child before he is conceived or born? Are you interested in creating your own custom-designed preconception and prenatal birth plan? This book can help you prepare for your child in ways you may never have imagined.

Before we take this journey into parenthood together, I would like to share with you my personal experience, which clearly showed me that parenting begins before conception.

In my early twenties I began individual therapy to deal with issues raised when my parents divorced after thirty years of marriage. It was during this quest for personal growth that the seed of my life's work was planted in me. During therapy, vivid birth and prenatal memories spontaneously occurred to me. In these sessions it became clear to me that the origin of some of my lifelong beliefs as an adult had begun in the womb. I know my mom did her very best with the limited knowledge she had regarding my prenatal needs. Like most women of her generation, she had no understanding that consciousness existed in the first trimester. Yet in spite of her love, I was affected by some of her subtle unconscious choices. In healing several experiences of my intrauterine life and of my birth experience, my present life became healthier.

In 1979 I learned about the Rebirthing Method, which was being introduced around the country. Rebirthing offered adults simple techniques to consciously access their prebirth memories. I studied and followed the work of one of the method's international pioneers, Sondra Ray. As I explored her method, I began to recall primal sensations of my physical conception experience. In addition, I occasionally glimpsed what appeared to be memories of past lives, as well as impressions of my existence in the soul planes without a physical body!

I shared my process with my mother, hoping my memories—particularly about my prenatal life and birth—might correspond with her own. It was remarkable how many of my insights did agree with her recollections of that time. In 1980 my research became especially exciting when I learned of a new book called *The Secret Life of the Unborn Child* by Thomas Verny, M.D. Verny pioneered the educational movement in this country that introduced prenatal psychology to the mainstream public. In his book Verny offered many cross-cultural scientific studies supporting what I had experienced internally for years. He provided the scientific substantiation that the unborn child is a feeling, experiencing, remembering being who responds to, and is deeply influenced by, her environment. Verny revealed that our personalities and psychological predispositions can be influenced before birth, and he offered compelling case studies to illustrate his findings.

The creative seed in me was growing fast in the richness of my awakening inner life. I began to share my insights with friends, to whom I gave healing sessions based on my personal work; within several years I had a thriving counseling practice.

My growing business, however, proved not an end but only a means, leading me to an important discovery and my real work. One afternoon, sitting across from yet another talented, competent, yet unfulfilled client, I had an "Aha." Many of the creative individuals I was working with were spending their adult years healing themselves from childhood trauma, which often began before birth.

The profoundly debilitating effect of childhood wounds on ego development was not an original insight; Sigmund Freud, William James,

Virginia Satir, John Bradshaw, and other great psychologists had developed numerous models to explain the cumulative effect of childhood experience on adult personality disorders. Yet many of these theorists did not consider that some psychological dysfunction can begin before the child is born—often, even at the time of conception. Nor did most human development models and psychological assessment procedures include the soul nature and those life lessons of the struggling adult originating in *past life* circumstances. Child development models were based on the evolution of the ego, with little regard for awakening to and integrating the soul identity with the human personality.

I began to realize that something fundamental was missing in the fabric of the family and education system. Why should most adults spend the core of their creative life *in reaction to the effects of their childhood experiences and traumas?* Most were identified with the pain of the past and had little, if any, understanding of their soul identity. Though I personally had very loving, educated, and concerned parents, I was not exempt. I was a memory bank of early-life experiences that were still creating dysfunctional patterns in my life. I intuitively knew that I was more than my limited sense of self, but all my years of education, including four years as a psychology major at Harvard University, never gave me the understanding that I was in fact a soul, experiencing life through a human personality. I identified with my human struggles, totally disconnected from my divine self. I had no notion that perhaps my life reflected karmic conditions that I had chosen to experience before I was even conceived by my parents.

In the American culture my experience was clearly the norm. What was profoundly lacking in our social consciousness, and within me, was an awareness that above all we are souls trying to radiate freely through our human bodies and minds. My own healing process, as well as my therapeutic work with many other intelligent adults, led me to develop a holistic model that can help prevent an incoming child from experiencing unnecessary trauma and can facilitate the awakening and integration of the soul with the human personality. Using this model, the child can remain connected to his spiritual identity throughout life. To care for a human life before it has even been created can become a realistic goal of prospective parents, and a basic building block to any holistic health care system.

Prenatal research has revealed that the child in the womb can be seriously endangered if the mother abuses her own health during pregnancy. Likewise, if the mother feels chronic ambivalence about having the child, this neglect and lack of prenatal bonding can have a significant negative impact on the child's sense of self for her entire life. Verny's studies, as well as numerous others, suggest that childhood abuse and neglect actually can begin in the womb, at the moment of conception. Thus, prospective parents who think their child is impervious to the prenatal environment need to understand the harm they may be doing their child in her earliest moments of ensoulment.

In this book you will read about some of your child's prebirth needs—for his body, mind, and spirit—as well as ways to address them during this early developmental period. You might, for example, consider that *parenting begins the moment you make any conscious effort to care for your own health* in preparation for enhancing your child's conception. Your preparation for parenthood will support the overall health of the soul who has chosen you to nurture its life on earth.

As the holistic health movement continues to gain momentum and the wisdom of preventive medicine is finally being recognized, we cannot afford to overlook health care surrounding the beginning of life. My passion for developing a holistic *preconception* health care model is further inspired by a clear vision that it will have a profound impact on the health care system at large. If a child begins life with parents who care for her whole health, she will innately know the elements for creating a life of well-being. And since each and every human being is conceived and born, this potential crosses all cultural barriers. It is the ultimate in holistic preventive medicine.

The PreSeeding Birth Program

It is every child's birthright to have a family and culture that support his essential nature. But how do we create this? Many years ago I began inquiring: When does consciousness begin? Before or after conception? When does human life begin? Can parent-child bonding begin before conception or birth? What can parents specifically do to prepare for their child before he is born? Can a parent assist in the child's emotional and mental health before he is conceived? Do children "choose" their parents? Are there practical applications to the ageless wisdom teachings about reincarnation? Who or what is responsible when a prebirth or early-childhood dysfunctional pattern is experienced by a child—is it genetics, karma, parents, the soul, society? And then I asked the most exciting question: *If unhealthy parenting has such a negative impact on adult personality, is there, conversely, a preventive holistic model for parenting that can produce positive, healthy children and adults?* The answer for me was the program I developed called PreSeeding Birth. This program offers parents ways to honor the full potential of the child and inspires them to begin this process *preceding birth*, ideally before conception.

The PreSeeding Birth Program integrates the psychosocial concerns of the past decade's recovery movement, which work to heal transgenerational patterns within family systems, into a holistic prebirth health care approach so that children need not be wounded at all. Aided by the universal guidelines of the PreSeeding Birth Program, prospective parents—both couples and singles—have learned how to optimize the physical, psychological, and spiritual health of their future children before or soon after conception. Nearly all have given birth to beautiful and healthy newborns who continue to radiate love and life because they are born to parents *who have already been caring for and loving them.*

In 1984 I founded the Center for Creative Parenting, where I shared my work with hundreds of women and couples who wanted to explore preconception and prenatal health ideas with me. Many of their stories are told in this book. In my work at the center I was challenged to find reliable resources that could explain, for example, the soul's journey; how a soul actually experiences reincarnating; how spirit moves from the soul to human cells. I wondered what were the ideal conditions that a soul might require from its parents to support the unfolding of its magnificent divinity. I sought detailed understanding of what a soul does to influence the development of its new human personality when it chooses to incarnate for another human life. And I really wanted to know whether a soul incarnates alone, or is assisted by other spiritual forces or entities such as angels, as it begins its descent into the human dimension of expression and experience.

Although exceptionally progressive in their perspectives, most Western prenatal researchers of the 1980s were not stating (or discovering) that consciousness exists before conception, because it is difficult to prove the subjective realms of the prephysical state. Therefore, I went to study the esoteric scriptures in India, where the subjective reality of the soul is commonly known and accepted by the entire culture. Talking to Vedic scholars in India, as well as Kabbala scholars in Israel, confirmed what I intuitively sensed: consciousness does indeed exist before physical conception. According to the Kabbala and Taoist, Vedic, and Theosophical texts, the soul evolves through multiple incarnations. I include this transpersonal perspective in my health care model.

This book, the natural child of my personal journey, my studies, and my work with many beautiful parents-to-be, includes both modern and ancient perspectives on preconception and prenatal health care. Each chapter explores the natural phases of becoming a parent—from preconception preparation to the moment of conception, then through the pregnancy, birth, and postnatal experiences. I will share with you how to prepare your own body, mind, and spirit before conceiving your baby. Then you will read about how to nurture the development of her physical, emotional, mental, and spiritual bodies—before, during, and after conception.

The book will help you clarify your purpose for preparing for parenthood, as well as the benefits of perceiving your future child as a multidimensional being. Like all creations of art, you and your child are unique. Being a fulfilled and healthy parent is a dynamic process of intentionally unfolding your inner wisdom and loving nature, and those of your child. You have many choices in how you conceive, perceive, and nurture your child. My hope is that this book offers some new understandings and useful guidelines to help you consciously and creatively prepare for a precious new life who will choose you as his parents. I invite you, even before conception, to prepare for and care for your child in ways that will honor his divine nature. Let this book be a companion in the beginning of your journey as a parent.

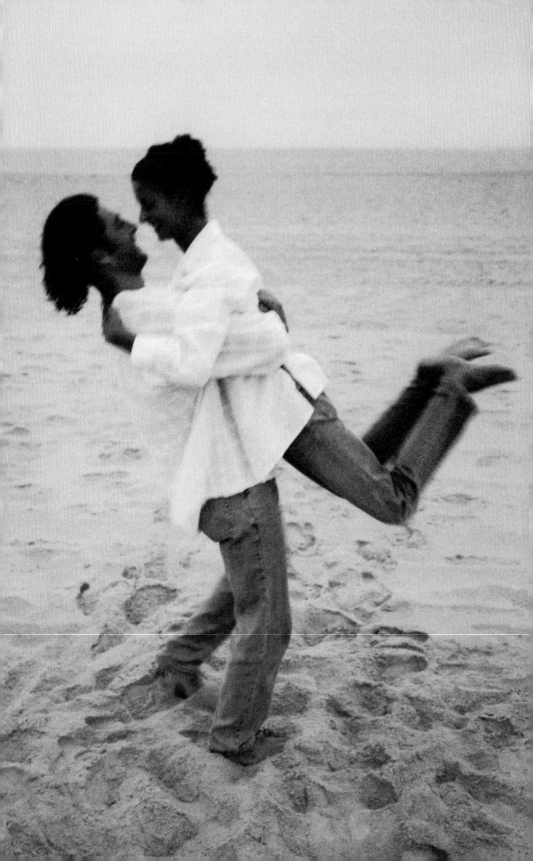

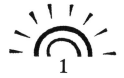

1

Why Prepare
for Parenthood?

*And what a splendid support for your child's wholeness when
you will recount to him with the smallest details the Great Story
of your preparation for him: running, singing, praying . . .
months or years before he came into the world!*

Laura Archer Huxley and Piero Ferrucci

For the past twenty years I have had the great honor of sharing with women and men specific ways that they can prepare for parenthood. In that time I have found that one of the greatest concerns of prospective parents is the dramatic stories they've heard from new parents about the overwhelming changes they had to make in their personal and professional lives after their child was born. Loss of freedom, changes in sexual patterns, and sleep deprivation can challenge the healthiest of couples, and the lack of a reliable support person can certainly exhaust a new single parent.

When my parenting center began offering New Baby and Mom support groups, I heard a recurring lament from the new moms: "Why didn't anyone tell me it would be this way? Why wasn't I told to *prepare* for becoming a parent?" Since in our culture it's not unusual to enter parenthood without any feelings of readiness, we could be led to think that preparation is unnecessary or even, perhaps, self-indulgent.

Yet those who began to explore their parenting concerns with me before or soon after conception have a noticeably different response. As JoEllen remembers:

> Johnny and I had looked at so many of our fears about parenthood before giving birth to our Miles that by the time he was born, we could more easily enjoy the wonder of his presence—unlike many of our friends, who were often on the verge of emotional breakdowns.

By knowing what to expect—first and foremost a major upheaval in sleeping, eating, and work routines, as well as in your intimacy and recreation patterns—you, as a *prepared* new parent, will be able to welcome the demands of your newborn as a natural progression of your life, rather than an overwhelming reality.

You do not know who your child may turn out to be. All the potentials of personality, the great virtues of love, wisdom, and creativity, as well as the potential for less endearing characteristics, exist in your future child. The seeds of consciousness that you plant at the time of conception and nurture thereafter can profoundly affect the incarnating soul's personality. During the hubbub of the twenty-four-hours-a-day responsibility of parenting, your baby will need you to remember that she has recently come from a heavenly realm. She will be an extraordinary miracle of life who has chosen you to be her primary physical, psychological, and spiritual provider and guide. Are you and your partner prepared to provide your child with healthy conditions that will allow her to harmoniously express and embody her true self from the first moments of life? There is so much you can do—even before conception—to become a confident and conscious parent.

The Link between Heaven and Earth

The soul that rises with us, our life's Star, hath
had elsewhere its setting, and cometh from afar.
Wordsworth

In our highly technological society great numbers of people are seeking to get more closely in touch with their inner spiritual beings. Many have discovered that the paths of Eastern and Western mysticism can offer useful guidelines for self-actualization and spiritual understanding. It is exciting that now many of us are beginning to see the experiences of pregnancy and parenting as opportunities for our own psychological and spiritual growth. Parents can not only integrate their personal spiritual development with their own relationship but also see it color the everyday events of relating to their child—before and after birth.

The conception of your child occurs at the moment a sperm fuses with an egg. Yet remember that this biological union is imbued with sacred mystery. It is at the auspicious moment of fertilization that the soul of your child will begin its descent from the subtle levels of the spiritual realms into its unfolding mortal body. For the spiritually oriented couple, conception can be a divine experience, a union with God.

You, the chosen parents, are re-creating the act of divine creation that has occurred throughout eternity. You are the link between heaven and earth for your destined child, as you reproduce the miracle of spirit to matter. It is your sperm or egg, your body and soul, the relationship and home environment that you have created, that allow the soul to transport itself into your world.

I wrote in my journal after the conception of my daughter:

> Holy temple, am I, as egg-woman ovulates to meet in sacred dance with sperm-man. Weaving their ancestral tapestries of life as DNA merges with Spirit, and Eternal Life springs forth in my belly like a pure Fountain of Youth. Primordial oceans wash across the shore of my womb as my blood becomes the lifeline for a Holy One who resides both in Heaven and on Earth simultaneously. My breath softens into my rounding body as I unify my every action to nurture this consciousness who has entrusted me to perfect the quality of my life so that it can grow its human form to match its Essence. . . . I blend and unify with the Universal Mother within me. The woman within knows it is okay to be human—to fear, tire, and feel nausea. This experience called pregnancy has been lived by countless women before me. . . . I am not the first to realize my own essential nature in the reflection of motherhood.

Since the subconscious mind of the fetus will store prenatal experiences, it becomes vital that the mother provides what I call "heavenly conditions." As the vessel for the soul, she can contemplate the gift of grace that her child is bestowing upon her. By the time the incoming soul is conceived as a physical being on earth, it has already been on a long spiritual journey from the heavenly realms.

During pregnancy, the mother shares her body with the developing fetus. The child within demands physical, psychological, and spiritual nutrients if he is to fulfill his potential from the beginning of life. Her mate is offered the opportunity to perceive the pregnant woman as an embodiment of the Divine Mother. For him, initiation into fatherhood is a psychological and spiritual rite of passage that forces him to redefine himself and reprioritize his goals. Jerry, for example, experienced a powerful identity shift when he learned that his wife was pregnant:

> During that initial moment when we discovered *we* were pregnant, I remember looking at my wife and seeing her in a totally new way. She instantly became the expression of the universal mother. . . . Her job was to nourish and protect our growing child within her sacred belly, while my responsibility was to nourish and protect her. From that day onward my own needs have remained important, but I always embrace those of my wife and child as equally important— frequently even more so. Becoming a family man has given me a new purpose in life.

Committing to parenthood means a willingness to be an ever-present source of love and wisdom, as well as a commitment to the right use of will. Your relationship as a couple will have many opportunities to transform and mature as you learn that accepting responsibility for the care of a soul demands continual reevaluation of your choices—before, during, and after conception. Your purpose will be to assist the incarnating soul in the creation of its personality by empowering your child to express the Divine, and by nurturing your child's special qualities and capabilities to succeed in the world.

Throughout your preparation for conception and pregnancy, and even after the moment of birth, the incarnating soul of your child will be dispensing myriad blessings to you. Opportunities to express and embody unconditional love, patience, sacrifice, and health are infused in each moment of your child's development. Your child, an unfolding human being, is primarily a child of God, lent to you for a single lifetime. Therefore, both parents and child may be perceived as divine, and as the family emerges, the virtuous nature of each person is supported and encouraged.

As you prepare for parenthood, you will be invited to become consciously aware of the mysteries within conception, pregnancy, and birth. As spiritual guides to the incoming soul, it is your consciousness and conduct that will enable your child to maintain an innate link to heaven while on earth.

The Benefits of a Psychologically Healthy Parent

It need not be said that preparing for parenthood is a major life initiation. It is a personal and provocative journey and involves much soul searching. When combining a holistic health perspective with preconception health care, your psychological wellness is as important as that of your body and spirit. Standing on the threshold of parenthood creates a powerful opportunity to explore the unresolved psychological themes of your own childhood, as well as a precious time to contemplate the future emotional and mental concerns of becoming a mom or dad.

This is an invaluable moment to explore your sense of yourself as a person, a partner, and a potential parent. It is important that *both* partners evaluate their psychological preparedness and the identity challenges of becoming a parent. All children greatly benefit when both parents respond to them as mature adults, rather than having to negotiate a psychological or emotional maze of one parent's inappropriate behavior.

To optimize your future child's whole health, it's important that you consider the soundness of your own self-esteem and self-expression. In addition to consistently wholesome dietary habits, you should have equal regard for the psychological nutrients you expose your child to as soon as she is conceived, and throughout her life.

Revisiting the Past

Your own personal history and that of your partner will color and shape your child's ability to develop a positive sense of self. For your child to achieve understanding of such issues as dependency, individuality, right use of will, self-love, and self-care, your guidance will be required.

Unless you develop the habit of acting consciously and with clarity, you may at times react to your child out of your own childhood wounds, embodying the same dysfunctional behavior that your parents may have expressed to you. When you respond to your child *consciously*, you are passing along behavior that is healthy and empowering.

Some confusion is natural. For example, the first time you consider disciplining your child, you may wonder whether you are controlling your child or your child is controlling you. The more you explore your own emotional temperament, as well as your and your partner's ethical beliefs, the less unhealthy psychological tendencies will be part of your relationship with your child.

Raising your child will constantly force you to revisit and reevaluate your own childhood. I am moved to share an experience that happened to me a few years ago. My sixteen-month-old daughter, Kylea Sophia, had been expressing her budding will more forcefully every day. She had taken to pulling herself onto the couch, where she jumped up and down with great glee—a stunt that was adorable, yet dangerous if she lost her balance and fell. She could not understand why I said *"no"* every time she had a joyful urge to stand up and bounce on the couch. It was painful for me as her mom to restrict her happy impulse, yet I felt she needed to learn that certain activities are too risky. As her parent, it is my responsibility to discipline her. But I was unclear how to assert my adult will without stifling her newly unfolding will. It was distressing to be stern with her, yet when I was gentle she just smiled at me and kept jumping.

I remembered, as a child, that there were times when I was disciplined by my parents without an explanation. Now, as an adult, I understand that my parents would never have intentionally hurt me; they just didn't know a better way. Yet as a child it was painful for me to not understand why my self-expression was being limited. I realized that this wound accounted for my resistance to disciplining Kylea with a firm no. When I took the time to explain to Kylea why I was restraining her—that I loved her delight in jumping, but I did not want her to hurt herself—she responded in a receptive way, and I felt clear and at peace with my no.

As you change your attitudes to embrace your child's point of view, the entire dynamic within yourself—and thus between you and your child—transforms, and your child will more easily be able to honor certain limitations requested of him. Your insights into your own childhood experiences become lessons you can use in parenting.

When you decide not to repeat your own childhood experience in your parenting, you need to separate your past from your child's present. For example, if you feel you were emotionally neglected as a baby by your mother and father, you may be emotionally overbearing with your child if your sole focus is on healing your own past. Remember that your child's emotional requirements are not the same as yours. They are unique.

For most of us, childhood was a mixture of positive and negative emotional input. Now, before you conceive your child, is the best time to consciously evaluate what qualities you hope to pass on to her and what you hope to leave behind. What unhealthy patterns do you hope to transcend? Which beneficial ones would you like to re-create? Many of your own psychological issues will not reveal themselves until your child is actually in your life and you hear yourself parroting your parents' hurtful words or are pleasantly surprised when an "inherited" attribute can be called upon to soothe.

It is your willingness to examine your personal history and make substantial changes to meet the authentic needs of your child's true self that will determine the quality of your parent-child bond and your child's sense of self. You will have endless opportunities to deeply heal some childhood wounds that you never knew needed your attention until you became a parent. Parenthood will be a continual journey into your past, a daily evaluation of your present responses, and a clear commitment to explore, heal, and transform future conflicts within and between you and your child.

Fusing and Separating Identities

Your child's identity will mingle with yours for the rest of your life, just as your parents' identities are integral to your sense of self. Numerous subconscious memories of yourself as a child will be activated unexpectedly in your daily experiences with your own son or daughter; you will probably see yourself in your child, and your parent in yourself, time and time again. Psychologically healthy parents do not misuse their child's life to settle their unresolved wounds. Rather, attentive parents are committed to using any remembered pain to remain consciously loving with their child, while seeking help from each other, friends, counselors, or support groups to heal reactive patterns that could potentially harm the child.

Many parents claim that their children mimic their moods; this emotional interdependency shapes not only the child's experience of the parent but also the parent's feelings about the child. Occasionally, an urge to unify with your child's emotional state will be totally appropriate, while at other times it can create confusion for one or both of you. You cannot depend on an infant to establish for himself the boundaries between healthy and dysfunctional behavior. He needs you to be consistent in your role as the adult, so if you feel childish in your communication with your child, be aware of how this may affect his ability to trust you as a reliable parent.

Being silly and expressing delight while playing with your child is a healthy expression of your childlike qualities. However, your own tantrum in reaction to your child's tantrum is not. It is part of human development for a toddler to express dissatisfaction or frustration—often loudly—as she explores her newfound personal will. But a mother or father who uses this technique leaves a child feeling unsafe and often frightened. Upset or anger with a child must be expressed so that her sense of security, trust, and unconditional love is not threatened. Make a commitment to being responsible in the way you express your emotions to your future child. Seek professional counseling if you sense that you will not be able to lovingly care for your child.

Tom's early parenting experience was an awakening for him and his wife:

> The first few months Sara and I parented Eric, it was a nonstop experience of love, love, love. Even the lack of sleep did not mar our feelings of absolute joy caring for his needs. Then, when he started to roll around, our control patterns got pushed. By the time he was crawling, and especially when he began to walk, I began to feel frustrated when he didn't listen to me or when he needed to be restrained from hurting himself.
>
> One day he tried to go out the front door, and he just cried and cried when we kept redirecting him. Then Sara expressed her fear that he was not learning to respect us, and I got upset with her. We were all out of control, bouncing off each other's anger. All of a sudden I looked down at Eric and he looked terrified—he had lost the emotional security of both his parents and he looked like an abandoned pup.
>
> Knowing Eric was showing us our own wounds, the very next day Sara and I returned to our couples therapist and discovered that we had all kinds of unresolved feelings about our parents' misguided discipline of us during our childhood. . . . Now, if Sara and I get triggered by Eric's reactions, we go to each other to work it out, while protecting him from our misplaced feelings.

A psychologically healthy parent can be responsive to a whole range of emotional highs and lows. For some, preparing to conceive is predominantly an intellectual experience. Once pregnancy has been confirmed, however, the emotional reactions can vary from elation and wonder to shock, disbelief, and anxiety. For the pregnant and postpartum mother, physical and hormonal changes will also continuously affect her mental state; feelings are often magnified, and her sensitive condition can directly affect her partner's moods. For both partners, having a baby will offer a full spectrum of feelings—losing control, feeling blessed, being consumed with fear, and feeling overwhelmed with love are all normal.

Bearing this in mind, the following questions can help you assess your psychological preparedness for all the emotional and mental nuances and upheavals you'll experience with the arrival of your child:

- How capable are you of loving a child under stressful conditions such as sleep deprivation, money challenges, lack of support from your partner, work deadlines, or social isolation?
- What will you do if you cannot resolve emotional conflicts with your partner that are affecting the health of your relationship, and your child?
- What are your choices if your childhood wounds cause you to react inappropriately to your child or partner?
- What is your capacity to distinguish beneficial from harmful behavior with your child?
- Based on your present habits, is your future child vulnerable to being physically or psychologically wounded by you? Be specific.
- What parts of your own relationship with your parents do you need to remain conscious not to repeat with your child?
- In what ways are you psychologically healthy to love and care for your child?

Even when you are a concerned, loving, and emotionally involved parent, there is no guarantee that your child will become the person you envision. Yet as the primary role model and guiding force for his formative years, it is your responsibility to evaluate and invest in your psychological health so that you can be counted on to preserve and protect his psychological well-being from the beginning of his life in the womb.

Endless Phases: New Opportunities to Learn and Grow

The first weeks after my daughter, Kylea, was born, I was overwhelmed with the many changes and challenges of parenthood, as well as the many adjustments that my baby was experiencing. Then I received a note from my older brother, who had become a father three weeks earlier. "Try not to take parenting so seriously," he wrote. "Everything is just a phase." This simple yet enlightening remark is a good reminder to all new parents. You and your child will continue to go through changes, and there will always be something new to learn.

Indeed, life as a parent is filled with many different phases, from the moment a child is conceived through each adjustment during pregnancy, birth, infancy, and beyond. Some of these conditions are brief, others more long lasting. Just when you master one, a growth spurt in your child will require you to explore and expand your parenting wisdom once again.

Let's look at some of the major phases that you can be aware of and prepare for as new parents.

- **Conception:** Your conscious exploration of the optimal conditions and time to conceive your child can include a complete review of your past relationship with your own parents, the strengths and weaknesses of your partnership, and the physical and psychological health of you and your partner. You may want to include the spiritual needs of your child as well.
- **Pregnancy:** Physical changes in the mother, such as nausea, sporadic body aches, astonishing food cravings, and broken sleep cycles, will have a profound impact on you and your partner as you readjust sleep and workloads (both professionally and at home) and give all due consideration to mood swings from intense hormonal fluctuations.
- **Giving Birth:** While this generally lasts no more than a day, the conscious preparation will take many weeks or even months. Discussing options—midwife, hospital, or a combination of both; breast-feeding; immunization; and circumcision—will present many learning opportunities. As you educate yourselves, you may find previously held philosophies challenged.
- **Coping with Fatigue:** One of the least-considered changes, which has an impact on both partners, fatigue can begin during pregnancy and frequently lasts throughout your child's infancy. Being aware of the likelihood of fatigue allows you to plan the sharing of necessary tasks accordingly.

- **Re-balancing Your Relationship:** Commonly, once your baby is born, sexuality and relationship changes as well as possible career and financial challenges will comprise a new phase that may shift and require continual conscious adjustment for years. Just as you have learned what your child needs to support one phase of his development, this knowledge will become obsolete as he changes his eating, sleeping, and playing requirements constantly.

It's important to remain flexible—that is, don't become attached to what you learned in one phase, which may not carry well into the next. And as my brother pointed out, remember that *everything* is a phase, so try not to take your parenting too seriously. There will be creative solutions and life lessons for all family members each step of the way. Even the most challenging phase, whether it lasts a moment, a day, a month, or years, will present you with new opportunities to improve the physical and psychological well-being of both yourselves and your child. One phase that will never end—that only grows each day—is experiencing the wonders of giving and receiving love.

Anticipate Lifestyle Changes Now

Once a child is born, changes are swift and may be overwhelming. Parenthood, partnership, career, and self-care become a balancing act. You'll find yourself trying to be your true self while being a reliable source of love for your family, a beloved to your partner, a friend to your community, and an effective professional in your career.

Making Things Work

Some employers are very supportive in offering flextime, while others are resistant to considering their employees' family responsibilities. Self-employed people have their own concerns; they commonly struggle to budget enough work time separate from their endless domestic responsibilities. Personal and professional routines often seem to blend into one large list of tasks whose priorities need to be continually assessed.

Keys to balancing your work with your new family will include:

- Considering your **willingness to sacrifice** some of the activities and behaviors of your previous lifestyle.

- **Prioritizing** goals and commitments: family, personal, and business.
- Anticipating the ways in which you will have to **reorganize** your personal and professional time and space.
- **Rebudgeting** your finances.
- **Revising** your work-related and most cherished personal interests.
- Knowing that you will be continually **considering the essential needs** of your child, partner, self, and work, over and over again, as new requirements unfold.

Often a baby demands immediate and urgent attention at the most inconvenient moments of your already overcommitted day. Frustration is predictable on days that hold both deadlines and a needy child; on the other hand, you'll feel fulfilled and strengthened on the days you gracefully complete your goals. The more flexible and objective you can be, the more likely it is that you will not only endure but also enjoy the radical changes in your daily routine that will begin the moment your child is born.

Penny appreciated her twin sister's warning to begin making changes in her work commitments before her son was born:

> After twelve years of devoting myself to a successful home business with a part-time employee, I suddenly found myself spending the same quantity of time I used to spend on the phone changing diapers and feeding my newborn. If I had not set up other people to run my business while I took a four-month maternity leave, I would have had to shut it down. There's no way I could have spent more than a few minutes caring for my clients. I was lucky to have time to make a quick phone call to my family or friends. I was so glad I had learned how all-consuming a newborn is before I had my baby. And even if I had miraculously created time to work those first few months, I had no desire to. . . . My baby needed a full-time mother.

What Will I Have to Sacrifice?

Sacrifice implies relinquishing something highly valued for the sake of a greater value. When you're responsible for a young child, you need to make specific choices concerning what is most essential for her and for you at any given moment. In the days ahead you will certainly have to let go of doing some things that are very important to you because your child's needs are even more essential. Prioritizing in advance can give you clarity when a tough decision must be made. Claire's story will be familiar to many young parents:

> I will never forget the time my husband's company gave us an all-expenses-paid, first-class vacation to Hawaii as part of his promotion. The dates for the tickets were fixed, and they happened to be during the week before our son's christening. Our families already had their plane tickets. We were so in need of a break and had very little extra money due to my extended maternity leave. It was a difficult opportunity to let go of, but Hawaii is always there, money is always coming in and out of our lives, and our son is only given this blessing once in his life. Our priority was "family first" so there really was no indecision.

In preparing for parenthood, no hard rules govern when and what to sacrifice. Your own values, principles, and priorities will be your guide. Some of the sacrifices that new parents commonly make are lengthy dinner preparations, frequent restaurant dining, daily exercise, going to the movies or parties, keeping a tidy house, making love, spending time alone, pleasure reading and writing, visiting with friends, and traveling. Family or work tasks will often take precedence over self-care.

The stronger your desire to be a parent, the easier it is to let go of past ways so you can devote your time to nurturing a child. If you are ambivalent about the huge responsibility of caring for a new life, you may find it difficult to release the commitments and pleasures of your previous lifestyle.

Your child's age will determine how much time you need to devote to playing, teaching, and feeding. Some children are innately very independent and enjoy some brief periods of time playing alone, while others need the constant presence of someone to interact with and care for them. Even though your child may be born with a particular temperament and personality, his needs will change constantly, and your own lifestyle will continually "morph" to adapt.

Stephanie recalls:

> My first son, Todd, was very dependent on me and would not let anyone else feed him for the first year. He would starve himself

before he would eat from my husband or caregivers, so I always had to be around during his frequent feeding times. I had to let go of a lot of my previous commitments. Then, at thirteen months, he learned to feed himself, and I had much greater freedom to do other things.

Gerald, our second son, would play with mirrors on his changing table for long periods and loved to watch objects while lying on his back the first six months or so. I could get much more done around the house than with Todd. Then, when Gerald began to walk at ten months, he completely switched, and for several months his separation anxiety was so high that it was stressful for me to leave the room.

Prioritize Your Life Goals

Each day you'll need to prioritize where to commit your limited time and energy. It helps to revise your personal, financial, and business goals as part of your prebirth planning. Are they compatible with parenthood? Making an inventory of personal and business interests before you have a child gives you a set of general guidelines for making future choices. For example, most new parents have difficulty deciding how to allocate their money in anticipation of child care expenses. Both the short- and long-term costs of having a baby will determine how much you'll invest in assets, personal belongings, vacations, education, and the exigencies of daily life. Inventorying these items with your partner and assigning them different values provides a basis for the choices you will make. But stay flexible and expect these initial values to change, especially in the first few years, as with Pamela and Ira. Pamela explains:

> Neither of us makes a lot of money, but we have plenty to pay our bills and take a vacation or two each year while maintaining a gentle increase in our savings. When we were planning for our baby, I knew that I wanted to take six months maternity leave. I was self-employed so this meant no income during this time. We decided to move to a smaller place with lower rent so that I would not feel pressure to return to work so quickly. We also simplified our food and entertainment needs during this time. Our first priority was time with our child. Then, after a year, we realized we wanted to have part-time child care. This required me to work part time as well, but by this time our goals and our child's needs had changed.

Work plans that require a lot of time and effort may be complicated to pull off when caring for a new baby. Consider completing large projects before your child is born. Once you become a parent, be open to postponing unnecessary or stressful work commitments until you become familiar with child care. For example, my client Tara decided to complete her doctoral dissertation before becoming pregnant, because "I knew I could never sit in front of a computer for hours on end if I had morning sickness. Also, I could not imagine having school deadlines while needing to attend to my new baby."

Some couples will wish to further their educations or to fulfill a travel dream without having to tote children along. Some women prefer to be in top physical shape before they become pregnant, while other couples want to secure a home that is large enough for future children. Take some time to list your goals and prioritize them. Note which are important to complete *before* having a child, and clarify the length of time it will take to fulfill each of these.

For most adults, balancing personal and professional goals is already difficult. When the responsibilities of parenthood are added, there are many more variables to juggle each day. Personal projects get relegated to naptime, when the child is not present to distract their attention. But be warned: many newborns have irregular nap patterns throughout the first few months, and infants and toddlers can resist scheduling as well. The most productive attitude is to understand that, at least for a while, your former productivity may be just a memory.

Organize Home and Workspace

Having a baby will require major changes in your environment. A once natural placement of your personal belongings will most likely need to be rearranged to allow space for your baby's clothes, furniture, toys, and accessories. For some new parents, this can even mean a move to a bigger home before the baby's arrival.

Do not underestimate the stress of moving during your pregnancy. Many pregnant women and their partners wait until the last trimester to change residences, contrary to the natural impulse to nest at this time. You will feel reluctant to pull up roots just when home should be supporting you. If you know that you must move before your child comes, try to do it before you conceive. Morning sickness is very common during the first trimester, so you will not be very happy about moving at this delicate time. If you must move or even remodel your existing home during your pregnancy, the second trimester is the best time to do so.

Anticipate any changes you'll need in your work environment as well, particularly if your workplace has stressful components that could jeopardize your prenatal health or that of your baby. Exposure to any type of toxic substance in the environment must be avoided prior to conception and thereafter. This includes secondhand smoke and all chemicals; noise pollution (frequent loud sounds) can harm the fetus as well. Even if you have a healthy pregnancy, your newborn will appreciate environmental conditions that support her sensitivities. The first three months after the birth are really equivalent to a "fourth trimester" of gestation for the infant. The quality of light, sound, and air will affect her sense of security and well-being.

Before you conceive, make a personal inventory of your surroundings. Is it a baby-friendly climate? Clarify the specific changes you need to make before or after conception.

Dara remembers sitting in her rocking chair, five months pregnant, during a humid summer day:

> I had spent the day at work in a small room with no windows, and I came home to the sound of city traffic and a house full of smoggy air. I thought to myself, "Here I am caring about my child's womb life, yet I am totally stressed by the conditions of my job and home." It was up to me to create a safe world for my baby. Within a month of that realization, we were moved into an apartment on a quiet street next to a park, and my boss gave me a room with air-conditioning and windows. All I had to do was recognize the importance of my physical circumstances to know exactly what changes to make.

Imagine what kind of world you would like your prenate and newborn to experience. Now—before you conceive—is the time to evaluate and make the necessary lifestyle changes.

Keeping a Prebirth Journal

On my daughter's first birthday I pulled out the diary I had begun for her several years before she was even conceived. Reading all of the reflective entries as I relived my journey to motherhood was deeply moving. The years of yearning to be a parent and the longing to meet my baby were captured in the spontaneously written expression of my emotions. I had captured my happiness, fear, passion, excitement, and pensiveness about becoming a mother. I was able to read a full spectrum of emotional intensity. And I was surprised by how accurate my intuitive insights about the soul of my daughter were, before she was even born! The perceptions I had of the unique qualities of her spirit essence now radiate through her personality as a child.

Days after I had confirmed that I was pregnant, I wrote:

> It has been a week since I learned I am a full-fledged mom with a baby *inside* of me! . . . Every physical change excites and concerns me . . . my primal instinct continuously asking whether I am offering healthy conditions for this little embryo. I concern myself about my blood—is it nourishing? I concern myself about my emotions and thoughts—am I flooding this child with virtuous patterns of divine consciousness . . . or the unhealthy stresses of living in a modern world? I feel so protective of my baby's heart and nervous system this week, and my commitment to create a field of pure light and harmonic vibes.

I had written a poem to the spirit of the little embryo growing steadfastly within me. I called her Kylea Sophia—the name that had come to me intuitively before she was conceived.

> Kylea, week four begins for your developing body . . . gathering cosmic lines of light from opalescent streams of Heaven. . . . I weave your essence into my body, mind, and Soul. Fiberoptic spirals imprinting perfection into my womb . . . you. My love-filled heart chakra dripping life into the etheric web of my child incarnating. I love you, Mom.

Imagine if your mother and father had kept a journal while they were preparing for your conception and throughout your prenatal life. How would you feel if you could read about your parents' deep desire for you, and their commitment to prepare their life for your arrival? A prebirth journal can remind you and your child of all the details of this special time as the years go by. However, I suggest not sharing your journal with your child until she is mature enough to understand the emotional complexities of being a parent. First and foremost, your journal is your private space.

Jared, Kylea's father, wrote in his journal as he sat in the sun, contemplating her presence:

> The heat is soaking into the hillside and you are setting into the watery world of Mommy's belly now that you are ten weeks old. We are clearing our fears of "not having enough money" to care for you. I know that you will have everything you need and everything you desire that is healthy for you. I feel blessed to be your dad and serve you. You are my first Guru. I will learn about love like never before. Daddy loves you.

Two weeks later Jared's journal reflected his evolving process:

> Today is Father's Day. I sense you swimming in Mommy's belly. I am feeling strong and clear about my ability to care for you. All will be provided for you—joyfully. You and Mommy and I will have many memorable moments sharing Father's Day together.

The primary purpose of keeping a journal is to record an open, honest, and sensitive expression of your evolving consciousness of becoming a parent. By exercising the least restraint of your feelings, you will discover your own deepest truths. Give yourself permission to ride emotional waves, deeply moved by the surges and tides of your unfolding inner life. Express yourself freely and forget about spelling and grammar. This journal is for you to discover yourself as a developing parent. It can also be for your partner to share the inner awakenings you are experiencing—individually and together. Or it can be for your future child to read when he is older if you feel that he'll delight in discovering the care that you devoted to him. Whatever your personal reasons for keeping a journal, remember that those precious moments of early parenthood go quickly; if you don't capture the confusion and wonder of your experiences as they happen, you may never be able to recall the intimate thoughts or profound revelations you had at this significant passage.

Buy yourself a special blank notebook or sketch pad that will be your prebirth journal. Begin each entry with a date so that you can keep track of your age and that of your child. Consider beginning your journal by examining your fear as well as your excitement about becoming a parent.

Let your journal be your confidante, and be truthful about your inner-most desires and concerns. Exploring fears can be therapeutic. Memories of your own childhood may impel you to examine the feelings that surrounded those experiences. Concerns about changes in your relationships, career challenges, and the burden of parenthood can often be worked through as you write—and in the process become conscious of them. Other times inspiration may pour through you that will generate a poem or even a letter to the spirit of your child. The mysteries of conception and pregnancy may find you pondering the meaning of life, or becoming aware of primal instincts that motherhood or fatherhood may unleash within you.

As you write in your journal or meditate and reflect on becoming a parent, you may find that a name for your child-to-be comes to you spontaneously. Some people prefer not to use a gendered name for the fetus because the child may turn out to be the other sex. Prior to conception, when I perceived my daughter's essence and her name was intuitively revealed to me, I was never certain if her feminine quality was her soul essence or her physical form. I was not attached to the idea that she was a girl. Rather, I was writing to her spirit nature as it was communicating with me, knowing that although she seemed feminine, the soul could still choose a male physical body for this incarnation. When writing to your child in your journal, remain open to the mystery of her eventual physical form. If a name is revealed by the soul or chosen by you, consider it a spirit name that you may or may not use once your child is born.

During my preconception and prenatal journey, I documented many of my inner awakenings by drawing pictures in my journal using crayons, pencil, or paints. You can use drawing or any art form to focus your feelings about having a baby. Sometimes a pattern or picture will capture deep subconscious feelings in a simple abstract image that writing cannot easily portray. For example, for more than a year before I conceived Kylea I was in a dynamic phase of conscious preparation and documentation of my preconception process. During each ovulation period, I drew a picture. Upon reflection, I could perceive numerous emotional messages from my subconscious in the images each picture contained.

At the end of each chapter you will find Creative Exercises to inspire you to clarify your own truth about many of the notions discussed in the chapter. Consider using your journal as a place to record your responses and thoughts. Whether you use writing, drawing, or a combination of both, your journal will capture the transformation of your identity and lifestyle as you creatively prepare for parenthood.

Creative Exercise:
Your Personal Plan to Prepare for Your Baby

Answer the following questions as fully as possible:

1. What are some of the benefits of preparing for parenthood? Consider the benefits to both yourself and your future child.
2. How can you be a healthy link between heaven and earth for your baby before birth? After birth?
3. What are the benefits of being a psychologically healthy parent for your child?
4. How do you feel about the endless phases of your child's growth? Does one phase feel more interesting or overwhelming or exciting than another?
5. What are the specific sacrifices in your life that you feel prepared to make upon conceiving your child? In what ways do you feel resistant to making any changes?
6. In what ways do you sense that having a child will create positive changes in your lifestyle?
7. What are the areas of your life—personal and professional—that you will be challenged to balance with the responsibilities of parenthood?
8. Specify your work-related and personal interests. Then revise and prioritize your goals and commitments to include parenting your future child.
9. Begin a prebirth journal by examining the insights you have gained from this chapter, including the Creative Exercise. Also, begin to clarify in these pages your personal plan to prepare for your baby. You may wish to include:
   - Physical health concerns you have, and changes you want to make.
   - Psychological health concerns you have, and changes you want to make.
   - Financial concerns you have, and changes you want to make.

- Career concerns you have, and changes you want to make.
- Relationship concerns you have, and changes you want to make.
- Concerns you have about your partner, and changes you want to make.
- Other concerns you have, and changes you want to make.

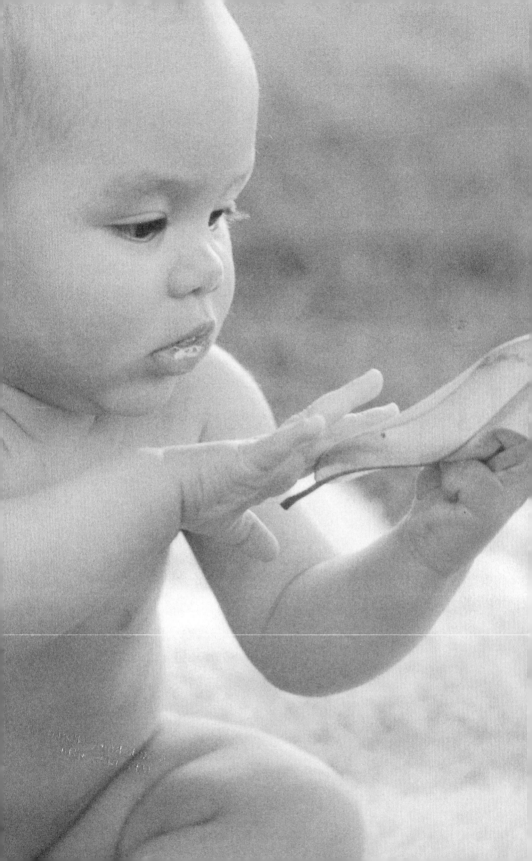

2

Your Child:
A Multidimensional Being

Man's Essence has a spiritual nature for which
his body serves only as an outer cloak.
Gershom Scholem

Consider a Holistic Health Approach

Have you ever considered how a holistic approach to parenting can benefit you and your future child? Holistic health care takes into account the whole person. Most of us think of preconception and prenatal care as optimizing the *physical* health of the child and mother. We rarely consider the father's health, the psychological health of the parents and their relationship, and the whole health—body, mind, and soul—of the unborn child. Your own prebirth holistic health care plan, however, can include all of these aspects in preparing to conceive your child.

Although the term *holistic health* has been defined in many ways, common among them is the concept that each of us is a multifaceted being with complex physical, psychological, and spiritual needs for achieving a state of whole health. Every individual has a physical, emotional, mental, and spiritual body, and the well-being of each of these bodies is equally important. If one or more of these bodies is in dis-ease, the health of all of them is affected. When all of these aspects are in balance and integrated, we are in optimal holistic health. A holistic perspective also includes environmental influences that contribute to our health—social, economic, political, and educational.

Whereas traditional allopathic health programs tend to focus on the symptoms of a condition, holistic health care addresses the *reasons why a symptom is appearing*. Instead of medicating a condition to get rid of it, a holistic practitioner will assess what needs to be physically or psychologically altered within your lifestyle to naturally improve your life. When you practice holistic living, you may discover that many of your health challenges are resolved intuitively, as Sandra's experience illustrates:

> David and I had been trying to conceive a baby for almost three years. Our doctor recommended strong fertility drugs, and so we tried that for another year with no results. I was becoming more and more depressed and our relationship was suffering. I finally began to address the emotional fear about not being able to have a baby. I discovered I had a lot of sadness about my abortion six years earlier, and a tremendous amount of pain regarding my mother's death following my birth. It suddenly dawned on me that I was stewing in a belief that I or my child would die if I became pregnant. I realized I was subconsciously giving my body the message that it was safer for me to stay infertile. Once I acknowledged and worked through the unresolved grief from my past, I realized that I could create a different outcome for my life. Two months later I became pregnant without the assistance of any drugs. The fertility drugs never worked because it was not a physical problem; it was a psychological one. Our doctor had never even asked me about my past, or my beliefs about becoming a mother. All of the answers to my fertility challenge were in my mind.

Another holistic health axiom is *prevention*. Holistic living asks you to create lifestyles that enhance well-being for its own sake. You do not need to be in a health crisis to make daily efforts to improve your health. As a holistically oriented person, you can create a daily life of exercising and eating well to nourish the physical body; meditating to maintain emotional, mental, and spiritual balance; and working and living in environmental and social conditions that support you in maintaining a positive attitude about your life. If you apply these holistic principles to the preparation for and care of your unborn child, you will contribute greatly to her first experiences of human life. Before and after conception, you can consciously nurture your child's whole being.

Cultivating Your Child's Whole Self from the Beginning

"What is the life that brings us here?" asks Richard Grossinger in his book *Embryogenesis*. "How is the loose energy of the cosmos snared in our tissues and our personalities?"[1] The Western medical model offers a biological understanding of exactly how your future child will develop his physical body. All human beings, we can agree, need a heart, lungs, blood, bones, and so on to exist. But there is more to caring for your child's life than just his physical development.

As a soul incarnates into a new human life, a holistic approach to preconception and prenatal health care includes many variables besides the essential contribution of DNA from the sperm and egg. In addition to the microcosmic contribution of you and your mate's DNA blueprint, holism recognizes your child's presence within the universe at large, including macrocosmic influences, such as cosmological and celestial forces that will directly affect the pattern of life created at human conception and throughout prenatal development. For example, according to the five-thousand-year-old science of astrology, the position of the stars in the heavens at the moment in time when a child is conceived and born affect many of that soul's life lessons. There will be a dynamic interplay between both the biochemical and the heavenly causes that influence your future child's life.

Traditional Western physiological and psychological models do not inquire when spirit begins its influence on the development of human life; nor do they include the reality of spiritual influences on an unborn child. The foundation of holistic prebirth preparation, on the other hand, considers the many biological and spiritual forces initiating fertilization of human life. The holistically oriented parent does accept the inviolable laws of matter and science but combines this perspective with an understanding of archetypal forces that precede matter.

In the biological development of a human being there are measurable constants and variables as each biological system develops sequentially. The process of incarnation, however, cannot be pared down and reproduced at will in the controlled conditions of physical science experiments. Many aspects of human development cannot be objectively measured—particularly the presence of your future child's soul, or the qualities of her emotional and mental expression.

Incarnation requires that the soul integrate psyche with physical form, the human embryo. The human cells need the life force of the soul, and the soul needs the physical cells, if human life is to exist. *The cells and the soul cannot isolate their unique function one from another if there is to be a living human being.*

Because there are so many collective forces that influence consciousness and human existence, there is no precise moment at which it can be said that your child is primarily matter, or primarily spirit, or even when his spirit merges with human fluids and flesh. Paradigms describing only the development of the physical body have not solved the mystery of life or the secrets of the mind. Subatomic particles, biochemicals, family, society, the stars, consciousness, and spiritual forces all contribute to an incarnating soul's human embodiment.

Your unborn child will use extrasensory forms and forces to create herself. Yet it would be narrow-minded to idealize her wholeness as if she were solely angelic or metaphysical. While you can perceive your future child as a soul who is descending into matter and organizing it to create a human body, remember that, as William Blake stated, "Man has no Body distinct from his Soul."[2] The soul needs the body to express itself in human form, just as the body needs the life force of the soul to exist.

The Design of the Personality and Soul

The human personality is an embodied expression of a soul process.
Corinne Laughlin

In many holistic models a human being is composed of two major aspects: the human personality and the immortal soul. In the early 1930s the Italian psychiatrist Dr. Roberto Assagioli created a human development model called *psychosynthesis* that included the soul identity. Psychosynthesis recognizes that the person *is* a soul, but *has* a personality. "I have a body," Assagioli stated, "but *I* am not my body. I have feelings, but I am not my feelings. I have desires, but I am not my desires. . . . I use these. I am the Soul."[3]

The aspect of the consciousness that exists, infinitely, independent of your child's human personality is called the soul. *The soul is the spiritual and immortal part of a human being.* The soul's consciousness is the accumulated fruits of all past lives—especially in the realms of knowledge and ability. Through many lifetimes the soul unfolds the qualities of love and wisdom as it develops and learns to refine virtues such as will, truth, selflessness, service, honesty, power, cooperation, and peace.

The soul's goal is to freely express its divine nature through the human personality without distortion.

As you can see in the diagram on page 36, your future child's personality is composed of four different bodies: physical, etheric, emotional, and mental. These four aspects interpenetrate each other, and when a soul incarnates it functions simultaneously in all four of these realms of consciousness. This distinctive personality is the vehicle used by the soul to experience unfolding its evolutionary potential during a life cycle on earth. Let's take a closer look at your future child's human design.

The Physical Body: This is the aspect of the personality that is composed of the densest matter. All of the biological and biochemical systems belong to the physical. Without a physical body your child cannot express her emotions, thoughts, or intelligence in a three-dimensional plane. All five physical senses are experienced through the body. Your future child will depend on you to help her develop a healthy body to express her activities and abilities.

The Etheric Body: This is the most esoteric (or least widely understood) aspect of the human personality. Although most Western systems of depicting the human constitution do not include the etheric body, Eastern medical and metaphysical systems (such as Ayurvedic medicine from India and acupuncture from China and Japan) do. The etheric body is a link between the spiritual, mental, and emotional bodies and the physical body. It is not a body of consciousness, but rather one of activity, focusing life force to energize the physical. The etheric substance gives the physical body warmth, motion, and sensitivity. "Every form has its etheric counterpart."[4] Since it is the energy field that organizes, powers, and maintains the dense physical body, it is often referred to as the "physical-etheric" body. In her book *The Chakras*, the Theosophist C. W. Leadbeater wrote: "This invisible part of the physical body is of great importance to us, for it is the vehicle through which flows the streams of vitality which keep the body alive, and without it as a bridge to convey undulations of thought and feeling from the [emotional] to the visible denser physical matter, the ego [the individuality] could make no use of the cells of his brain."[5]

The Emotional Body: This body "is the vehicle through which all emotions, passions, desires and appetites act on the physical body, and find their expression in the physical world."[6] In esoteric healing models this emotional aspect is often called the astral body. The two terms are synonymous. The emotional body is the vehicle for the consciousness

A SIMPLIFIED DEPICTION OF THE ENERGETIC FUNCTION BETWEEN SPIRIT, SOUL, AND PERSONALITY

Although spirit and soul interpenetrate all of the four personality bodies, each personality body has a specific function. The spirit and soul are immortal, whereas the personality is created anew each lifetime the soul reincarnates as a human being. A purpose of reincarnating is to learn to refine and align the personality bodies so that the soul can embody its spiritual consciousness in dense human form.

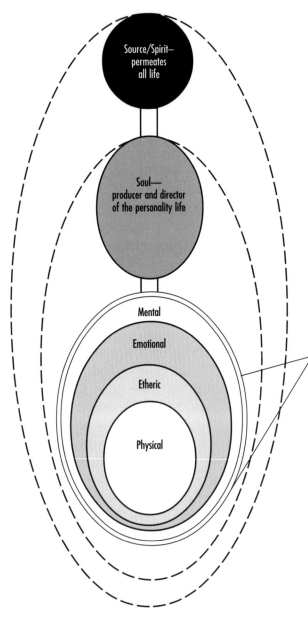

Source/Spirit—permeates all life

Soul—producer and director of the personality life

Mental

Emotional

Etheric

Physical

Source/Spirit:
A unified source of universal love, intelligence, and will permeates all creation (including the soul and personality, as depicted by dotted lines).

The Individual Soul:
It has the capacity to radiate divine attributes, virtues, or qualities. The soul evolves by creating human incarnations (a new personality each life-time) to experience itself in matter and perfect its expression of consciousness through a human form (it permeates the personality as depicted by dotted lines).

The Personality:
Composed of four bodies that create the specific character nature of a single human life cycle on earth.

The Mental Body:
Thoughts, values, beliefs.

The Emotional Body:
The full spectrum of feelings ranging from hate to love.

The Etheric Body:
The energy blueprint for the chakras, acupuncture meridians, and physical body.

The Physical Body:
Densest substance of matter for soul consciousness to express itself through a human form.

and for the expression of personal emotions and desires; it governs the feeling nature. By asking yourself, your partner, or your child what or how they are *feeling*, you are focusing attention on the emotional body. Your future child will need your guidance to appropriately express his feelings, ranging from fear to love.

The Mental Body: This is the vehicle for consciousness; it governs thought, concepts, and the use of memory. By asking, "What are you thinking?" you will be activating your child's mental body. All attitudes, beliefs, and thought-forms are functions of the mental body. Your child will need you to teach her how to use her thoughts to express her creative intelligence.

While the soul is the aspect of individual consciousness that remains constant throughout numerous incarnations, the personality is newly created with each incarnation. Through successive incarnations the soul continually withdraws and rebirths itself, accumulating the essence of subsequent personalities. This process is the foundation of reincarnation theory. "The soul overshadows the personality and connects with man by a thread of energy [the 'silver cord' referred to in the Bible] during the entire span of earth life. The personality is its instrument of expression."[7]

The purpose of incarnation is the evolution of the soul. Although the human experience offers opportunities to develop the personality, all your future child's life challenges are to assist his soul in perfecting its ability to experience and express its divine consciousness and virtues in human form. In each new incarnation the soul is challenged to perfect control of its personality nature through continual conscious adjustment of its physical-etheric, emotional, and mental bodies. Daily life experiences offer feedback for the soul to evaluate its progress. As prospective parents, your challenge is to provide healthy conditions for your child's soul to develop, balance, and integrate its personality with its divine consciousness. Ideally, this awareness begins before conception, and certainly once the baby is growing in the womb.

Your child's soul will express itself through the use of its bodies to move (physical-etheric), feel (emotional), and think (mental). Only when the physical-etheric, emotional, and mental bodies are unified as one consciousness can they be used effectively by the soul in everyday living. Therefore, holistic parenting is concerned with the constant *integration of the personality and the soul.* One student, Fran, told me:

It was not until I was in your Preconception Health Care class that I realized what I needed to do to be ready for motherhood. It is not just my physical diet that I have to change. I need also to be acutely aware of the emotional, mental, and spiritual nutrition that I feed this soul. It is depending on me to positively nourish its feelings and thoughts about itself and life.

Reincarnation: The Past Is Present

Before I formed thee in the belly I knew thee; and before thou camest forth out of the womb I santified thee.

Jeremiah 1:5

Reincarnation means literally "the process of coming into flesh again."[8] The phenomenon of reincarnation has generated innumerable cross-cultural religious, academic, and philosophical explications. But simply put, reincarnation is the understanding that the life force animating the physical body does not cease with the body's physical death but goes on living in the subjective spiritual etheric realms for a specific period of time. It is then reborn into a new human body and repeats this cycle hundreds, sometimes thousands, of times until the life force, the soul, has perfected itself.

Reincarnation is the foundation of a number of major world religions, including mystic Christianity and Judaism, Hinduism, Buddhism, and Sikhism. Its teachings have appeared as Taoism in China, Vedanta in India, Gnosticism in the classical Mediterranean world, Kabbalism among the Jews, Sufism among the Moslems; it holds that "we are part of a great, ordered plan of physical–intellectual–spiritual evolution, stretching back to the primordial beginnings of things and moving forward to a final state of perfection."[9]

Evidence of belief in reincarnation appears in numerous religious texts. In the Hindu text, the *Bhagavad-Gita,* Krishna tells his student, Arjuna, "As a man throweth away old garments and putteth on new, even so the dweller in the body, having quitted its old mortal frames, entereth into others which are new." Krishna continues, "Both I and thou have passed through many births. Mine are known unto me, but thou knowest not of thine." In a well-known biblical reference to reincarnation, Jesus asked his disciples, "Whom say the people that I am? they answered, 'John the Baptist; but some say Elias; and others say, that one of the old prophets is risen again'" (Luke 9:18–19). Likewise, the Kabbalist and medieval Sufi philosophers talked about "metempsychosis, 'the monad's insouling after insouling' through its progressive expressions in various physical forms."[10]

A present-day understanding of rebirth is reflected in the Tibetan tradition. Upon the death of the Dalai Lama, who is considered by his devotees to be the authentic embodiment of a Buddha, his soul returns to incarnate as it overshadows a living person or enters the body of a child who died at birth or soon after. When the child recognizes objects formerly used or treasured by the previous Dalai Lama, the new Dalai Lama is proclaimed. This rebirth is referred to as a *tulka* or the incarnation of a "living Buddha." Bernardo Bertolucci's film, *Little Buddha,* clearly illustrates this ancient phenomena.[11]

Nor is reincarnation absent in Western historical and philosophical writings. Hundreds of historical and contemporary world figures have written or spoken about this ancient view of life and death and consciousness.

Rabbi Berg, one of the world's foremost authorities on the Kabbalah, "the inner soul of the Torah," has written a contemporary book called *Wheels of a Soul* exploring the concept of reincarnation and Judaism. Rabbi Berg states that "the Hebrew word for reincarnation is *Gilgul Neshamot,* which means literally 'wheel of the soul'. . . Gilgul Neshamot is a wheel constantly in motion, and with its turning, souls come and go again and again in the cycle of birth, evolution, death and birth again." Like the wheel, growth and evolution have no beginning and no end, and life is a progression of experiences from one incarnation to another.

Rabbi Berg cites examples in support of the case of belief in the ways that reincarnation is not a religious issue "dependent on faith or doctrine, but [one] of logic and reason [with] the Bible its fountainhead." For example, he describes how "The Book of Exodus provides the full explanation, not only of reincarnation, but also of its effects [on] parents and children, brothers and sisters, and how all interrelate in the immediate environment." He suggests that reincarnation is relevant to each of us and believes that we can "use its precepts to enhance the fruits of our lives." He writes: "The soul of man is no more dependent upon the existence of the brain than a musician is dependent upon the existence of his violin though both instruments are necessary for musical expression in the physical world. Only when we can fully grasp this viewpoint can we begin to approach the study of reincarnation."[12]

Among the Greeks, Pythagoras, Hippocrates, Aristotle, Plato, and many others have referred to reincarnation in their writings, as did Romans such as Julius Caesar, Virgil, and Cicero. Even Dante speaks of reincarnation in his *Divine Comedy*.

Numerous European philosophers, artists, and writers have theorized on reincarnation, including Sir Francis Bacon, Henry Moore, William Blake, William Wordsworth, Robert Browning, Aldous Huxley, Charles Dickens, Oscar Wilde, George Bernard Shaw, Rudyard Kipling, H. G. Wells, Somerset Maugham, Voltaire, Napoleon Bonaparte, Victor Hugo, Count Lev Tolstoy, and Fyodor Dostoevsky, to name just a few. And in America Thomas Paine, Ralph Waldo Emerson, Henry David Thoreau, Louisa May Alcott, John Muir, Oliver Wendell Holmes, Walt Whitman, Emily Dickinson, Robert Frost, Kahlil Gibran, Mark Twain, Louis Bloomfield, William Faulkner, and J. D. Salinger all entertained the notion of immortality and reincarnation in their writings. This strong belief has found some unusual proponents, including William Randolph Hearst, Charles Lindbergh, and even Harry Houdini, who wished all his life to believe.[13]

On the humorous side, Benjamin Franklin wrote his own epitaph at the age of twenty-two: "The body of B. Franklin, Printer, Like the Cover of an Old Book, Its Contents Torn Out, And Stripped of its Lettering and Gilding, Lies Here Food for Worms, But the Work shall not be Lost, For it Will as He Believed Appear Once More In a New and more Elegant Edition Revised and corrected By the Author."[14]

Science and psychology offer their own contributions, which may open the minds of skeptics. The great Swiss psychiatrist Carl Jung, for instance, posits that "rebirth is not a process that we can in any way observe. We can neither measure nor weigh not photograph it. . . . The mere fact that people talk about rebirth, and that there is such a concept at all means that a store of psychic experiences designated by that term must actually exist."[15]

Although not directly writing about reincarnation, Albert Einstein and Charles Darwin wrote about immortality and the soul. Darwin stated, with a certain darkness, that "to those who fully admit the immortality of the human soul, the destruction of our world will not appear so dreadful." Einstein said, "It is enough for me to contemplate the mystery of conscious life, perpetuating itself through all eternity."[16]

A belief in reincarnation is a manifest reality in every culture—East and West—and on every continent. Many of the greatest minds of the world have written of their convictions about the continuity of soul and immortality. I have found the Theosophical interpretation of reincarnation to be the most practical and universal for prospective parents seeking to integrate this perennial philosophy into their preparation for conceiving a child. The term *Theosophy* refers to the beliefs and teachings of the Theosophical Society, which was founded in the United States in 1875 by Madame Elena Petrovena Blavatsky and others. The founding Theosophists combined the teachings of various religions, with Hindu and Buddhist doctrines most prominent.

The Theosophical Society describes itself as a worldwide organization that is nonsectarian, nonpolitical, and nondogmatic. It is devoted to cultural understanding, human solidarity, and self-development. It seeks to bring people together; to reconcile religions, philosophies, and sciences of both East and West; and to increase awareness of the inner reality inherent in every human being.[17]

Theosophy embraces a spectrum of doctrines in philosophy, science, and ethics with the intention of furthering our understanding of the essential underlying truths of all philosophies striving to penetrate the mysteries of nature, including the embodiment of spirit in human form. Theosophical teachings resonate with me because they are centered around the ageless wisdom teachings, a large and varied group of texts from Buddhism, Hinduism, and Christianity, including the Bible. Theosophists explored these writings and created an explanation of reincarnation that included the essential esoteric teachings of these basic religions. The teachings hold both a worldview and a vision of human self-development eventually leading to enlightenment.

I invite you to consider whether reincarnation is a basic assumption you wish to include in the perceptions you hold of your future child. Because it is a *metaphysical* reality, there are no empirical techniques to objectively investigate reincarnation. Still, who has really been able to objectively prove the existence of the soul, of spirit, of God, of the angels? And although they cannot be scientifically proven, do they not exist? While reincarnation is not established fact, it is a valid and useful philosophical and spiritual perspective about the process of human life. As prospective parents, it is up to you to decide whether or not the concept or metaphor of reincarnation enhances the process of preparing for and caring for the human being that you will be conceiving.

A fundamental teaching of reincarnation is that a soul does not attain perfection in one life on earth but requires many cycles of experiences. For this purpose, the soul assumes a succession of personalities who are born into the different periods of history, different cultures, different astrological signs, different degrees of wealth, and often different physical conditions—all carrying various emotional and intellectual experiences that offer a range of lessons until the soul is perfected. In addition, the soul lives many years between incarnations in the etheric realms, processing knowledge attained in its last life in preparation for its next incarnation. All phases of our life cycle are affected by the laws of reincarnation, but I will focus on only the evolutionary states of preconception through birth as you prepare for parenthood.

The mysteries of human life are limitless. Part of your preparation as new parents of an incarnating soul might be to explore the following questions:

- When does a soul choose to incarnate in a human personality?
- At what moment does the last incarnation end, and the new one start?
- Can you contribute to the soul's well-being *before* it is physically conceived?
- What can you do to assist the development of the emotional and mental bodies before and after conception?
- What determines the design of the physical body and the nature of the personality? Is this design genetic only, or are there influences from the soul?
- Are there specific steps and experiences that occur for each soul as it incarnates?
- Are some souls more evolved in consciousness than others?
- Does an incarnating soul choose its parents, culture, religion, race?
- Who determines the life purpose of the incoming soul?
- Can astrology help you understand, appreciate, and support your child's soul purpose?
- Is there value in knowing past-life information about your incoming child to help you improve and understand her present life? If so, are there practical ways you can learn to access this information?
- Assuming that soul consciousness exists on etheric levels prior to conception, can you learn to intuitively communicate with your child before he is conceived?
- How does karma affect the process of reincarnation?

Suzanne and Alan felt very empowered as they learned about reincarnation theory. Suzanne says:

> I had a miscarriage three months into my pregnancy after trying to conceive for more than a year. I never felt anything had died, I just felt the soul decided to drop its physical body and return to the spirit world. I felt sad I would never meet it as a human being, but I felt its soul presence never left me. I feel connected to this being to this day, even after I successfully gave birth to my son, Paul, thirteen months later. Sometimes I feel this soul is a guide for me, who taught me that we are more than our physical bodies, and we do not need them to give and experience love. I am grateful to this soul. It also taught me that my son is more than just my child . . . that he existed before he chose me as his mom and his real self has a reason why it decided to be born while the other soul has a reason why it did not incarnate through me. I feel I am the mother of two children, although I am grateful to have Paul to care for every day in a human way. I just never want to forget that Paul is a magnificent soul, not just a little boy.

Religious and philosophical writings from both East and West have concerned themselves with the intricate and multidimensional processes involved in the generation of the human species. Many esoteric schools concealed their knowledge to protect their membership from persecution. The Rosicrucians and Kabbalists, for example, veiled their teachings in symbols during the unenlightened ages.

Today's metaphysical philosophies probe the ancient mysteries. Metaphysics does not dispute the findings of scientific investigation, "but maintains that so-called physical causes are secondary to superphysical causes."[18] Metaphysical perspectives provide the knowledge of the invisible world and recognize that each body is a universe, organized according to universal laws. Metaphysical doctrines are not inharmonious with the evolutionary theories of the Western world. In fact, they can provide a spiritual context for our worldly pursuits. Automotive pioneer Henry Ford once confided, "When I was a young man I, like so may others, was bewildered. I found myself asking the question . . . 'What are we here for?' I found no answer. Without some answer to that question, life is empty, useless. Then one day a friend handed me a book. . . .That little book gave me the answer I was seeking. . . . It changed my outlook upon life to purpose and meaning. I believe that we are here now and will come back again. . . . Of this I am sure . . . that we are here for a purpose. And that we go on. Mind and memory—they are the eternals."[19]

You as a potential parent can optimize the integration and embodiment of your future child's multidimensional aspects by considering metaphysical viewpoints. Imagine if your own parents had perceived you as a lovable and wise personality, as well as a brilliant soul with divine consciousness. (See appendix D, From Soul to Cell, to explore this topic in more detail.)

Your New Child Is an Old Soul

The body of a woman who is to conceive is being chosen as a channel for the expression of divinity into materiality.

Edgar Cayce

As a prospective parent, including the perspective that *your future child is a soul who is reincarnating* will offer your child's personality a spacious opportunity to consciously discover a meaning and purpose for human life. Descent into incarnation is never forced upon a soul by an external power against its own will. Rather, the soul has its own timing and responds to an innate impulse to descend into human form. As the soul chooses the specific opportunity to further its evolutionary progress through incarnating with you, you as the parents can support your child's soul by pondering why you were selected as parents—as the guardians of its development this lifetime—and how your present conditions may affect your child's soul journey to perfection.

What might be the specific reasons a soul chooses to be cared for by *you* this incarnation? It may be fun for you to make a list. For example, if you have artistic or scientific inclinations, or you are a humanitarian, a soul may choose to use these qualities for its own evolution. Possibly your love of nature or sports, or your skill with cooking or gardening, will be an important example for the child's personality development. Some souls need to develop their social awareness and will choose a parent who is very confident with people. Parents may also be chosen for their inherent weaknesses or challenges. For example, in the most extreme case a soul may choose a parent who is abusive because the soul needs to balance its tendency to misuse power in past life actions; it is incarnating to master love, right use of will, and forgiveness this lifetime. Although you may never know for sure why your child's soul has chosen you, you'll find it useful to remain aware of the ways your and your partner's personalities and abilities can be positive models for your child's developing character and life purpose.

Pamela is very clear about why she chose her parents:

> I came into this world to minister to people. I had a mother who loved to serve anyone and everyone she had the opportunity to help. My dad was a deeply philosophical man who loved to teach me the connection between all forms of creation, and always talked about the presence of spirit in the most mundane aspects of daily life. I knew it was my life purpose to be a minister, and even though my parents never sent me to a Sunday school, their unique personalities were the best education I could have had to prepare me for my soul's mission this lifetime.

Two children of the same parents raised in the same household with the same environmental and hereditary conditions can be very different in their character and nature. We all are profoundly affected by our inherited genes, transgenerational patterns, and family and cultural factors. Yet reincarnation suggests that there are additional causes behind our inclinations and predispositions that have been developed during past lives (and obvious differences between siblings seem to bear this out). The Buddhists use the term *skandhas* to describe these innate behaviors, which are the fruits of our actions of our previous incarnations. Child prodigies—like Mozart, who played the harpsichord at age three—are examples of such possibilities. Yet these highly gifted children cannot develop their precocious talent without a supportive family environment or the appropriate genetic conditions. All factors from past lives and the present one need to align if the full potential of a child is to be unfolded.

How do you know if your child is incarnating with specific *skandhas*? A vigilant desire to discover who your child really is (including her past life heritage) and to care about her soul's highest destiny in this lifetime will naturally shape how you care for your child. Her talents may reveal themselves in her general abilities and propensities early on in life, so these abilities can be nurtured if she is destined to develop them in this lifetime.

Optimally, a child is conceived, nurtured, birthed, and parented in a spirit supportive of his continual unfolding potential. Often the conditions of caring for the *skandhas* can begin prior to birth. For example, during pregnancy a woman may suddenly find herself inspired to cultivate an artistic talent or academic pursuit that she had no previous personal inclination for. A Mozart type of soul may telepathically impress upon his mother a desire to listen to classical music during pregnancy.

Janice became very artistic during her pregnancy for the first time in her life. After her child was born, she lost interest again, but her child showed a passion for art very early in his life. It is impossible not to ask whose interest was being pursued during the pregnancy:

> It was a bizarre feeling . . . to find myself four months pregnant and to suddenly not only have a passion, but the skill to be painting like I was a professor of art. Paintings poured out of me throughout the rest of my pregnancy . . . styles I would not normally like . . . and then, as soon as George was born, the entire urge went out with the placenta. No kidding! His artistic abilities took over my life during that time, and now I have the wisdom and sensitivity to provide him with what he needs to express this gift of his. From the time he was able to hold a crayon, he was fascinated with drawing. Art has always been his favorite interest, starting in preschool.

It is possible that the soul of your child will be more mature and wise than either you or your partner. Therefore, it is important that both of you maintain a humble and honest attitude, allowing your child and her consciousness to explore and embody her own unique gifts, expressions, needs, and abilities. Recognize the incarnating soul as divine in its real nature—a unique, immortal spiritual being. You as parents are guardians, protectors, and guides of the soul's child body. The child belongs to the evolving consciousness of the soul, not to you as the parents. As you needed your own parents to support your growth, you now need to assist your child. Experience your child as incarnating for the purpose of evolving a spiritual self in human form, to perfect the expression of a divine consciousness and attributes in a human body. Experience the honor of being chosen to be parents for this lifetime of your child.

Creative Exercise:
Perceiving Your Future Child's Whole Self

1. How can a holistic approach to preparing for parenthood benefit you? Be specific.
   - Physically:
   - Emotionally:
   - Mentally:
   - Spiritually:
2. How can a holistic approach benefit the whole health of your future child? Be specific.
   - Physically:
   - Emotionally:
   - Mentally:
   - Spiritually:
3. If an incarnating soul needs a body to express itself in human form, and the body needs the life force of the soul to exist, what is your responsibility as a parent to your future child?
4. What is your personal understanding of your future child's whole self? How can you use this perspective to prepare for parenthood?
5. How does the notion of reincarnation contribute to your perception of your future child? What are the limitations of including reincarnation principles into your parenting experience? What are the benefits? Be specific.
6. What special qualities might attract a soul to choose you as its parents this lifetime?
7. Consider writing or drawing in your journal. You might:
   - Write a letter to the soul of your future child, integrating many of the insights you have gathered from reading this chapter.
   - Draw a picture of the soul of your future child. Then draw a picture of the human personality and the soul integrating before birth, and another picture showing their dynamic after they have been born.
   - Make a collage (using magazine images and words) exploring any of the above themes.

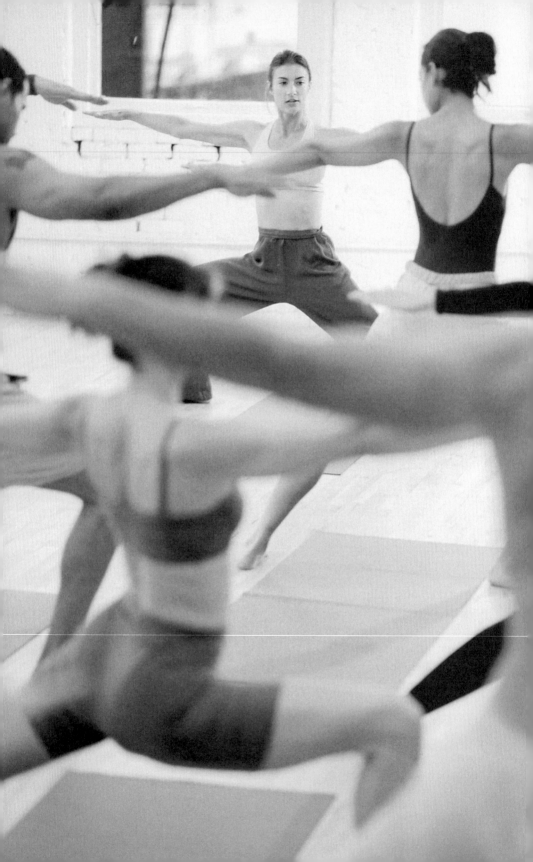

3

Preparing Your Body for Conception

From a material . . . point of view, it would seem that some of the teach-
ings concerning the timing of conception and prenatal care are unrea-
sonable curtailments of our individual pleasure. . . . But human activ-
ity is imbued with a certain spiritual responsibility. If we recognize the
tremendous creative power inherent in the human condition as being
co-equal to the power of Heaven and Earth, then perhaps we can accept
the responsibility that goes with that power.

Bob Flaws

Preparing Your Physical Body

For the holistically oriented couple, the moment of conception is filled
with mystery. Both parents know that the incoming soul exists apart
from matter, yet during their physical union the woman and man
transfer their genetic heritage to their child, creating the potential for a
spirit to embody in flesh. The sperm and egg unite to become one cell.
Each parent's chromosomal patterns merge to create the new zygote.
This fragile ball of unfolding cells will miraculously become a fully
formed baby within nine months.

How you prepare your physical health will impact how your sperm
and egg will carry the life force for the soul's optimal expression of its
divine essence in a human form. There is so much you can do to prepare

the sperm and egg to be their absolute healthiest before trying to conceive your child's physical body.

A child's physical body does not begin at conception or birth. It actually begins when the mother is in her own mother's womb. This is because the egg that will become her child is created at that time.

Between the fourth and fifth months of uterine development, the ovaries form in the female fetus; by the sixth month, all of the eggs she will ever have for her whole life are formed. The number of eggs is finite, and a particular egg may be twenty, thirty, forty, or more years old when finally used to create a human being. Because the stresses of life affect a woman's hormonal system, her eggs become less potent as she ages. Lifestyle choices also may expose the genes to harmful elements. In a very real way the egg that will create your future child has lived through all of your life conditions and has been exposed to the same toxins and environmental influences that you have experienced.[1]

Although the father's sperm cells are newly made each day, the male reproductive system is as delicate as the woman's. Extended immersion in water hotter than 101 degrees Fahrenheit, for example, as well as innumerable environmental influences, can disrupt a man's functional sperm for months. As the sperm matures, its quality and ability to move effectively through the female reproductive tract are affected by many conditions. Sperm motility, count, shape, and size all can decrease under various internal conditions.

The point is this: do not wait until the time of conception to focus on your physical health and that of your partner. This chapter will focus on how your diet, exercise, environment, and lifestyle patterns can endanger or optimize your egg or sperm and your ability to conceive, as well as jeopardize or promote your child's lifelong physical well-being.

Fertility Awareness

The time period of ovulation—an essential factor for conception to occur—is brief, so I recommend that you come to fully understand the miraculous mechanics of conception as part of your prepregnancy planning. Synchronization of both partners' reproductive systems is key for physical conception to occur. It is essential that a woman become knowledgeable about when she is most fertile, how the ovulatory cycle functions, how the body prepares to release the egg, how the sperm fertilizes the egg, and how the zygote implants and begins to develop in the uterus. Remember that the "average" cycle may not be your cycle.

Jake and Sally tried to conceive for more than two years without success. Jake recalls:

> Sal and I had been devoted to making love on the fourteenth day after the first day of her menstrual cycle every month. We had been on a radical preconception preparation program for a year before we even started, so we felt really healthy and ready for nature to gift us with life. One day our friend Hannah told us about how her infertility condition had been resolved. Her doctor thought she might be ovulating earlier than the average day fourteen that you read about in most fertility books. She was actually ovulating earlier than the norm. After Hannah's first month of determining her actual ovulation time, she conceived. That led Sal and me to question our assumed ovulation timing, and lo and behold! Her ovulation time was later than we had believed. Once we discovered Sally's unique timing, all three of our children were effortlessly conceived. I wonder how many "infertile" couples are ovulating early or late and don't even realize that conception is within their control. No one should take for granted knowing about timing and mechanics in making a baby.

Since the timing of ovulation is different for each woman, it is important for you to know your own cycle. Each month, once the egg has been released into the fallopian tube, it usually lives for twelve to thirty-six hours; only during this time can it be fertilized by the sperm and grow into a viable embryo. After ejaculation, it is estimated that sperm is capable of fertilizing an egg from the time of ejaculation up to seventy-two hours later. Given all the possible variations—especially for those with irregular menstrual cycles—appropriately timed sex can be a major factor in becoming a parent. There are numerous books on fertility awareness that will help you take advantage of your reproductive cycle. With your partner invest some time in your local library or bookstore to find a resource that illustrates in detail each partner's reproductive role.

Assess Your Physical Health

While planning for your baby, both parents can benefit by beginning to improve physical health at least three to six months prior to conception. It is never too soon to care for your health. Evaluating your health before pregnancy can minimize potential problems during and after the pregnancy.

There are no absolute rules to optimizing preconception and prenatal health care. The basic principle is to be as healthy as possible before a baby is conceived to ensure that your child is healthy from the beginning of his life. For some, optimizing health may mean stopping a destructive food, drug, or alcohol addiction. For others, it may mean a comprehensive evaluation and transformation of their diet, their body weight, or any harmful behavior. Potential parents who choose to sustain an addiction are putting their child at risk of developing abnormalities before or after birth. Similarly, those who continue to eat a poor diet should not feel victimized by a high-risk pregnancy or a malnourished newborn. By consciously improving your health habits before conceiving, you give your child the best opportunity to bloom with health.

Potential Risks

You can reduce risks during pregnancy by evaluating both your and your partner's reproductive health before conception. Each of you should begin by writing down your medical history. Identify potentially risky existing conditions, then work with your physician to keep a potentially high-risk pregnancy low risk. You may need to make major changes in diet and lifestyle, including professional obligations that can aggravate any unhealthy condition. Focus on solutions, not problems.

Divide your medical history into four parts:

1. The woman's general health.
2. The woman's reproductive health—birth control methods, past sexual diseases, previous miscarriages or abortions, menstruation patterns, infections, operations, past births, difficulty conceiving, past pregnancy or childbirth complications.
3. The man's general health.
4. The man's reproductive health.

Specify chronic conditions that may need to be controlled or monitored before, during, and after pregnancy, such as obesity, underweight, diabetes, heart disease, cancer (or a precancerous condition), other organ disease, genetic risks, and so on. Next, share this health inventory with your regular doctor or reproductive specialist and request a comprehensive physical exam and consultation.

Before trying to become pregnant, make sure your weight, blood pressure, hormonal system, and organs are in optimal health for fertility. A blood test can reveal any major deficiencies or imbalances that could prevent conception or a healthy pregnancy. Women should also get a Pap smear as well as a comprehensive evaluation to detect possible sexually transmitted diseases (STDs), especially if either partner was recently sexually active outside the current relationship. STDs such as herpes, chlamydia, syphilis, gonorrhea, and AIDS can cause miscarriage, birth defects, and infertility. Undetected venereal disease can endanger and even prevent your ability to conceive.

You may want to ask your health care provider whether you should have a mammogram several months before trying to conceive because pregnancy hormones can aggravate some precancerous and cancerous conditions. You do not want to get a mammogram once you are pregnant, or may be pregnant, unless medically advised. Also, some doctors suggest waiting to perform a mammogram until a mother is completely finished breast-feeding, so it may be a while before you can receive a mammogram once you do get pregnant. Talk over your concerns with your doctor.

One out of four women miscarries, and 70 percent of these women carry a pregnancy to term after two miscarriages. There are numerous reasons why a woman miscarries—genetic abnormalities, poor diet, excessive psychological or physical stress, or excessive exercise, to name but a few. Alice Domar, M.D., director of the Women's Health Programs at Harvard Medical School, states that "animal and human studies have [also] linked extreme stress and emotional upset to miscarriages."[2] A woman with a personal history of miscarriage can explore alternative as well as allopathic medical solutions. Learning conscious relaxation techniques and nourishing your own body, mind, and spirit will greatly help the fetus grow to full term once you conceive.

Consider your genetic makeup before conceiving. It's important to assess the genetic health of recent generations of both partners for any history of unhealthy genetic patterns or diseases within the family system. Get a genetic consultation prior to conception, or at the beginning of the first trimester of pregnancy. Genetic anomalies in either partner can give the appearance of extended periods of infertility because of spontaneous abortions or miscarriages that go undiagnosed. In *Before You Conceive* John R. Sussman, M.D., and B. Blake Levitt suggest that your child is vulnerable to genetic risks if any family member of either partner has a history of muscular dystrophy, cystic fibrosis, Down's syndrome, mental retardation, bleeding disorders, birth defects, skeletal deformities, spina bifida, anemia, epilepsy, limb abnormalities, liver or kidney disease, chemical imbalances, congenital heart defects, some forms of blindness, two or more miscarriages, long periods of infertility, or siblings who are stillborn or die at a young age. "Even slight mental deficits or mild facial irregularities," according to Sussman, "can indicate a recessive disorder that may manifest itself more severely in other family members."[3]

A holistic perspective takes these common medical facts into account but considers metaphysical influences as well. In chapter 5 you will learn that many physical abnormalities and disabilities are actually chosen by the incarnating soul as a part of its lessons in a particular lifetime. Thus, who or what determines whether a particular child will have a genetic disorder is unclear. Although you cannot know your future child's karma, gathering information regarding potential genetic challenges can reveal any red flags that indicate a need for testing. And remember that even if a genetic predisposition is transmitted to your child, it does not mean that the condition will manifest.

Some researchers now believe that your nurturing qualities can affect the genetic patterns in your prenate or child. According to cell biologist Bruce H. Lipton, Ph.D., the concept of genetic determinacy has traditionally held that "our lives are *predetermined* by the hardwiring of gene programs." But his cell research, and that of others, suggests that "the regulation of gene expression, that is the switching on and off of genes, is *not* a property of the genes themselves, but is controlled by environmental signals. Organisms under stress, are able to actively alter their DNA and create new genes in an effort to accommodate environmental challenges. Rather than being genetically 'predetermined,' organisms develop in balance with their environment, and purposely select, or if necessary rewrite, what they *perceive* to be appropriate gene programs to ensure their survival." Thus, the expression of specific genetic patterns in a child is now recognized to be regulated by nongenetic factors, including prenatal influences. Lipton notes that the "mother's [chronic] emotions, such as fear, anger, love [or] hope, among others, can biochemically alter the genetic expression of the offspring."[4] As I'll discuss more fully in chapter 4, your psychological health and your ability to love and nurture can therefore have a direct effect on the health of your future child.

If you feel your child is vulnerable to genetic disorders, I urge you to choose a holistic approach that includes genetic counseling as well as an understanding of the role psychological and metaphysical influences may play.

Glands and Hormones

Reproductive vitality requires balanced glands and hormones. Hormones—which are secreted into the bloodstream by glands—stimulate specific bodily functions and are the building blocks for reproductive health for the mother, as well as essential for the prenatal development of the child in utero. Even a minute imbalance or deficiency can affect fertility. Prior to conceiving, a qualified nutritionist or a doctor of traditional Chinese medicine who specializes in fertility issues can assist you in learning the appropriate diet for your unique physical constitution to optimize gland and hormone health.

Since the body and mind are interconnected and interdependent, here, too, psychological stress can trigger chemical and neurological changes, imbalancing the delicate hormonal system nourishing your reproductive system. Your childhood and emotional history—including both conscious and subconscious feelings, thoughts, and beliefs—can create adverse responses in your body.

Alice Domar, M.D., a leading pioneer in the field of fertility, states in her book *Healing Mind, Healthy Woman*, "We already have clues that stress and depression do contribute to infertility. On the female side, emotional upset has been shown to cause tubal spasms, irregular ovulation, and hormonal shifts, all of which can impact fertility. On the male side, stress has been associated with significant drops in sperm counts and quality." Given that the hypothalamus both controls the flow of reproductive hormones and regulates our emotional responses to stress, Dr. Domar concludes that "stress can alter the way the hypothalamus orchestrates these hormones, leading to irregularities that interfere with fertility. Stress can affect the levels of estrogen which is essential for normal ovulation and progesterone which is necessary for the embryo to implant."[5]

Improving the Health of Egg and Sperm

It is not uncommon for couples to conceive a child while remaining unaware of the complex and delicate factors involved in sustaining both a healthy reproductive system and healthy sperm and eggs. However, it increases your chances for a happy outcome if you optimize the vitality of these precious packets of DNA before they meet to create your future child.

For Future Dads: Optimize Sperm Health

Many potential fathers would be surprised to learn that, in cases of infertility, men are the infertile partner 40 percent of the time, and a contributing cause 20 percent of the time.[6] It is essential that a man produce enough sperm during ejaculation. But quantity is not the only criterion for a viable fertilization to occur. Men need to create *quality* sperm as well—defective sperm will challenge a man's ability to conceive naturally.

As a future dad, consider the many ways you can protect your sperm count and quality during your preconception preparation time. At the time of ejaculation you'll have just one auspicious moment to make your genetic contribution to your future child. Now is the time to optimize your offering:

- Care about your diet. Junk food and refined sugars are not good for the health of your reproductive system. Avoid products that contain cottonseed oil (often found in fried foods). Cottonseed oil is rich in gossypol, an antifertility agent that can affect sperm count. Protein-rich foods increase sperm vitality, as do whole grains and fiber. Follow a diet similar to the mother's pregnancy diet.

- Consider foods high in zinc. Zinc plays a significant role in the development of healthy sperm, because sperm cells have a greater zinc concentration than any other cells in the body. Zinc deficiency can cause decreased testosterone levels and sperm production. Food sources of zinc include seafood, meat, nuts, pumpkin and sunflower seeds, dairy products, whole grains, and brewer's yeast.

- Question your use of alcohol and tobacco. Cigarettes have a well-documented adverse effect on fertility.[7] And a man who drinks regularly during the month prior to conception (two drinks a day or five drinks at one sitting) may father a baby with low birth weight.[8]

- Research the health impact of recreational drugs. Marijuana and recreational drug use can affect sperm production.[9]

- Be aware of side effects of prescription drugs. Certain medications may decrease sperm production. Among these are some antidepressants and anticancer medications, as well as large doses of aspirin. If you experience fertility challenges, consult your doctor. Remember to read the label of your prescription drugs to see if there are warnings against side effects on fertility.

- Avoid steroid use at least three months before trying to father a child. Steroids can damage sperm and chromosomes.[10]
- Sexually transmitted diseases can create infertility, so you might want to get tested for these before attempting to conceive.
- Guard yourself against excessive X rays and radiation sources and against exposure to heavy metals. Some X rays can damage sperm production. In the body, the organs most sensitive to radiation are the male and female reproductive organs. Both radiation and many heavy metals can damage sperm and chromosomes.[11]
- Research workplace toxins that can inhibit sperm health. Fertility challenges have been found in workers who handle lead, pesticides, radiation, anesthetic gas, polystyrene, xylene, particular solvents, benzene, plutonium, arsenic, boron, cadmium, dioxin, and mercury.[12] Many of these substances also contribute to birth defects. If your vocation exposes you to any of these chemicals, consider ways you can safeguard yourself. Research the nutrients, such as antioxidants, that can protect you against some of the harmful effects of dangerous chemicals.
- Avoid pesticides such as DDT and Dens, which are known to lower fertility in men.
- Minimize heat and obstructions to your testicles. Excessive heat and obstruction to the testicles can harm fragile sperm. Studies show that higher body temperatures can reduce sperm production in the testes; this can affect your ability to conceive even if the mother is healthy. Although the normal core body temperature is 98.6 degrees Fahrenheit, sperm cells do not develop or function well when their temperature is higher than 93 or 94 degrees. Therefore, nature has put the testicles in a sac outside the body to allow sperm production.

Sitting in hot tubs, saunas, or Jacuzzis for long periods of time is not advised because the sperm cells can literally become cooked. Men who are experiencing infertility problems should wear looser pants and 100 percent cotton boxer underwear to increase air circulation, thus keeping the testes cooler.

This also applies to men who sit or straddle at work. Be sure to get up and move at regular intervals.

At least three months before trying to father a child, men should avoid hot tubs, saunas, electric blankets, hot water beds, and wearing bikini underwear. Fevers, infections, stress, and illnesses can affect sperm production for up to three months. This is because even though new sperm are produced daily, the cells take a little more than two months to fully form, and another several weeks to travel through the male reproductive system before they are ripe to fertilize an egg. So one fever or hot-tub exposure can completely wipe out a man's sperm count for months. And although it only takes one sperm to fertilize an egg, a count of twenty million sperm per cubic centimeter of ejaculate is considered low.

For Future Moms:
Optimize the Health of the Egg and Reproductive System

Ovulation occurs just once a month with a single egg. Considering the variables that must fall into place for pregnancy to occur, even under the best of circumstances a couple has about a 25 to 30 percent chance each month of conceiving. Age and lifestyle patterns affect ovulation cycles, which in turn can also affect the odds of conception occurring.

The growth and development of the follicles and egg during each ovulatory cycle are affected by two hormones, follicle-stimulating hormone (FSH) and lutenizing hormone (LH), which are controlled by the pituitary. In his comprehensive *Fertility Book* Dr. Richard Marrs explains that "emotional or other life experiences . . . may result in changes in the levels of hormones the pituitary releases, and ultimately a change in ovarian function."[13] He continues, "Anything that throws off the balance between the LH release and the response of the egg in its final maturity—be it stress, competitive physical training, or chronic illness—can affect fertilization and normal genetic competency."[14]

Since your eggs are present at birth, they are exposed to all of the toxic and environmental experiences of your life. Thus, the efficacy of your eggs may be affected over time, affecting your ability to produce a healthy baby. Anytime is always a good time to consider ways to reduce the deterioration of your eggs, and support the short- and long-term well-being of your reproductive system.

- Research and take a reliable daily prenatal vitamin that includes absorbable minerals and trace minerals for basic body building. You can begin taking a prenatal vitamin prior to conception, but it becomes crucial once you're pregnant. Make sure that any resource that you use to guide you about which vitamins to take also notes the essential quantities needed, as well as which amounts of certain vitamins are toxic to embryos. I suggest using several different sources to educate yourself, and then you can make an informed choice for you and your baby.
- Eat well before conception to store up specific nutrients. It is unclear how diet and fasting affect egg health, so why take the chance of depriving yourself of essential nutrients needed to keep your hormones balanced and your reproductive system well nourished? And once you're pregnant, your vulnerable fetus will be exposed to any detox reactions that can result from dieting or fasting. So refrain from dieting or fasting once you stop using birth control, especially diets that eliminate one of the four major food groups.
- Avoid overcooking; overcooked foods lose much of their wholesome value.
- Use whole grains and fibers when possible. Avoid junk food and refined sugars as well as processed foods that are nutritionally deficient.
- Cigarettes have well-documented harmful effects on a woman's fertility health. In addition, substances like tobacco and alcohol are associated with numerous obstetric complications for the fetus, as well as birth defects.[15]
- Certain medications may be detrimental to your reproductive system. If you plan on conceiving or experience fertility challenges, consult your doctor. Remember to read the label of your prescription drugs to see if there are warnings against side effects on fertility or pregnancy. And be sure to confirm that any herbs you are taking are not contraindicated during pregnancy.
- Research workplace and environmental toxins that can affect your reproductive health. Some hazardous biological and chemical substances can affect your eggs, ovaries, fallopian

tubes, and uterus and disrupt ovulation cycles. Fertility challenges have been found in workers who handle lead, pesticides, radiation, anesthetic gas, polystyrene, xylene, particular solvents, benzene, plutonium, arsenic, boron, cadmium, dioxin, and mercury.[16] Many of these substances also contribute to birth defects. If your vocation exposes you to any of these chemicals, consider ways you can safeguard yourself. Research the nutrients, such as antioxidants, that can protect you against some of the harmful effects of dangerous chemicals.

Choose Quality Food: A Healthy Diet for Fertility

Proper nutrition is a crucial component of preparing for your pregnancy because the food you eat becomes the building blocks from which your developing baby grows her physical body. Most women begin to actively care for their physical health once they know that they are pregnant, yet many are nutritionally careless before pregnancy begins. Adequate nutrition is important before conceiving your child, and it becomes essential from the very beginning of the delicate first trimester, when all of the organs are formed. For example, a lack of folic acid at conception can increase the risk of spinal tube defects; during the last trimester, poor protein consumption can affect brain development. Miscarriages and congenital defects, as well as high-risk pregnancies and deliveries (resulting in premature, underdeveloped babies), are more common among women who eat poorly either before or during their pregnancy.

Now is a perfect time to explore which foods are important for the developing fetus. If you can mamage it, a full year preceding conception is a healthy amount of time to make the necessary changes. Entering your pregnancy in an optimal nutritional state will give you some crucial reserves if you have morning sickness the first trimester and cannot eat much. According to Chinese medicine, your blossoming pregnant body will use the many nutrients you accumulated the trimester before you became pregnant. It is difficult to clinically determine subtle nutritional deficiencies, but you can improve your odds of having a healthy baby by taking charge of your diet and becoming mindful of the nutritional content of what you eat.

Begin to evaluate whether your nutritional intake is balanced among the food groups. There are more than fifty known nutrients needed for your body to function. These nutrients are divided into six categories: carbohydrates, proteins, fats, vitamins, minerals, and water. Minerals and vitamins are essential for many of the mother's body functions as well as the fetus's growth. Dieting or fasting before or during pregnancy can lead to nutritional deficiencies that can harm the fetus. As you prepare to conceive your baby, boost and nourish your body with nutrients rather than purging or eliminating them. There are some fasting programs that are scientifically designed to restore health. If you follow such a program, be sure you are clear about when you are planning to become pregnant.

Due to environmental and hereditary factors, everyone has a different basic constitution and caloric requirements vary from woman to woman. The same number of calories can be insufficient for one woman and yet excessive for another—and either case can be detrimental to the fetus. If you are either overweight or underweight, reevaluate your caloric intake before becoming pregnant. Seek a qualified nutritionist who specializes in fertility health to assist you in assessing your unique nutritional needs based on your lifelong biochemical history. If you have serious nutritional deficiencies, dietary changes and individual supplements should begin before you become pregnant. Although dietary requirements are different for everyone, some guidelines are useful to all:

- Learn about the amount of protein, carbohydrates, low- and high-fat foods, fruits, vegetables, salt, sugar, cholesterol, and fluids your baby will require you to eat as soon as you become pregnant. I used several pregnancy books that had been recently written or revised to educate myself, since recommendations may vary. Pay particular attention to discovering food sources that are rich in calcium, iron, vitamins, and minerals for proper fetal development and maternal health. Because at least two or three crucial weeks of fetal development occur before you can confirm that you are pregnant, begin this diet before you stop using birth control—optimally at least three months before you attempt to conceive, so you are on a healthy pregnancy diet at the time of conception. Future fathers may follow a prepregnancy diet that is similar to the mother's, adjusting the calories and nutritional requirements to their weight and health.
- Both men and women should make a detailed list of foods that are detrimental to health and can jeopardize the fetus, and make a conscious plan to eliminate these foods as soon as

possible. Read labels on any processed foods to identify questionable additives such as colorings, flavorings, preservatives, and "enhancers" such as MSG. Avoid foods preserved with nitrates and nitrites, including hot dogs, smoked meats, and luncheon meats such as salami and bologna. Fast foods and fried foods are seldom fresh and usually loaded with food additives and chemicals.

- Cook your own foods with fresh ingredients to obtain the greatest vitality. Overcooking can decrease nutritive value; freezing and canning food can also result in a loss of nutrients. Some processed whole foods that contain no chemicals can be nutritious; for example, preserved soybean products such as tofu and tempeh, cold-processed oil, honey, farmhouse cheeses, and nut butters are high in nutritive value.

When you eat organic produce, you are safeguarding the sperm and egg, and later the fetus, from toxic pesticide residue. If you must eat nonorganic fruits and vegetables, give them a detergent bath before using them. Foreign produce often contains higher levels of pesticides, since farming regulations are less strict than in the United States. Scrub and peel fruits and vegetables, especially right after you conceive your baby. What may not be toxic to you still may be harmful to the fetus.

- Eat complex whole-grain carbohydrates. Whole grains retain the outer husk or bran, which makes them nutritionally preferable to white and refined grains.

- Try to eat *certified-organic* meat, chicken, or fish, available at most health food stores. Inorganic livestock is given growth-stimulating hormones and antibiotics that can be potentially harmful to reproductive health. It is unknown what effect these additives may have on the developing fetus or the sperm and egg, so to avoid risks, make an effort to find a hormone- and antibiotic-free source of eggs, chicken, and meat.

Your local health department can inform you whether the fish in your area are contaminated with PCBs or other chemicals from polluted waters. PCBs are stored in fat tissue; there are birth defects classified as PCB syndrome. In general, ocean fish are safer than local fish from rivers and lakes, though dark fatty fish such as bluefish and striped bass can sometimes cause severe health hazards to the unborn child.[17]

- Eat iron- and calcium-rich foods to build nutritional reserves prior to conception. Once you become pregnant, you will immediately need to increase your intake of these minerals for the developmental needs of your child. Foods high in calcium include sprouted seeds and grains; dairy products; fish (salmon and sardines); soy products; dark green vegetables such as kale, collards, and broccoli; corn tortillas; some cooked dried beans; sesame seeds; almonds, filberts, and peanuts; dried fruit; and seaweed. High-iron foods include almonds, legumes (beans and peas), spinach, potatoes with skin, soy products, carob, blackstrap molasses, dried fruits, brewer's yeast, beets, green leafy vegetables, seaweeds, and eggs. Avoid coffee or tea with your meal or immediately after eating because these stimulants can inhibit the absorption of iron.

- Fats, carbohydrates, and proteins are basic components of any healthy diet. In particular, proteins provide the amino acids essential for the effective functioning of your hormones and antibodies, both key factors to your fertility health. Meat, poultry, dairy products, fish, and eggs are complete proteins. Beans and nuts need to be combined with grains for the body to get enough protein.

- Folic acid prevents neural tube defects as well as assisting the building of red blood cells and your child's nervous system. Dark leafy greens and root vegetables, brewer's yeast, whole and sprouted grains, whole milk, dates, mushrooms, and orange juice are great natural sources of folic acid.

- Strengthen your body's immune system with foods and, if necessary, supplements. This will support the health of your pregnancy, diminishing the chances of a miscarriage, stillbirth, or birth defects.

- Along with oxygen, water is essential to the creation and sustenance of life. The child will float in the water that you drink. Any substances that are harmful to the mother will be exponentially detrimental to the prenate, so make sure that your tap water is safe to drink before you become pregnant.

Some water in the United States is known to be contaminated with lead from old pipes. Some toxic sewer and chemical sites, factory wastes, dumping grounds, and underground

storage tanks can contaminate your local water source. Underground water wells are also vulnerable to contamination.
Check with your local health department about the safety and
purity of your drinking water. If you are not sure that your
water is chemical-free, invest in a reliable water filter before
you become pregnant.

- Women and men who are vegetarians will have different requirements and restrictions than those with more inclusive
diets. If you are a vegetarian, carefully assess your diet over a
considerable time before becoming pregnant. Once pregnant,
you will need more iron, zinc and B_6, as well as the protein
and calcium commonly obtained from meat, fish, eggs, and
dairy products. Health food products such as spirulina and
other "green foods" can supplement potential nutritional deficiencies. There are many books on being a pregnant vegetarian
woman that allow you to research specific dietary recommendations during your prepregnancy preparation. Begin to increase protein, calcium, iron, and vitamin intake.

Supplement Options

Supplements can resolve nutritional deficiencies and support metabolic
needs for virility and fertility. There are two main types of supplements
to support fertility health: herbal nutrition and vitamins/minerals.
Optimally, iron, calcium, folic acid, vitamins A, C, D, E, K, and all of the
B-complex vitamins need to be available to the mother's body from the
beginning of pregnancy. Some men and women struggling with infertility may be missing essential nutrients. Studies have shown that certain
concentrations of copper, evening primrose oil, and vitamins A and B_6
can benefit such women. To assist a man in creating healthy sperm,
vitamin C, arginine, and B_{12} in small doses have been shown to be
beneficial.[18] Inform yourself about possible proper prenatal supplementation for both parents before you try to conceive.

Once you're pregnant, illnesses, biochemical imbalances, and daily
supplement programs need to be treated differently. A megadose of
anything, even a natural supplement, can overload the growing fetus's
system. The fetus's small systemic capacity should be taken into account
when figuring dosages of all supplements, whether synthetic or natural.
For example, Dr. Sussman warns that "too much Vitamin C (as well as
other vitamins) ingested during the pregnancy may create artificial

dependencies in the baby . . . babies may have to be weaned from vitamins they receive in the womb much like babies of addicts must be weaned from drugs."[19] So if you are taking any supplements to strengthen your reproductive health before becoming pregnant, make sure you don't take large doses of vitamins once you stop using birth control. High doses of vitamins A, B$_6$, C, and D, and of iodine, have been implicated as potential causes of birth defects. A properly formulated prenatal vitamin will protect you from ingesting excessive doses of any one vitamin.

The best way to optimize your vitamin and mineral intake is to learn what foods are rich in the nutrients essential for fertility health, although there are some people who will benefit from supplementation because of their unhealthy lifestyle patterns or unknown fertility challenges.

Vitamin E is frequently mentioned as a way to improve the sperm's ability to impregnate. It also has been shown to prevent miscarriages because it strengthens the uterine wall and placenta. Whole grains, wheat germ, vegetable oils, green vegetables, seeds, and nuts—especially uncooked almonds—are great sources of vitamin E.

There is growing evidence that vitamin C has beneficial effects on sperm production[20] as well as assisting ovarian function and egg health. Vitamin C is not stored in the body, so a fresh dose is needed daily. Excellent fruit and vegetable sources of vitamin C include cantaloupes, citrus fruits and juices, berries, tomato products, papayas, mangos, avocados, pineapples, asparagus, peppers, broccoli, cauliflower, mustard greens, radishes, brussels sprouts, and red cabbage. Bioflavonoids assist the development of the uterine lining by improving the tone of veins and capillary walls, thus optimizing implantation. Broccoli, cabbage, green peppers, parsley, and citrus fruit rinds are great sources of bioflavonoids.

The B vitamins strengthen the nervous system and hormonal balance. Vitamin B deficiency can create an excess of estrogen, while too much of the B vitamins can cause an insufficiency. The B vitamins are found in unprocessed whole grains, and they are devoured by refined sugar, caffeine, alcohol, drugs, and stress. Yeast, eggs, fish, wheat germ, avocados, nuts, seeds, and soybeans are great sources for the B-complex vitamins.

It is worth repeating the importance of folic acid (found in the vitamin B family) in both parents' diets prior to conception to prevent neural tube defects. Excellent food sources of folic acid include dark green leafy vegetables, root vegetables, whole milk, mushrooms, orange juice, brewer's yeast, salmon, and dates. Although folic acid is readily available in the diet, many prenatal health books urge women and men to take a 400 mcg to 800 mcg folic acid supplement beginning several months before attempting to conceive. Most prenatal supplements provide the proper amount of folic acid.

Vitamin A has been linked to sperm production as well. Since this vitamin can be toxic in megadoses, use beta-carotene—a precursor to vitamin A with all its benefits. Many fruits and vegetables are beta-carotene rich, especially the yellow fruits and vegetables such as apricots, papayas, cantaloupes, carrots, sweet potatoes, winter squash, peas, and broccoli and some leafy greens like kale and spinach.

Food sources of vitamin D include eggs, fish liver oils, fortified milk, and butter.

Although most of these vitamins and minerals are beneficial when ingested as unprocessed natural food, be aware that some are toxic if taken as supplements. For example, vitamins A and D and zinc can be harmful in large amounts; vitamin C also can have side effects. Qualified nutritional counselors who specialize in prepregnancy health can help you determine safe dosages. They can also recommend specific nutritional supplements for increasing energy to the reproductive system, improving the vitality of the eggs and sperm, and tonifying the endocrine system by nourishing the glands, thereby enhancing proper hormone secretions. If you are unable to find such expertise, eat the foods that will offer you a well-balanced nutrient supply.

A good-quality prenatal vitamin has the appropriate quantities of essential nutrients. Take extra absorbable calcium and nonconstipating iron as supplements if daily dietary intake is low. If you do take an iron supplement, combine it with vitamin C to aid absorption. According to some sources, calcium is ineffective when combined with iron, so consider taking them as separate supplements at different times of day.

Medicinal herbs can be thought of as concentrated foods that work in conjunction with the body's own enzyme action. They are natural nutrients used to "inspire" the body to do its own work and restore natural balance. Herbs nourish the body because they are full of absorbable minerals, vitamins, amino acids, and precursors. They work best in combination with other herbs; formulas should be customized to meet the unique needs of each person. The vast majority of herbs are safe and are not addictive or habit forming.

However, not all herbs are beneficial for the prenate and some can be potentially harmful. Some commonly used herbs that are contraindicated (in medicinal amounts) once you're pregnant include: aloe vera (as a laxative), angelica, bayberry, black cohosh, blueberry, catnip, chaparral, coffee, coltsfoot, comfrey, dong quai, ephedra, fennel seed, goldenseal, juniper berry, kava kava, licorice, pennyroyal, sage, senna, shepherd's purse, uva ursi, and yarrow. Other herbs traditionally used for childbirth, such as blue cohosh, should be used only under medical supervision. Likewise, while some herbalists recommend ginger for morning sickness, practitioners of traditional Chinese medicine believe it is inappropriate for women who are vulnerable to miscarriage. The safest plan is to always work with a qualified herbalist who is experienced with pregnant women.

Dottie, a women's health care nutritionist, has seen many women with difficulties conceiving suddenly become pregnant when their nutritional and supplemental programs were redesigned. "I cannot tell you how naive most women are about the harmful effects of too little or too much supplementation. What is beneficial for one woman may be very harmful to another and her prenate. Even books and practitioners vary in their opinions, so women should get more than one perspective."

Exercise Can Help

Important note: Check with your doctor before embarking on any type of prepregnancy or pregnancy exercise if you have a known potential for premature labor, high blood pressure, heart disease, fetal abnormality, anemia, diabetes, or other chronic condition.

Pregnancy is a challenge for the body. Being in healthy physical shape before you conceive will contribute toward the health of your pregnancy, as well as increase your ability to give birth naturally and make a speedy postnatal recovery. Women who are less fit before they become pregnant are often unable to continue their routine activities without considerable fatigue. Before conception, increase your vitality and strengthen your cardiovascular condition to withstand the rigors of pregnancy. Develop an exercise routine that will tone and strengthen your muscles in preparation for carrying and giving birth to your baby.

Since the abdominal and lower-back muscles are the most stressed as pregnancy progresses, before conception is the time to strengthen them. In Chinese medicine it is suggested that using the abdominal muscles with too much vigor can strain rather than strengthen them. Overexertion or standing too long can be depleting for some women's reproductive energy. The Chinese perspective prescribes exercise that is gentle and nurturing; activities such as walking, moderate hiking, and swimming are recommended. For some women, excessive bike riding is not considered beneficial because it overstimulates the uterus. If you use weight lifting as part of your routine, you must be careful. Too much lifting can drain the vital reproductive life force that you need to conceive, implant, and maintain the growth of the fetus in the womb, especially during the first trimester. Avoid any activity that can lead to abdominal trauma. Avoid risky sports such as skiing, surfing, and horseback riding, which can precipitate miscarriage if you fall and jostle the embryo. Also, avoid aggressive, competitive contact sports. As soon as you stop using birth control, begin to enjoy gentler pastimes.

Excessive exercise can also interfere with ovulation. For certain women, regular routines that tighten the abdominal muscles can actually affect the uterine blood flow needed for conception and implantation to occur and be sustained. And although building stamina and muscle strength before pregnancy is advantageous, a strenuous and prolonged routine during the first weeks of your pregnancy can put undue stress on the embryo. Since most women are unaware of pregnancy for several weeks, it's important to adjust your workout once you stop using birth control.

A further concern is that during an intense workout routine, the mother's body temperature is elevated to levels that are unsafe for the embryo. The baby is unable to transfer excessive body heat throughout his system, which can result in organ damage or even miscarriage. It's important that you structure your exercise program accordingly. The standard preconception and pregnancy protocol for vigorous exercise is a fifteen-minute period with a cool-down interval of five or ten minutes before beginning again. A class designed for pregnant women, like prenatal yoga or prenatal aerobics, will certainly take the dangers of overexercise into consideration, but it's a good idea to question the teacher before signing up. Any type of yoga that emphasizes stretching and supporting muscle flexibility is beneficial preparation for your body to become, or be, pregnant. There are some yoga positions that are to be avoided during pregnancy. Find a class that follows the guidelines of the American College of Obstetricians and Gynecologists (ACOG) for prepregnancy and pregnancy exercise.

Men, too, should temper their activity when attempting parenthood. Too much stress before conception, according to Chinese medicine, can weaken the sperm. While it is okay to continue exercising around the time of your partner's ovulation, be gentle; choose more nurturing exercises, or exercise only for a length of time that does not drain your vitality.

Toby and Clay were both body builders and spent four years trying to conceive. Toby feels passionately about the impact this had had on her ability to conceive:

> It was not until I discovered that not all exercise is good for me and my reproductive health that I stopped my compulsive exercise and switched to a gentler stretching routine. Not only did it enable me to become pregnant with twins, but it helped me feel more self-nurturing and, because of that, more maternal toward my children in utero. I realize in retrospect that until I dropped my obsessive need to be physically toned, my body (and mind) were too wired for any fetus to feel I was open and receptive to it.

Ideally, prepregnancy exercise is oriented toward opening, releasing, gentle toning, and joyful movement. Here are some guidelines that will be appropriate for most women to follow:

- Get in condition before pregnancy to build stamina and muscle strength.
- Engage in light aerobic-type exercise at least three times a week for twenty minutes minimum before conception to prepare for the endurance, flexibility, and strength you'll need for pregnancy and childbirth. Brisk walking, bicycling, and swimming are safe exercises. Strenuous jogging can stop ovulation for some women.
- Strengthen abdominal muscles and lower-back muscles before pregnancy if possible. These muscles are the most stretched by the growing fetus.
- Enjoy safe sports. Check sports equipment for safety.
- Do yoga postures beneficial to the pituitary, ovarian or testicular, and glandular systems. Check with a qualified yoga teacher about the safety of any yoga postures that you practice.

The Biological Clock and Fertility Challenges

Most women can become pregnant naturally only during a finite period of time, usually between the ages of twelve and forty-five. The tension of a ticking biological clock can increase the stress of a couple's preconception preparation experience. Many couples who have waited until their late thirties or early forties to attempt becoming pregnant experience fertility problems. Those who pursued careers, waiting to establish financial security, or who have had personal reasons to defer parenthood might feel the pressure to become pregnant before they get too old. Everyone knows people who have encountered fertility challenges and been told that they were "too old" to be fertile. Commonly referred to as infertility, this crisis can tax the best of relationships.

Who determines when a man or woman is "too old" to become pregnant or give birth to a child? While women face the biological reality that their age can defy their desire to have a child, no natural age limit has been placed on men who want to become fathers. Assisted Reproductive Technologies (ART) such as fertility drugs, artificial insemination, in vitro fertilization (IVF), and sperm or egg donation has extended the potential window of pregnancy for both women and men. If you are feeling the reproductive clock ticking, first determine whether your concerns are based in reality or are in reaction to a stubborn cultural mythology that women over thirty-five have a hard time conceiving.

For a natural conception to occur, the woman's ovaries must produce a viable egg, the fallopian tube must be open to receive the egg, the lining of the uterus must be healthy enough to allow and sustain the implantation of a fertilized egg, and the woman's own hormones must be balanced, producing the proper amount and kind of hormones to support ovulation and then implantation and growth of the embryo. The man must produce enough healthy sperm capable of reaching and fertilizing the egg while it is in the fallopian tubes.

It is true that the incidence of infertility is increasing with every decade. Presently, one in six couples is considered infertile. The rise in infertility has numerous causes. Many women from the baby-boom generation postponed motherhood in favor of establishing careers. Often these women have put off childbearing past the optimal time of "effortless conception," increasing the incidence of age-related infertility. And this is not just a female problem: The average sperm count has decreased about 30 percent since 1950. Male infertility prevents conception 40 percent of the time, while 40 percent can be traced to women. About 10 percent of infertility is the result of health problems of both partners, and 10 percent is designated "unexplained."

The medical definition of *infertility* is an "inability to conceive after a year of unprotected sexual intercourse," assuming that you are ovulating normally and having appropriately timed sex. Normally, about 25 percent of all couples attempting to become pregnant will conceive the first month, and about 80 percent within a year if they are having intercourse two or three times a week, and particularly when the woman is ovulating. It is common for couples to try to conceive for six to twelve months before succeeding.

If you and your partner have been experiencing fertility challenges— that is, if after twelve months or more you have not been able to conceive—you may want to explore the matter further. If you are near forty, you may want to take action after six months. Hundreds of variables can affect the reproductive synergy between you and your partner. Delayed childbearing and environmental factors can create many health challenges for both of you. However, many imbalances and abnormalities that disrupt the intricate reproductive process can be healed with holistic treatments.

The innumerable causes of challenged fertility, commonly referred to as infertility, are beyond the scope of this book. Recent breakthroughs in high-tech fertility medicine have given hope to many couples who thought that they could never have children. If you are experiencing difficulty in becoming pregnant, consult your doctor or contact Resolve, a national educational organization devoted to the resolution of infertility.

If you eventually choose to seek medical treatment for infertility, including the holistic approach offered by this book can increase the effectiveness of those procedures. Most traditional Western fertility therapies address the condition by offering medical drugs or technological procedures to rectify the depleted or injured reproductive system; a holistic approach will nurture and strengthen the innate physical and psychological weaknesses that may be causing infertility. Chances for positive outcomes are improved when necessary medical and technological fertility treatments are combined with holistic and body-mind approaches. It is important to know that even though the physical body may be ready, lifestyle patterns and unconscious psychological conflicts may still prevent a successful conception and pregnancy. Those who choose to implement the holistic approach will enhance their whole health, whether or not they conceive.

Reality and Myth about Time

The contemporary trend is to discourage women from feeling confident that they can conceive as they near or surpass the age of forty. This can be misleading for those who are in excellent physical and reproductive health. Your biological age (determined by the year you were born) can be quite different from your reproductive age (most commonly determined by the condition of your eggs or sperm, as well as your hormones and reproductive organs). Some women have a biological age of forty or more, but a younger reproductive age. Conversely, there are women who are twenty-five but, due to hormonal imbalances, are pre- or perimenopausal like women in their late forties or fifties. The forty-year-old in optimal health has a much better chance of becoming pregnant than the twenty-five-year-old who is addicted to drugs or alcohol, or who has lived her life eating junk food and smoking cigarettes.

Although age-related infertility does destroy many couples' dreams of having their own biological child, another factor is more often responsible. As I mentioned previously about Dr. Alice Domar's research, stress may affect the levels of a woman's estrogen (essential for normal ovulation) and progesterone (necessary for an embryo to implant), as well as a man's sperm count and quality. Since either partner's hormonal system can be affected by many types of physical and psychological stress, a couple experiencing fertility challenges, or those who just want to be as healthy as possible before conception, should examine how their lifestyle or work situation may be adding to their stress levels.

Rather than listening to the stress-producing tick of your reproductive clock, you can use the holistic perspective to optimize your reproductive health so that as you continue to age, your reproductive system becomes younger and healthier. Even younger couples should bear in mind that it is never too early to learn how to defy age-related statistics. Though for many couples infertility is an authentic condition, there are many others who have learned how to redesign their lifestyle to prevent premature reproductive aging—and some have even reversed their reproductive aging.

My own experience is a good example. At the age of thirty-five I was told by a fertility specialist that my biological condition was too weak to conceive a child and sustain a pregnancy. I was devastated to learn this, for my life calling was to be a mother, and I had never dreamed that this destiny of mine could be threatened. It seemed absurd to me that as a thirty-five-year-old woman, I was unable to become a mother. Choosing to empower the very core of my identity, I refused to consider myself infertile. I began to describe my condition as a "fertility challenge," giving myself the suggestion that I faced the formidable task of discovering the elements that were weakening my physical and psychological capability to be fruitful. I was up for the challenge.

As I muddled through the mainstream infertility books, I was overwhelmed by the pessimistic statistics. But when I learned that there was a difference between reproductive and biological age, I became determined to learn what I could do to heal my weakened reproductive state. I pored through dozens of alternative-medicine books, searching for guideposts that could point me in the direction of hope and renewal of my birthright as a fertile woman.

It was through my own fertility journey that I learned that the biological clock is both reality and myth. For by the time I conceived my daughter—naturally, at the biological age of thirty-nine—I was reproductively much younger and healthier than I had been at thirty-five. I had discovered the key to the restoration of my reproductive health in blending the best of Eastern and Western approaches. And I learned, through direct experience, the power that self-awareness had to reclaim my physical heritage as a mother.

Negative labels such as *infertility, unproductive organs, old eggs, poor sperm quality,* and *inadequate hormones* disempower women and men in their journey toward parenthood. According to Niravi Payne, creator of the Whole Person Fertility Program, "The 'too oldisms' that currently are prevalent in our culture are a smoke screen for much larger family and personal issues that affect your mind and body."[21] I invite you to explore the power of the mind-body connection over your fertility health. No matter what your age, your preconception planning will benefit if you include the mind-body link in it.

Stress and Reproductive Vitality

During the past several decades, as holistic care has been increasingly accepted by the mainstream, the term *mind-body medicine* has become respected in Western medicine. Rather than depending exclusively on drugs or invasive procedures to treat medical conditions, mind-body medicine recognizes the importance of psychological and behavioral care to treat the whole person. Mind-body approaches suggest that our physical and psychological imbalances can be transformed by applying an intentionally developed self-awareness to the resolution of our suffering.

Scientific research demonstrates that the stress in our lives can create havoc in our body. Alice Domar, M.D., explains that "our hearts get overstimulated, our hormonal output becomes unbalanced, and our immune systems—those inner networks of healing and defense—are weakened. We now have evidence that women's reproductive systems can be affected by stress and ongoing emotional upset."[22] Domar's health programs for conditions that predominantly affect women show that managing physical and emotional stress can improve physiology, including the reproductive systems of both women and men. Domar considers mind-body medicine to be any method in which we use our mind to change our physical or psychological health. The mind-body effect also occurs any time we align our behavior with ways that promote health, with or without the use of a "technique."

Nonetheless, devote some time to exploring some of the more common techniques that induce a mind-body connection, such as meditation, yoga, deep breathing, or any activity that elicits a state of relaxation and mindfulness. Stress management, including coping skills, emotional exploration and expression, problem solving, and effective communication skills, also should be embraced for its value in reducing levels of stress. Domar and others advocate individual or group cognitive therapy, which assists you in evaluating and changing limiting thoughts and feelings that undermine your health. Biofeedback and hypnosis are also useful techniques, although they do depend on the assistance of a qualified practitioner.

Niravi Payne challenges the use of the term *stress* to describe a state of being. She believes that your "current responses to tension-provoking situations are often related to your family conditioning and early childhood experiences."[23] When you feel angry, sad, anxious, lonely, or even depressed, she recommends that you name the feeling rather than blame the stress. Since suppressing emotional reactions to past experiences can affect the delicate balance of the hormonal system necessary for conception, do not deny the psychological realities that may be adversely affecting your reproductive health. Consciously consider and acknowledge where you may be holding your feelings in your body.

Although we often think of stress as only negative, a state that drains our creative energy, remember that what is stressful to one person may be invigorating or inspiring to another. There is positive stress that can challenge you to unfold your full potential. Effective stress management thus goes beyond coping with your daily tensions; it is better understood as the ability to experience the stresses of life while maintaining the positive and healthy quality of your inner and outer world.

The Mind-Body Connection to Your Fertility Wellness

The term *mind-body* suggests that the physical, emotional, and mental states of your being are interconnected and interdependent. The mind-body approach to preconception and prenatal health care addresses the effects of anxiety and stress on fertility outcomes. Your feelings and thoughts trigger physiological responses in the body that can affect the chemical, hormonal, and neurological balances in your reproductive system. For example, you may consciously feel ready to have a baby while subconsciously remaining ambivalent, perhaps because of unresolved memories from your past. The biochemical effect of suppressed emotions can confuse the hormonal system. In her book *Women's Bodies, Women's Wisdom* Christiane Northrup, M.D., explains that "the mind/body approach to fertility is based on the premise that knowledge is power and that a change in perception based on new information is powerful enough to effect subtle changes in your endocrine, immune and nervous systems."[24] While psychological well-being will be explored at greater length in the next chapter, you should be aware of how psychological stresses can affect your physical state, particularly your ability or inability to conceive.

Psychoneuroendocrinology is the study of the relationships among emotions, the nervous system, and the endocrine (hormone) system. Scientific evidence verifies that emotions do affect the body's delicately balanced hormone functions. Depression, stress, and other forms of psychological trauma can set off chemical processes in the body that interfere with ovulation.

Dr. Alice Domar has explained how stress and emotions can affect fertility outcomes for women and men. Niravi Payne concurs as she describes "how emotionally laden experiences are transmitted biochemi-cally and electrically to the hypothalamus, ultimately negatively affect-ing the pituitary gland's output of LH and FSH, affecting ovulation and spermatogenesis."[25]

Many scientific findings suggest that psychological support can improve conception and positive birth outcomes. Dr. Northrup states that "you need to know that your ability to conceive is profoundly influenced by the complex interaction among psychosocial, psycho-logical, and emotional factors, and that you can consciously work with this to enhance your ability to conceive."[26] Consciously addressing your feelings and thoughts is essential to optimizing your fertility health. Now is a great time to evaluate any potential psychological barriers to conception.

Holistic health modalities can relieve physical and psychological stress and empower you to open up to new possibilities. Anne remembers:

> I was not able to conceive after a year of consistent effort. My childhood sexual abuse experiences were literally shutting out my chances of becoming a mother. The shame, the fear that I might restimulate these past memories, the suppressed anger, grief, and confusion that had been stored in my belly for three decades were literally telling my womb, "No way life can grow in me, and no way do I deserve to be a mother." I was afraid that having a baby would bring back all the suppressed pain. After months of intensive coun-seling, I felt my self-respect restored and my body excited to have a baby, and I even had positive thoughts about my childhood. My body went from being run by a deep subconscious no to mother-hood to a wonderful yes to life growing inside me. I will never again underestimate the power of the mind-body connection.

Repatterning lifelong beliefs about sexuality, conception, pregnancy, birth, children, parenthood, and family relationships will increase your ability to conceive and nurture a healthy pregnancy to fruition. You can change your personal and professional life so that your mind-body responds positively to the challenges of your life.

Which holistic modalities can best increase your chances of concep-tion? Each person has unique needs. Some need to pay more attention to physical health considerations, while others need more psychological or spiritual support. Since the physiological, psychological, and spiri-tual factors related to reproduction are interconnected, it's beneficial to work with a practitioner who addresses your whole health. A holistic prebirth evaluation session can clarify which areas of your inner and outer life need care. In addition, most natural approaches will increase the effectiveness of medical fertility interventions.

Some couples may benefit from counseling. For those with continual and unresolved feelings of anxiety, self-judgment, resentment, guilt, shame, anger, longing, depression, ambivalence, disappointment, or any unresolved emotions—or if you feel emotionally out of control, reactive, detached from life, or ambivalent about having a child—I strongly recommend including counseling as part of your prepregnancy program.

Prepregnancy Self-Test

Your custom fertility program should be designed to meet your unique needs as well as those of your partner and your future child. Whether you are able to consult a professional preconception counselor or not, begin by writing a comprehensive examination of your personal and professional lifestyle. Include:

- History of your fertility health treatments
- Your diet
- Social and professional lifestyle
- Stress patterns (define)
- Unresolved past traumas
- Preconception preparation ideas
- Early-childhood memories
- Psychological concerns
- Relationship challenges
- Ambivalences, fears, and doubts
- Exercise and self-care routines
- Other fertility concerns

Bringing this information into your conscious awareness allows you to draw on it when deciding which issues need the most attention and nurturing in your prepregnancy planning.

A holistic program will combine the best of all modalities—Western and Eastern medicine, nutritional and herbal education, psychological counseling, body-oriented therapies, homeopathy, acupuncture and Chinese medicine, and, for those who desire it, spiritual support. By investing in pregnancy wellness, you will also improve your overall health.

Using Eastern Medicine in Your Prepregnancy Program

The wisdom of traditional Chinese medicine (TCM) can be a valuable asset while you prepare for a healthy pregnancy. Historically, Chinese society has placed a great emphasis on the birth of children and the healthy continuation of the family lineage. Chinese medical practices related to conception and prenatal health care have been used for more than two thousand years. Eastern medicine is founded on a conceptual model of the human body that's significantly different from modern Western medicine's. Yet rather than invalidating one another, the two systems are complementary when applied knowledgeably.

Yin and Yang

Yin (negative, feminine) and yang (positive, masculine) are the two qualities of the universal force that exist as primordial energy within all forms of creation. In all aspects of life there is a continual dance between these two opposing yet interdependent forces as life and death, light and dark, female and male arise and disappear. In humans yang is represented by fire, yin by water. Any biological or psychological state or energetic change that is similar to the qualities of fire or water is described as yin or yang. Nothing is innately yin or yang; a condition that is yin in one situation may be yang in another, since things are yin or yang only in relationship to something else.

"Within the body, yin and yang must remain in dynamic, harmonious balance. Yang must quicken yin; yin must nourish, cool, and root yang. Life requires them both, as the seed sprouts in spring only with nourishment of the soil and melting snow (yin) and the warmth of the sun (yang)."[27] If this harmonious relationship of yin and yang is not sustained in the body of a woman or man trying to conceive, the imbalance may prevent conception from occurring.

According to Chinese medicine, climate can affect the yin or yang essence of the body. For example, wearing short skirts or going outside with a wet head on a cold day can create an imbalance, especially when a woman is menstruating. Excessive physical work, strenuous exercise, or improper diet can weaken an organ's yin-yang balance.

Janet recounts her joy in discovering the wisdom behind applying principles of Chinese medicine to preconception health care:

> For years I tried to become pregnant, and people kept telling me to change my diet and my stressful lifestyle. It was not until I started

reading about Chinese healing principles that I realized there were ancient guidelines I could use to repattern all of my habitual "burn-out" patterns. Now I am forty-four years old and have a newborn. Understanding how to revitalize myself and consciously stay on an even energy keel has kept me from premature aging and allowed me to have a child so late in my life.

Chi

All forms of Chinese medicine, including the most popular forms of acupuncture, acupressure, and herbology practiced in the West, are based on the concept of chi, the vital energy force flowing through the body. Chi is the basic principle behind most Eastern philosophies. It is the "activating energy of the universe . . . that condenses and disperses in alternating cycles of negative and positive (yin and yang) energy, materializing in different ways, forms and shapes."[28] Our thoughts and feelings are temporary manifestations of energy, as is the human form—our physical matter. Chi maintains all of the biological systems of the body and keeps all of the parts united until death, when the chi is withdrawn from the physical body.

Chinese medicine is founded on the understanding that health is dependent on the quality and quantity of chi, and how it either circulates or stagnates in the body. The healing arts that recognize chi as a causal factor will diagnose a deficiency or excess of chi in an organ as the cause of a physical or psychological imbalance. By releasing blockages and increasing the flow of chi, we can often heal ourselves.

In their book *Body of Light* John Mann and Larry Shore note that forty-nine different cultures around the world recognize chi or a parallel concept to describe the original energy within creation. Hebrews called it *ruach* in Genesis, meaning "divine breath." The Japanese call it *ki,* the Hindus refer to *prana* in Sanskrit, and the Tibetans use the word *lung.* The Islamic use *barraka,* to the Lakota Sioux it is *neyatoneya,* and to Russians it is *bioplasma.* Considering how widespread this concept is, it is strange that most mainstream medical science in the West shows slight interest in understanding chi. Only with the advent of holistic health theory has this idea of subtle energy life force, sometimes referred to as "etheric energy," been included in health care models.

Chi flows through twelve pairs of energy channels, commonly referred to as meridians, which are linked to our different organs. In addition, two channels run down the front and back midlines, and six extra meridians link the entire energy system. Every part of the body is animated by this energy.

For optimal preconception health of both parents, as well as prenatal harmony for mother and child, the chi must flow freely. For example, the spleen, stomach, and kidney meridians nourish the uterus, placenta, and baby from the moment of conception until the baby is born from the mother's body. If these pathways are blocked, an acupuncturist can use very fine needles to stimulate specific points along the meridians that will encourage reproductive vitality and realign physical imbalances to their innate healthy state. Those who are reluctant to accept the use of needles can visit an acupressure practitioner, who will use finger pressure to stimulate acupuncture points along the meridians. Since certain points should not be used during pregnancy, it is important to work only with a well-trained practitioner who regularly cares for pregnant women.

Reproductive Essence: The Red and the White

According to traditional Chinese medicine, the sexual essences of the parents combine to form the fertilized zygote. Healthy female (red) and male (white) essences create a healthy baby.

In Chinese diagnosis, the red essence refers to the quality of the mother's menstrual blood. Healthy blood has the consistency of liquid paint. It should be bright, fresh red, and free from clots, with a full three- to four-day flow unaccompanied by menstrual pain. If there is dark color, heavy flow, or significant clots, the blood is considered deficient in chi and is often diagnosed as the cause of difficulties with conception and miscarriages. Also, in a case of insufficient blood, fertility challenges may occur because of the blood's inability to flow freely to and through the womb.

Because menstruation is the clearest indication of the quantity and quality of blood, a first step in preparing for motherhood is to adjust the menstrual symptoms if they are not reflecting reproductive vitality. Some common menstrual conditions that justify the attention of a doctor of traditional Chinese medicine are early or late menstruation, irregular menstrual and ovulation patterns, premenstrual breast disten- tion, excessive bleeding and cramping, and intolerable PMS.

The white essence refers to the father's semen. Healthy semen is white, heavy, sweet, and abundant. If a male's semen does not fit this description, it could be diagnosed as the cause of difficulty in conceiving a child.

"The Chinese classics teach that strong parents usually produce strong offspring. The nervous system, spine and bones are inherited from the father and the digestive system, flesh and organs from the mother."[29]

Evaluating the red and white essences of each parent requires a simple diagnostic technique—in contrast to Western medical tests and procedures, which can be invasive and expensive. So part of your preconception preparation can be to consult with a qualified TCM doctor who specializes in reproductive health care. Sara believes she could have been saved from three miscarriages:

> I do not understand why our teenage sex education classes never taught us this simple way of tracking the health of the reproductive system. So many women and men would save themselves years of wondering "What could be wrong?" if they checked their essences and knew when to seek professional help to correct obvious imbalances. A woman has the chance to evaluate her well-being every month from her teenage years, and a man can check his status anytime, rain or shine.

Kidney chi, another specific marker in Chinese medicine required if conception is to occur and stabilize, is the flow of chi through the kidney meridian of each parent. Acupuncturist Leslie Ann Oldershaw writes about how Chinese medicine specializes in the treatment of male and female fertility health. She describes how strong kidney essence, with a healthy balance of yin and yang properties, creates a highly functional menstrual period in the woman and healthy sperm and sexual function in the man.

Oldershaw notes that patterns contributing to fertility challenges and sometimes infertility are broken down into two categories—deficiency and excess. When a man or woman is deficient, they "lack the vital substances that are essential for conception." Female deficiency frequently appears as a poor uterine environment. "'Kidney yin' deficiency affects the menstrual blood and the nourishment needed for the uterus, and 'kidney yang' deficiency appears as not enough 'spark' in one's reproductive ability. An 'essence deficiency' can affect a woman's capacity to reproduce."[30]

Patterns of excess kidney chi are even more varied. Excess conditions can occur because pathogenic factors obstruct the reproductive system. An excess, called *cold* in Chinese medicine, impedes the circulation of chi and blood; a blood *heat* excess means the blood is too hot and may threaten the embryo. Dampness may involve an accumulation of phlegm blocking the fallopian tubes, which can be a reflection of pelvic inflammation. Stagnation of chi can block the flow of vital force through the lower abdomen, especially the uterine area. Blood stasis obstructs the flow of blood through the uterus and is associated with fibroids, endometriosis, ovarian cysts, and painful menses with blood clots.

Male essence deficiency implies reproductive challenges including poor sperm production and sexual dysfunction. A kidney yin deficiency means lack of nourishment for the sperm. A kidney yang deficiency suggests not enough metabolic spark to drive sperm production or sexual function. Whereas excess heat can cook the sperm, excess cold can inhibit proper sperm production while also inhibiting healthy sexual function.[31] "Cases of low sperm count (less than 640,000 per mil.) [are often a] kidney yin and yang deficiency."[32] Excessive ejaculation can also cause kidney deficiency, which affects sperm count and motility and makes the sperm thin, according to Chinese medical principle.

For these reasons, it is important that you assess your kidney essence. Stress and poor diet will adversely impact the quantity and quality of the kidney chi. Feeling tired or wired is a clue that your reproductive life essence might be depleted or stagnating.

Chinese medicine considers diet a very important health factor. An irregular diet can lead to undernourishment and depletion of the precious life force needed for conception, implantation, and prenatal development. Not only can caffeine and stimulants create a depletion of the kidney essence, but excessive consumption of cold and iced foods and drinks can also lead to coldness in the uterus. For some women trying to conceive, excessive consumption of greasy foods, dairy products, and citrus juices is very aggravating to the reproductive system as well. These foods can significantly affect a woman who has blockages in the fallopian tubes.[33] Whereas a Western fertility specialist may suggest an invasive technological procedure to resolve such a condition, a Chinese doctor will treat the woman using acupuncture and Chinese herbs and will strongly recommend that she eliminate the foods that are weakening her system.

Regulating Your Ovulation Cycle

In traditional Chinese medicine the first concern is assessing, and if necessary regulating, the woman's menstrual cycle. This means fine-tuning any organ or hormonal imbalance for the purpose of stimulating ovulation. Different methods are used to balance the hormones in different stages of the menstrual cycle. The preovulation, ovulation, and postovulation phases of a woman's cycle each requires a different treatment protocol to support uterine blood flow and nourish the blood, tone kidney function, support the vital essence chi used by the reproductive system, and warm the organs and meridians in order to support the fertility phases of a woman's cycle.

Your Reproductive Organs

Chinese tradition teaches that five solid organs are primarily involved in reproduction: the liver, heart, spleen, lungs, and kidneys. These organs are responsible for creating, receiving, and storing the pure substances of blood, fluids, and chi. They store rather than discharge—which is the function of the "hollow bowel" organs of the intestines, stomach, and bladder that transport and eliminate pure substance and waste materials. The uterus functions as a solid organ in that it receives the mother's reproductive essence and stores the growing fetus for nine months; it is also seen as a bowel organ in that it discharges menstruation and the fully formed baby at birth.[34]

In Chinese medicine the body and mind are recognized as interdependent, with each organ being affected by a specific emotion. Taoists believe that we each are born with specific virtues—higher aspects of our emotions that are derived from the positive energies of our organs. When we abundantly embody and express our virtuous nature, our life force flows through us effectively. For example, a person who expresses love and respect will have a greater abundance of life force than those who express anger, fear, sadness, impatience, or grief, risking detrimental effects on their internal organs and glands. The Taoist master Mantak Chia suggests that "if we neglect to nurture our good emotions and just work on bringing more energy into the body, we may energize our negative emotions, making them more powerful and more difficult to control and transform."[35]

The Kidneys: In traditional Chinese medicine the kidney is the primary organ controlling a man's or woman's reproductive health. Strong, balanced yin and yang kidney essence is essential for optimal fertility conditions. The yin essence is cooling and nourishing, while the yang is warm and active. A car cannot run without fuel in its tank; similarly, a reproductive system cannot create healthy sperm or sustain a growing fetus without enough vital energy created by the kidneys. An embryo requires substantial amounts of the mother's vital essence to develop, and the kidneys are the storehouse of this essence. Acting like a lifeline, the kidney chi maintains the fetus's life essence throughout the pregnancy. This is why, according to Chinese medicine, many women entering their forties have difficulty conceiving or sustaining a pregnancy. Their kidney chi is depleted from the stresses of life and poor dietary habits.

Fear is the emotion that most affects the kidneys. Chronic patterns of suppressed fear can weaken the supply of kidney chi. The virtues of gentleness, faith, and trust support the kidneys by restoring their innate vitality.

The Liver: Because blood nourishes the fetus, the liver—which stores the blood and oversees the flow of chi throughout the body, ensuring a healthy and consistent supply of blood to the uterus—is important to reproductive health. Congested liver chi can cause morning sickness and make labor more difficult. Therefore, a healthy and relaxed liver can benefit you and your baby from conception through birth. Moderate exercise, a proper diet, and a balanced emotional state can help the liver sustain a smooth flow of chi.

The liver is depleted by anger; kindness and forgiveness are healing for this organ.

The Spleen: This organ serves several functions once the child is conceived. Healthy spleen chi supports the reproductive organs against gravity, preventing miscarriage. In addition, the spleen manufactures the blood from the purest parts of the food that we eat. "This pure substance is sent to the heart where according to the classical literature, it is turned red. It is the heart's job to then send the blood down to the uterus."[36] Once you conceive, your developing child will be nourished by blood created by your spleen.

The spleen is weakened by excessive worry. Openness and trust are healing qualities that will replenish it.

The Heart: The heart and uterus are considered interdependent, as chi and blood flow between them through an internal channel at different times of the woman's cycle.

Hate and resentment are emotions that harm the health of the heart. An emotionally constricted heart can restrict the uterine blood flow, affecting implantation of the embryo. Since the heart also houses the spirit, it is vital that the mind rest peacefully if the heart and uterus are to function properly.

There is a strong emphasis in Chinese medicine on the pregnant woman being as relaxed and as free as possible from any anxiety that could unsettle her and affect communication between the heart and uterus. Likewise, a woman preparing to conceive should try to create pleasant and uplifting emotional and spiritual experiences, which can have a positive effect on her ability to conceive. A conscious effort to relax every day, and setting aside time for quiet meditation, will greatly benefit her future baby.

The Lungs: These are responsible for circulation of chi and the proper dispersion of bodily fluids.

Sadness, grief, and depression deplete lung chi, while the virtues of courage and joy can assist in healing the lungs.

You can begin to self-diagnose how your reactive patterns may be impacting your reproductive health. Consider viewing your chronic emotional reactions to your daily circumstances and relationships and clarify for yourself which organ is being affected.

Chinese Herbs and Acupuncture

There are more than ten thousand herbs documented in the *Materia Medica* published by the Chinese Ministry of Health, and several thousand herbal substances used extensively in fertility treatments. Herbal formulas are prescribed, according to a person's unique fertility condition, for their therapeutic and strengthening effects. Most of the herbal formulas prescribed by Chinese doctors have been used clinically for hundreds and in many cases thousands, of years.

In his article "Research on the Mechanism of Ovulation Induced by Acupuncture and Chinese Herbs" Dr. Yu Yun Chu stated, "The mechanism of inducing ovulation with Chinese herbs is based on tonifying the kidney and adding herbs to activate the blood. . . . Laboratory experiments proved that kidney-tonifying herbs can increase the function of the hypothalamus-pituitary-gonad axis [which regulates normal ovulation]."[37]

Properly prescribed by a qualified practitioner, herbs can tone the system prior to conception and strengthen the bodies of both mother and fetus during pregnancy. Once you are pregnant, however, some herbal medicines may be too difficult to digest if you are experiencing morning sickness. Alternately, acupuncture can alleviate many prenatal problems as well as being a great support for initiating or hastening labor that is slow or delayed.

For the future father, Chinese herbs and acupuncture are used to treat and enhance sperm count, shape, and motility, as well as seminal fluid. Donald claims that Chinese medicine granted him his fatherhood:

> As a painter who has worked with toxic paints all of my life, I never knew I was painting away my future as a father. But I received the horrific news that my sperm count was almost nil at the ripe old age of thirty-two. I consider the six months of acupuncture and herbal treatments I underwent as essential "gifts of renewal" to the sperm that created my son.

Eastern Nutrition

Proper nutrition is considered fundamental to maintaining reproductive health as well as preventing infertility. According to traditional Chinese medicine, the growing prenate "feeds on the mother's blood," and her diet must support blood production for both herself and her baby. Generally this implies supporting the spleen, whose function is to produce chi and blood from the purest parts of daily food. Foods that support the spleen are mostly warm and nourishing. Easily digested organic animal proteins are beneficial for making more blood and can be eaten in soup or broth for those who do not prefer much meat in their diet. If you are a vegetarian, classic Oriental foods that nourish the blood are found in most health food stores—mochi, amasake, sweet rice, litchi, and yellow vegetables such as carrots and winter squash are ideal.

Foods must be at least body temperature before the stomach and spleen can transform the nutrients into the chi and blood needed for conception and healthy pregnancy. A woman needs a reserve of blood after the child is born for her postpartum recovery, and an abundance of blood is also needed to make milk. For most people, cold foods should be kept to a minimum. Chilled and raw foods have a cooling property and overwork the spleen and stomach, leaving less energy to create chi and blood for fertilization and implantation. Cold foods to be avoided are juices, especially citrus. Fruits, too, are considered cooling but can be eaten in small quantities. If you are experiencing fertility challenges, a

TCM doctor may urge you to avoid most foods that are cold in temperature and property.

Most fish and fowl are good, but chicken and turkey can be questionable for certain preconception conditions. Dairy products are to be eaten in moderation. Because they have damp and cold properties, especially straight from the freezer or refrigerator, they are considered unsupportive for most women who want to create a warm womb for their future child. Each individual's dietary patterns may create excessive heat or coldness in the reproductive system, so it is best to consult a qualified Chinese medical doctor who will custom-design your diet to optimize fertility.

Fertility and Womb Ecology

Nothing can guarantee a healthy baby, but two adults who consciously choose to eliminate risk factors enhance the possibility of a healthy outcome for each stage of their child's life and maximize their chances for co-creating a balanced and whole child. Any couple attempting to conceive should behave as if conception has occurred until they get reliable verification so that the crucial initial weeks of developmental growth for the embryo are not compromised. A fetus is most vulnerable to harm during the first weeks of gestation, when all of its primary biological systems are starting to develop. Unfortunately, many women do not even seek prenatal care until after the first or second missed menstruation. A prenate is at a much higher risk at this time if the mother is still living with bad health habits.

Before a woman misses a period, she is already two weeks' pregnant. During the first few weeks, the central nervous system, heart, lungs, liver, limbs, and kidneys are actively developing. Because of the extreme vulnerability of the newly forming cells, most major and minor birth defects happen within this period and the weeks immediately thereafter, when the most complex cell divisions occur. During the first twelve weeks, some miscarriages occur due to unconscious negligence. For this reason, responsible preconception and prenatal health care practices strongly suggest that a woman assume she is potentially pregnant if she has stopped using birth control.

The most important action a woman can take to prevent birth defects is to withdraw from all toxic substances before pregnancy begins. Going from a nonpregnant to a pregnant state, a woman's body will experience extraordinary changes. Attempting detox while already pregnant is locking the barn door after the horse is out. Arleen's reluctance to trust her doctor's advice haunts her to this day:

> I will never know whether my daughter's chronic lung problems are because of my self-indulgent partying when I was not using birth control. I knew I was playing Russian roulette, but I didn't really take it seriously. I was so arrogant to think I could control all the forces involved in creating the tenderness of my child's prenatal life. Everyday I wonder if her lifelong suffering is my fault. She began having serious asthma attacks the first month of her life. I live with the fear that I'll have to tell her the truth someday.

Environmental Influences

We live on a very complex and radioactive planet. In a joint study, the Department of Health and the U. Mass Medical Center have "estimated that 14 million U.S. workers are exposed to known or suspected reproductive hazards each year." Between 3 and 7 percent of all children are born with birth defects, and in about two-thirds of these cases, the causes are unknown.[38] Many of the birth defects that result from exposure to toxic substances can be attributed to the father as much as the mother.

As prospective parents, you need to be concerned with the ecology of the future mother's womb, your child's first home. Since the sperm, egg, and womb can be affected by harmful environmental influences that both parents experience, now is the time to review your lifestyle. Environmental toxins can cause birth defects and miscarriages during any phase of a pregnancy. They can also create infertility in both men and women, affect ovulation cycles, contaminate breast milk, and sometimes even instigate early menopause. Also, certain chemicals may be more detrimental to a fetus, so do not underestimate the danger of exposure to a particular product simply because it causes you, an adult, no apparent harm. In some cases low-level exposure to toxins may be even more dangerous than high exposure, since higher levels may activate the immune system to fight off the damaging effects of a substance. If you have been exposed to an environmental contaminant, allow your body to cleanse itself before pregnancy begins. If you are not sure whether something is harmful, err on the side of caution.

Learn what environmental toxins cause infertility and birth defects, and educate yourself about your own workplace hazards. *Do not depend on employers to notify or protect you from occupational hazards that may harm your reproductive health.* Now is the time to explore what contaminants you may be exposed to on a regular basis. Consult your local library for a more complete list of specific chemicals to avoid, since hundreds of new chemicals, especially household cleaning products, are made available to the general public each year. Many of these products have not been fully tested, so it is always safer to use natural cleaning substances found at health food stores.

Remember, there may be a long period of time between your exposure to hazards and the appearance of a health problem in your child. The following guidelines briefly describe some of the concerns you need to address as part of your prepregnancy planning:

- Review with your partner and colleagues insecticides, household or industrial cleaners, other chemicals, weed killers, gases, and lead-based products—especially paint. Even regular exposure to loud noises can produce a toxic effect on the body.
- Evaluate leisure-time toxins. If you paint, garden (using pesticides), or do photography (using darkroom chemicals), or if you are an artist using chemicals, gaseous contaminants, or lead-based paint, you may be exposing yourself to reproductive risks.
- If you are in a high-tech industry, learn how exposure to heavy metals, acids, radiation, and gases in your work can be detrimental to fertility and pregnancy.
- Protect yourself against exposure to unsafe levels of radiation.
- Evaluate your exposure to infectious diseases.
- Avoid extreme temperatures at home or work; extreme heat can adversely affect fertility for men and is not safe for pregnant women.
- There has been much debate over whether the monitor or video display terminal (VDT) of your home or professional computer releases significant radiation. Be aware of any co-workers' screens as well as your own. Position screens with their backs against a wall and use a model designed to emit lower levels of radiation, or get a laptop that is battery or

electrically operated and radiation-free. The Service Employees International Union suggests that a pregnant woman request reassignment to a non-VDT job, and that one not pregnant restrict exposure to a monitor to 50 percent of the workday, with fifteen-minute rest breaks every two hours.[39]

A recent study of almost sixteen hundred women by the Kaiser-Permanente Medical Group in northern California found that women who worked at a computer video display terminal for more than twenty hours per week had twice as many miscarriages in the first trimester of pregnancy as nonusers. Also, those women who used a computer for just five hours a day were 40 percent more likely than nonusers to have babies born with a congenital birth defect.

Since most of the radiation escapes from the transformer at the back of your computer monitor, avoid standing within ten feet behind your computer, or sitting near the back or side of anyone else's computer. It is safer if the back of your monitor faces the wall. A monochrome monitor emits one-quarter to one-third the radiation that color monitors do, and most newer computers release less than older models do. Keep the monitor at arm's length to minimize radiation exposure. A laptop or portable computer will also emit lower levels of radiation.[40]

- Give serious thought to whether a home or work situation is so potentially hazardous that changing jobs or relocating is necessary to protect your reproductive health. If you have clearly been exposed to a hazardous substance, it is advisable that you make a change at least three months before conceiving. If a change is impossible, take extra precautions—wear approved protection such as a mask, goggles, respirators, radiation screens and aprons, and so on. Keep as much distance as possible between you and the source of any toxin. Good ventilation is helpful.
- If either partner works in any of the following occupations—all at high risk for toxin exposure—precautions are worth considering: airline employees exposed to X rays and radiation; hospital and health care workers including doctors, dentists, nurses, lab technicians, and medical assistants exposed to anesthetic gases, X rays and radiation, infectious diseases, and

chemicals; photographers who use film-processing materials; plasticsworkers; printers; textile workers; transportation operators; farmers and gardeners; firefighters; mechanics and drivers who breathe in toxic fumes; all artists, including jewelers and typesetters, who breathe in toxic substances; builders who use any kind of chemically treated materials; clothes cleaning services, especially dry cleaners; office personnel who work without proper ventilation; homemakers and domestic assistants who use solvents or industrial cleaners; nuclear industry employees; electronic workers who use epoxy and other hazardous substances; cosmetologists who use hairspray aerosols and dyes and polishes.[41]

If you live near any of these workplaces, you may also be at risk of exposure to these toxins. To learn more about these environmental and occupational risks, contact the Occupational Safety and Health Administration; the National Institute of Occupational Safety and Health; or the American College of Obstetricians and Gynecologists. Ask them for specific lists that identify which chemicals and toxins are hazardous to your reproductive health.

Ending Addictions

The foundation of prepregnancy planning is doing everything that you can to create maximum health. The pregnant mother and baby do not exist in separate worlds. How you treat your own body before and after you conceive your child can impact her lifelong health. If you smoke or consume alcohol, it is as if you are giving your developing baby a cigarette or drink before she's even born. The most precarious time for the delicate embryo is between the seventeenth and fifty-sixth days of development, or weeks five through ten after your last menstrual period.[42]

Your use of alcohol, nicotine, or caffeine can cause learning disabilities in your child. Nicotine constricts the flow of oxygen to the placenta, creating lower birth weight in the baby. It strips the baby of essential nutrients and vitamins and can result in premature birth. Fetal lung growth can also be affected, leading to lifelong breathing problems for the child. A pregnant woman can reduce her nutrient, vitamin, and mineral levels with just one cigarette a day.

Fathers need to quit smoking as well, since secondhand smoke is detrimental to the pregnant mother as well as to a newborn. And studies suggest that cigarettes also affect the prospective father's fertility. Bruce Ames of the University of California at Berkeley believes that cigarette smoking along with bad diets (not enough vitamin C–rich fruits and vegetables) are the biggest culprits in sperm damage.[43]

A hopeful father-to-be may want to take a "paternity leave" to clean up his sperm; during the sperm cells' three-month development in the testes, they undergo many cell divisions that can expose their genetic material to chemical assault. Bernard Robaire of McGill University has discovered that "drugs and ingested chemicals can readily invade the testes from the blood stream. Other toxic agents can ambush the sperm after they leave the testes . . . half of 100 agents studied so far—including byproducts of cigarette smoking—appear to harm sperm." Robert Yazigi of Temple University has offered new evidence that suggests that cocaine can reach the testes as well.[44]

There is no safe level of alcohol consumption for the mother during pregnancy because alcohol crosses the placenta and immediately affects the baby. Fetal alcohol syndrome (FAS) often results in low birth weight and other complications, including facial, skeletal, and organ malformations; mental retardation; and other growth problems. Even subtle learning disabilities that appear in later childhood or adulthood can be traced to FAS. Mild FAS can occur in pregnant women who drink only 1 ounce of alcohol a day, whereas full FAS can occur in women who drink 2 to 2.5 ounces or more a day. Studies have shown that pregnant women who drink only 1 ounce of alcohol twice a week increase the risk of second-trimester miscarriages. Drinking alcohol at any time—from conception through birth—acts as an intense toxin to the prenate. It is important to remember that the amount of alcohol is more important than the volume. Even if you dilute hard liquor, the alcohol amount remains the same.[45]

Again, the father's habit with alcohol can also affect his future child. "Animal studies have long shown that offspring sired by fathers exposed to alcohol are fewer, smaller, and weaker than those sired by alcohol-free fathers. A recent study found that babies of human fathers who drank regularly during the month prior to conception in amounts that equaled two drinks a day, or five drinks at one sitting, weighed approximately 6.5 ounces less than other babies."[46] This was true even if the mothers did not drink or smoke.

With this awareness of the potential dangers of drinking before and during your pregnancy, consider making a no-drinking policy part of your prepregnancy planning. An informal drink for you or your partner may become a lifetime disability for your child.

Surprisingly, caffeine is a risk far greater than most people realize. Who would think that coffee or tea or any caffeinated product such as cola could create birth defects? Begin reading labels to discover which products you use contain caffeine—chocolate does, for instance, and even aspirin.

Like alcohol, caffeine is known to cross the placenta. "Several studies show more birth defects in the children of women who consumed high amounts of caffeine during pregnancy than in those who did not. Animal studies show the same patterns. While some of the studies have been criticized for poor design, the results are indicative enough to warrant the FDA recommendation that a high intake of caffeine (more than four cups of coffee a day) may not be safe during pregnancy."[47]

Even decaffeinated coffee is controversial in its impact on the growth of the fetus. If you are a caffeine consumer, try herbal teas or some of the grain beverages that are offered as coffee substitutes in health food stores. If you are tired and need the caffeine buzz, try redesigning your lifestyle so that you can rest or get more sleep at night or even take short rest breaks throughout the day so that your exhaustion does not need to be relieved with caffeine "enhancers."

Recreational drugs of any kind pose too much risk to the embryo to justify even the smallest amount of use. Stop all such drugs before you become pregnant. Cocaine is suspected of causing birth defects and pregnancy complications, as is marijuana. Some sources state that males who use marijuana frequently risk harming their sperm. Pregnant women who are marijuana smokers expose the fetus to the same effects as cigarettes. Heroin also crosses the placenta and enters the system of the fetus within an hour of intake. The baby will experience the same withdrawal as the mother and sometimes dies in the process. Downers such as codeine and Quaaludes, as well as uppers including diet pills and amphetamines, can also cause birth defects. Hallucinogens, such as LSD and PCP, can cause anatomic abnormalities in babies exposed in utero. In addition to possible birth defects, all addictive substances can lead to life-threatening fetal distress from conception onward and may lead to miscarriage.[48]

If you are addicted to any substance, quitting can produce withdrawal symptoms, so take care of it before you become pregnant. It is particularly critical that you not expose the embryo to any detox reactions you may be experiencing during the second to eighth weeks after conception. Drug components can accumulate in the body and may take a while to break down and be excreted. Try to be drug-free for at least two to three months before trying to conceive. Find natural ways to alleviate stress. Layla found relaxation tapes helped her kick her habits:

> I am glad I read books before I got pregnant that told me the blatant truth that my recreational habits could harm my baby. I found my local bookstore had books and audiotapes to teach me how to relax and handle stress. I have learned to prefer the peace of my own clear mind to the noise of a chemical addiction irritating me throughout the day. I tell all of my girlfriends to get sober before they get pregnant.

If you are taking any prescription drugs, now is the time to review side effects with your doctor, and be sure to mention that you are preparing to conceive or are pregnant. Some prescription drugs are very harmful to the fetus. Certain drugs can lead to higher rates of miscarriage and birth defects, or to your baby being born with a dependency or addiction.

Although many couples do ingest addictive substances such as caffeine or nicotine and have healthy children, why take the risk? If you cannot change habits that can harm your child, you may want to evaluate whether you are ready to be a responsible and loving parent. If you become pregnant while ingesting harmful substances, you may always wonder whether you could have prevented an early- or later-life health problem for your child. Why not protect both yourself and your child from such unnecessary worries?

Technological Procedures

If you've tried to work with mother nature by using a noninvasive approach to fertility and have yet to conceive, you may find yourself exploring Assisted Reproductive Technologies (ART). As you have learned, the holistic approaches that suggest natural methods to improve your reproductive health sometimes do not yield a healthy pregnancy and baby. At what point do you start to consider yourself infertile or in need of medical assistance?

Interventive procedures can be expensive and overly prescribed but sometimes they are effective. If you are concerned about being able to conceive naturally, explore many different resources to gather a spectrum of opinions about your options. There are low-tech and high-tech procedures as well as many choices of fertility drugs. Since one out of six couples these days experiences fertility problems after long efforts to conceive, there are naturally numerous books, physicians, resource groups, and Internet contacts available to offer you a wide variety of support. If you want to blend Eastern and Western medicine, or include a holistic mind-body approach, make sure your physician is supportive of your orientation. Beyond being competent, your doctor should understand your needs and philosophies.

Infertility treatments are changing rapidly as new discoveries are made; old procedures are updated almost monthly. So this book will offer no specific recommendations because they may well be obsolete by the time you read it. When you do your own research, check for the most current data regarding short- and long-term effects—on both mother and child—of using reproductive technologies and fertility drugs.

If you want to include ART as part of your fertility experience, contact Resolve, a national nonprofit group offering the latest information and educational support to couples struggling to have a baby. Its national helpline phone number is (617) 623-0744.

Whether you're using natural or technological approaches, it should be clear that preparing your body for conception is a step you need to take. Review the information in this chapter, as well as other resources particular to your unique situation, and begin to clarify your own prepregnancy physical health care plan with your partner.

Ronda and Carl found that their commitment to becoming healthy has sustained them through the conception of four healthy children. Says Carl:

> If my therapist had not scared me by telling me that I could have a disabled child if I continued my addictions, I think my wife, kids, and I would have had a miserable life. Even if they had been born physically healthy, there would have been the emotional pain of having a dad addicted to his own self-destructive habits, rather than a dad committed to loving and providing security for the family. Ronda feels that even though she did not have any overtly harmful habits, her own prepregnancy health adjustments were partly responsible for our kids being "radiantly healthy," as she puts it, from their first breath of life.

Creative Exercise:
Preparing Your Body for Conception

I now invite you to assess your physical health before you conceive your child. How committed are you to preparing your body for your future child? Are you including your partner in your process? What is your plan? Here are a few guidelines to assist you in creating your own preconception preparation plan. Be specific with each step needed to manifest your plan:

1. What are your prepregnancy goals for your physical health, and when do you want to begin them and complete them?
2. Are there any people or resources you need to contact? When do you plan on taking action?
3. What steps do you recommend your partner take with you? Without you?
4. How do you want to change your diet and/or supplements?
5. Are there harmful addictive habits and/or environmental risks that may jeopardize your future child's pre- and postnatal health? Specify.
6. How do you want to improve the health of your eggs or sperm?
7. What prepregnancy exercise habits will be healthy for you and your future child?
8. How do you feel about the biological clock? Does the myth or the reality affect you or your partner? In what ways do you need to take charge of your reproductive life?
9. How willing are you to evaluate and change your stress patterns?
10. How can Western and Eastern principles assist you and your partner?

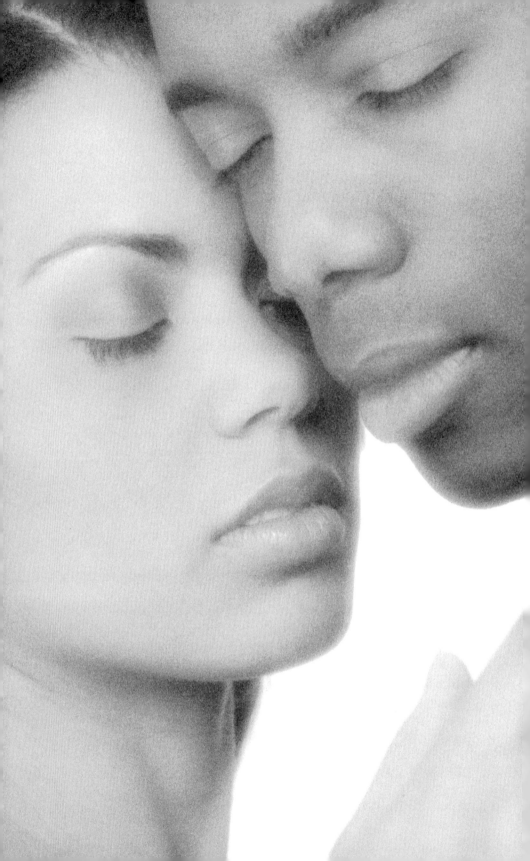

4

Preparing Your Mind
for Conception

Children are naturally predisposed to love and affection.
However, the child must first be loved before he can love.
John Bradshaw

Psychological Wholeness:
Emotional and Mental Well-Being

Your future child's ability to embody his soul consciousness will be dependent on the quality of his mental and emotional life. Discordant thoughts and feelings can hinder the soul's ability to express itself clearly through human form. Your child-to-be will need you to create harmonious conditions for him to develop his self-expression.

Our psychological health is made up of two major components: the emotional and mental bodies. Although deeply interdependent with the "dense" physical body, they are considered "subtle bodies." While we can see our physical form, most of us cannot easily see our feelings and thoughts. However, our thoughts and emotions do have form as well as unique functions. Understanding their distinctive purpose can assist you in optimizing your child's psychological development in the womb and thereafter.

The emotional body's primary function is to experiment, explore, and appropriately express *feelings*. The mental body is designed to experience

99

and express concrete and abstract *thoughts*. Both aspects can be felt physically, and they continuously influence each other. For example, you may *feel* happy that you are pregnant, *think* that your life is now blessed, and experience yourself so excited you cannot sleep. Or you may *feel* depressed that you are pregnant, *think* that your life is out of control, and find yourself becoming physically sick. And many new parents *feel positive* about having a child while having some *negative thoughts* about the many personal sacrifices they have to make, thus creating a psychological state of confusion and conflict, and bodily stress.

Prenatal Psychology

In his book *The Secret Life of the Unborn Child* Tom Verny, M.D., explains that our "personality characteristics and traits begin forming in utero. Our dislikes and likes, our fears and phobias—in other words, all the distinct behaviors that make us uniquely ourselves—are, in part, also the product of conditioned learning. And the womb is where this special kind of learning begins."[1] Understanding prenatal psychology helps you to assist your future child's soul in developing her emotional and mental well-being before she is even born. Self-identity begins in the womb. The messages a child receives from the mother in utero will begin shaping her attitudes about herself. If you have persistent ambivalence or anxiety about being a parent, you can injure your unborn child's personality. On the other hand, scientific studies demonstrate that loving desire and anticipation can positively affect the psychological development of a prenate.

"By creating a warm, emotionally enriching environment in utero," Verny says, "a woman can make a decisive difference in everything her child feels, hopes, dreams, thinks and accomplishes throughout life. During these months, a woman is her baby's conduit to the world. Everything that affects her, affects him."[2] The father's role in the prenatal equation is essential, too. How he relates to his partner has a direct impact on her emotional state. If the couple is in harmony, the prenate benefits because his mother is content. If the mother is agitated by chronic conflict with her partner, this affects her emotional stability, which in turn can affect the child's well-being. As Verny suggests, a father who abuses or neglects his pregnant partner is endangering the child in utero, because the baby will directly experience his mother's high levels of anxiety. The parents' behavior toward each other and the prenate during the pregnancy will be the child's foundational imprint as he unfolds his budding psychological qualities.

Raleigh regrets she and her husband were not more emotionally sensitive to each other:

> During the last trimester of my pregnancy, when Jerry and I would scream at each other, my baby would kick my ribs hard. I could tell she was distraught by the commotion. I felt she was telling me to stop being so upset, and that we were greatly disturbing her world. I could not help but think, "What are we teaching her about expressing feelings?"

Be aware of the need to heal any psychological problems between you and your partner before exposing the vulnerable prenate to unhealthy patterns. Your future child's psychological foundation is established through experiencing your emotional responses to life. The incoming soul is offering you an opportunity to transcend your reactive nature before it inherits your unresolved conflicts. Your lifestyle, personal character, behavior, and habits can create conditions that protect the prenate from negative influences. Consistently loving, empowering, and healthful actions safeguard the child from potential adverse conditioning.

The Soul's Need to Feel

When the soul begins to unite with the embryo during the first trimester in utero, it has an extraordinary sensitivity to its psychological surroundings. Both its emotional and mental bodies continually mature during the prenatal life. According to the ageless wisdom teachings, a child possesses the psychological tendencies of her last life in incarnation, and whether she develops the positive or negative tendencies depends largely upon the psychological condition of this lifetime's parents. It is the parents' responsibility to foster the healthiest psychological environment for the incarnating soul.

Beginning during the prenatal period and throughout the early years of the child's life, the soul has little control over his emotions and thoughts. A child's psyche is extremely responsive to his environment and receptive to all influences around him, whether good or evil. Yet although the emotional and mental bodies are easily molded in early youth, the patterns of expression solidify as childhood progresses. Thus, the child's future psychological health can be greatly affected by his parents' patterns of expression and thought before and after birth.

Psychological energies can be transformed and matured. Latent superconscious qualities such as intuition, inspiration, and mystical states of awareness can be awakened and activated. Parents who identify with their own soul natures will experience a regenerating influence on their own personality traits. Their behavior will also affect the child's ability to express and embody her human personality and immortal soul.

Brian recalls:

> Susie and I had a chronic tendency to bicker. Once we got pregnant and learned that the prenate could hear us argue, we would remind each other about our wedding vows to "love, honor, and cherish" one another. This intentional way of communicating supported us in caring for ourselves and our baby. When our discussions became heated, we learned to flash our wedding ring to the other, our signal to remember our commitment to speak kindly.

Even the best efforts of parents cannot fully protect a child from the inevitable negative influences, but they make a big difference in whether healthy emotional and mental qualities are stimulated first in the child. Positive tendencies that are nurtured before and for years after birth will establish a habit of positive response.

As you heal your own childhood and adult traumas, which are the foundation of your unhealthy reactive behaviors, you will offer your future child the best psychic environment to unfold his temperament. Honestly evaluate your own emotional health before having a child. For soul consciousness to embody, the emotional body must be trained to express positive qualities and feelings of love, harmlessness, and selflessness.

Meditation: A Practical Tool

Most people's thoughts and feelings are self-centered, and the personality is vulnerable to habit. A person in the habit of thinking negative or limiting thoughts usually creates a similar reality in the surroundings, while a person who has the habit of focusing on positive states of being has a more harmonious and fulfilling life. Meditation and relaxation exercises can support your psychological health by quieting your mind, allowing you to notice and eliminate negative feelings and thoughts so that the stream of divine life can flow through your body, mind, and soul. Since an incarnating soul uses the thought-forms of its mother and father to build its emotional and mental bodies throughout the prenatal life, parents can focus on beneficial thought-forms and express them to the developing child in the womb.

Many bookstores offer a wide choice of books to assist your meditation practice. When you meditate, keep as your goal the training of your thoughts and feelings to connect with the virtuous qualities of your soul, your true self.

Your Childhood Wounds

"Parenting forms children's core beliefs about themselves. Nothing could be more important. The future of the world depends on our children's conception of themselves. All their choices depend on their view of themselves. . . . There is a crisis in the family today. It has to do with our parenting rules and the multigenerational process by which families perpetuate these rules.

John Bradshaw

Your Relationship with Your Parents

From the moment you were born, you were a being with a complex cycle of changing needs and feelings. Even if you were fortunate to have parents who were committed to fulfilling your needs and caring for your feelings, you most likely have incurred subtle psychological wounds that may subconsciously affect your relationship with your partner as well as with your future child. Those who experienced the tragic childhood traumas of abuse, divorce, death of parents, or parents with substance addictions may have these wounds restimulated by the birth of a child if they have not begun to consciously explore their unresolved past. You may unconsciously re-create the conditions of your childhood with your own child in order to resolve the past frustrations and pain that you were unable to heal with your family members.

Each of us has the need to be nurtured. Yet so often this fundamental need is unsatisfied because our parents were never emotionally nourished by their parents, so they never learned how to love us in a healthy way.

In *Reclaiming and Championing Your Inner Child* John Bradshaw has said that "a child's healthy growth depends on someone loving and accepting him unconditionally. When this need is met, the child's energy of love is released so that he can love others. When a child is not loved for his own self, his sense of I Amness is severed. Because he is so dependent, his egocentricity sets in, and his true self experiences adverse conditions to full emergence. . . . The failure to be loved unconditionally causes the child to suffer greatly."[3]

Since an infant cannot take care of herself, her caretakers must be perceptive to her distress signals—the need to be fed, to have diapers changed, to sleep, to be soothed, to be stimulated, to be held, and then, slowly, the need to be separate yet connected to her mother, and eventually her father, her siblings, and the world. Her feeling of combined freedom and support affects all her later relationships. Often, those whose parents were unable to consistently provide healthy emotional and physical bonding either will overcompensate with their own children for what they did not have from their parents or will unconsciously re-create the same painful patterns with their kids.

Heidi's mother, Clara, was wounded from her own childhood because Clara's mom had completely neglected her. Because Clara recognized she had been emotionally abandoned by her mother, she embodied the opposite behavior with Heidi. As Heidi recalls:

> As far back as I can remember, my mother smothered me with attention. She watched me as I played with my friends until I was a teenager, and she rarely left me alone in my room without constantly checking on me. When I began to assert my independence, she accused me of not loving her and being selfish. I never got to feel her validate my own needs that were different from hers. As much as I want to have children, I am terrified to become pregnant because I sense the neediness of a baby will threaten my newfound independence—which I am reluctant to lose, since I never had it as a child. The baby's dependence on me could make me feel engulfed like I felt my whole childhood with my mom. I am also afraid of giving my child so much space that he might feel abandoned by me. I am committed to healing my low self-esteem and bonding issues before I become a parent.

Every developmental stage of childhood carries the potential for emotional pain and wounding. Parents who deny their child's autonomy harm the inner drive for independence. Parents who are physically and emotionally unavailable can raise children who fear rejection and have a driving need for intimacy. Most children learn to survive, but it's important that they authentically thrive. Childhood is not just about coping with each developmental stage; it is a time for the child to flourish in a world of consistent security and love, and to blossom into the essential self.

Even those parents who meet most of their child's needs cannot meet them all. And those parents who encourage their child to express her feelings may not understand all of them either. Difficulties are multiplied when there are siblings, who by their very existence imply divided parental attention.

Gerard and Layla describe their dilemma with four kids:

> Our first son, Jake, got the best of us because he had our full attention. Then Cara was born a little over a year later and our time was split between two infants with ceaseless needs. Jake was jealous of Cara and became resentful and competitive in a way he has never resolved. Then, when our twin boys were born two years later, every day at least one of the kids suffered by feeling left out and deprived of our time. With all our best intentions to provide our children with the bonding and independence they needed developmentally, we knew we could not completely control their painful early-life experiences, some of which we knew could become lifelong wounds. It made us realize that we had to let go of the idea that we could be perfect parents, providing our children with a painless childhood. Part of their character building was the daily struggle to give and receive enough love, and to learn when to let go and find other sources of security and safety.

Having a child can evoke memories within you of both the positive and negative characteristics of your parents, yourself, and your partner. This is because the feelings of primal love that you will feel with your baby can highlight the lack of love and care you felt from your own mom or dad. These forgotten hurts can overwhelm you as a new parent if you are not aware of your unhealed past. So part of preparing for parenthood is accepting that you will be healing your own childhood wounds as you develop a relationship with your child.

Before the child is in your life, you have the opportunity to openly acknowledge the "darker" aspects of your past, and to learn new ways to continue healing your self-esteem and unmet needs. By evaluating yourself, you can become a more loving and whole parent for your future child, less vulnerable to using your relationship to re-create your unresolved childhood issues. You can commit to exploring the dysfunctional behavior patterns that you internalized from your parents so that you can freely express your own divine nature of your self as well as empower the divine expression of your child and partner.

Beginning to Heal Neglect and Abuse

One of the most damaging experiences for a child is any form of abuse, whether physical, emotional, or mental. *Physical abuse* includes hurting a child, or misusing a child to fulfill your own sexual desires. *Emotional abuse* includes demeaning a child in any way, consistently neglecting or depriving a child of bonding experiences with either or both parents, or exposing a child to behavior that scares him or makes him feel unsafe. *Mental abuse* implies that the attitudes, beliefs, and thoughts of the child are discounted or harshly judged. This is a very important consideration as the child grows into his own unique personality nature. Parents need not agree with their child, but respecting his point of view is essential for the child's positive self-esteem.

So how can you tell if making an effort to heal your past wounds of neglect or abuse should be part of your prepregnancy planning? If you were raised with any of these experiences, or you and your partner behave in abusive ways toward each other, your child is a candidate to inherit the family pattern. This is especially true if you or your partner have a number of family members who modeled these behaviors for you. Even the most conscious people are still susceptible to unconscious reactions when they are under stress—and a newborn baby can be very stressful, if only for the simple fact that she can interrupt your sleep patterns for the first months or years of her life. If you feel that you are vulnerable to harming your future child in any way, get help in addressing patterns of abuse before you become a parent.

Make a Personal Inventory of Your Past

Those who want to deeply explore the impact of their childhood wounds on their life as part of preparing for parenthood can use the following exercises to reveal past experiences that may need attention and resolution before they can feel confident of their healthy parenting abilities. These questions are designed to reveal dysfunctional patterns with your parents, partner, or self that may need attention before you bring a child into your world. Evaluate your personal history honestly, then get the necessary personal or professional support to heal so that you do not unconsciously pass on to your child the pain of your past.

These exercises are not intended to judge anyone from the past. They are designed to help identify and heal reactive responses.

In her book *The Verbally Abusive Relationship* Patricia Evans defines verbal abuse in this way: when you are *frequently* "yelled at, snapped at, told that you are acting wrong, acting smart, acting dumb, trying to start a fight, imagining things, twisting things around, interrupting, trying to have the last word, going on and on, thinking wrong, looking for trouble, trying to start an argument, and so forth, you are being abused."[4]

Have you ever even considered that you yourself may be a verbal abuser, or have you been in a verbally abusive relationship with a family member, a friend, a colleague, a boss, or a partner? Does this style seem normal to you? Did you ever think to question the appropriateness of this communication pattern? Would you want to expose a newborn or child who is just learning to communicate to this style of verbal exchange? Take a moment to imagine how being exposed to this kind of expression might influence the self-esteem of a child. Consider how it might shape the way he communicates in his future relationships. On school playgrounds, for instance, parents can greatly influence whether their young children become bullies or peacemakers. Children are influenced by their role models at home. Creating either conflict or harmony is learned behavior.

The questions that follow are for the sake of knowing yourself better and preparing for the healthy life of your future child. The themes are rather provocative, and experiencing suppressed memories of the past may make you feel vulnerable. If you need to talk to a friend, partner, or counselor to be supported as you integrate your feelings and thoughts, please create that opportunity for yourself. If you are preparing to have a child with your partner, encourage him or her to review this list as well. Remember, an awareness of our weaknesses allows us to develop strengths. Every behavior pattern can be healed.

Allow your true feelings to flow through you as you write. Consider the first response that you become conscious of as carrying some message from deep within you. Allow all responses that come to you to be included. If you write in a stream of consciousness, you can edit later to discern your truth, as well as to notice where you may be holding back from being entirely honest. Include images that you see as well as feelings, thoughts, and memories. Feeling a strong emotional charge or resistance to a question can indicate that some part of you is repressing a truth that the question is evoking. Try not to skip over this question; instead, close your eyes and feel your resistance. Give yourself permission to be honest, at least with yourself. No one else needs to know. Be as specific as possible. The more detailed you can be, the deeper your understanding will be.

It can be just as important to discover that most of these questions are irrelevant to your life, and that you feel very little emotional response to them. Consciously realizing that you have a positive past and healthy role modeling can give you confidence in your ability to parent without abusing or neglecting your children. If, however, these questions assist you in recognizing that some personal growth may benefit you before you have a child, understand the gift you are giving your child by preparing for her arrival by first reviewing and healing your past.

1. When you were a child . . .
- Did your parents criticize, insult, or degrade you?
- Did your parents minimize your feelings or needs?
- Did your parents physically abuse you as a way of disciplining you?
- Did your parents threaten you?
- Did you fear your parents?
- Did they humiliate you in a way you felt had to be kept secret?
- Could you express sadness, fears, anger, hurt, or confusion with your parents?
- Did they control you with guilt?
- Did they disempower your acts?
- Did your parents make you feel unloved or unwanted? In what ways?
- Are your parents still exhibiting any of these behaviors with you?
- Did your parents use you to fulfill their unmet needs?
- Did you feel responsible for how your parents felt about each other?
- Do you still feel you need your parents' approval for your sense of self?

2. Are you ready to parent your own child . . .
- Are you able to express anger effectively without turning it inward and harming yourself? Are you able to express anger effectively without harming another by reacting with attacking rage?
- Do you feel that you nurture yourself—physically, emotionally, mentally, and spiritually?
- How do you feel when you are around other people's children?
- Do you have strong fears of responsibility for or rejection from a child?
- Do you have fears of being trapped by a committed love relationship with your child?
- Is providing your child with physical safety and security an important value for you in becoming a parent? Do you feel you know how to do this? What is your definition of physical (emotional, mental) safety?
- Considering your own childhood and your relationship with each of your parents, how prepared are you to parent your own child?
- Are you concerned or apprehensive about becoming a parent because you fear repeating your parents' pattern or overcompensating for it? Do you feel you have the ability to change? Do you need professional assistance to clarify this concern?
- Make a list of all the things you experienced with your parents that you fear you might pass on to your children.

3. Your relationship with your present intimate partner or past partners . . .
- Do you experience verbal abuse with your partner?
- Are you in an abusive relationship? How might this impact your ability to parent? If you do not make an effort to heal the relationship, how might this affect the development of your child?
- Do you or your partner refuse to discuss any stressful pattern or communication breakdown between you?
- Are you able to create mutual understanding with your partner? Do you respect each other's different points of view?
- Do you and your partner work through disagreements without guilt, blame, or emotionally hurting each other?

- Do you expect your partner to match your image of how you want him or her to be? Does your partner expect you to match his or her image? How concerned are each of you about being your true self with the other?
- Do you feel your partner cares about your physical, emotional, mental, and spiritual needs, or do those needs feel neglected?
- Does your partner judge, blame, invalidate, or criticize your personal qualities or personality?
- Does your relationship with your partner raise or lower your self-esteem? Does he or she empower or disempower you?
- Does your partner's behavior remind you of any negative behavior of either or both parents?
- How do you feel about the quality of intimacy with your partner? Does any behavior feel threatening or harmful?
- Does your partner own up to his or her inappropriate behavior with you? Are you each willing to forgive soon after you have hurt each other? What does this reflect about your relationship?
- Does your partner break agreements with you? How does this affect you? Do you trust his or her word? Do you feel betrayed?
- Are you feeling positive or negative about your relationship with your partner?
- Do you trust your point of view, or do you need your partner's validation?
- Does your partner try to overpower you, or do you overpower him or her in any way?
- Do you feel safe to express your truth with your partner?
- Are you re-creating or reexperiencing any childhood abuse or neglect patterns with your partner? Be very specific.
- Do you feel manipulated or controlled by your partner?
- Do you and your partner care how expressing anger might affect each other? Is expressing anger healing or harmful?
- Are you ignoring any unkind behaviors in how you treat your partner that you need to address?
- Have you ever questioned whether your relationship has abusive or neglectful or negative behavior in it that you do not want to pass on to your children? How does it feel?
- Have you ever been in or seen a healthy relationship with positive communication dynamics?

- Who are positive relationship role models for you?
- What have you learned about yourself, your partner, and your relationship by answering these questions? Be very specific.
- Are you feeling prepared to create a healthy parenting experience with your child? What do you need to focus on healing in your relationship with your partner to be optimally ready for any behavior you as parents, or your child, may express? Be very specific.

4. Owning your side of the dance . . .

Often when we withhold communications that need to be expressed, we begin to project onto our partner issues that actually belong to people in our past, and the relationship can become reactive. A variation of this is attributing behavior to our partner that is actually our own behavior. It is important that both partners own up to, and *own,* their behavior.

Very carefully, review your answers to the entire exercise above and consider: What do *you* need to own that you stated you experienced with your partner? Carefully make a list of the patterns you need to take responsibility for in the relationship. This will assist you in understanding some of the communication complexities of your partnership. It is not unusual for partners to discover that they have a wound in common. If you both have the same behavior pattern, it can be harder to see it, and difficult to heal it together. It can also explain why you may be highly reactive to your partner's behavior. Seek professional help if you do not feel you can heal it alone. Remember, becoming aware of a pattern is the first healthy step in transforming it. The more aware you are, the less likely it is that the pattern will be acted out through you unconsciously.

5. Your relationship with yourself . . .

- Are you abusive to yourself in any way—physically, emotionally, mentally, or spiritually? Be very specific.
- Do you neglect your needs, feelings, thoughts? If so, how?
- How do you disempower yourself? How do you empower yourself?
- Do you criticize, insult, or degrade yourself? Be specific.
- Do you minimize your feelings, thoughts, or needs? How?
- Do you acknowledge your feelings of sadness, fear, anger, or confusion?
- Do you freely express your inner truth to yourself?

- Are there any specific ways you harm yourself that are similar to how you were harmed by another person in your life (parents, family member, friend, lover, teacher, other)?
- Do you love yourself? Examine this fully.
- Do you have a positive sense of self—physically, mentally, and spiritually?
- Do you consciously own your behaviors or attitudes that are harmful to yourself or to others?
- Based on your present relationship with yourself, do you feel ready to parent a child? Explain in detail.
- Do you feel that you are a good role model for your future child? Examine your weaknesses and strengths.

6. Write a letter to the one who hurt you . . .

If you are experiencing any unresolved feelings from this exercise and there is no one available to share your feelings and thoughts with, or you want to clarify your reactions to this process before you talk with someone, you can write a letter. Freely express your truth in a stream-of-consciousness style without editing. Let emerge the feelings and thoughts that you withheld from the moment you were harmed or violated in any way, even if it may seem insignificant to the one who hurt you. It is important to know that many people who are abusive or neglectful to another are either unaware of their impact because they are not conscious of the influence their actions have on you, or are in denial, shame, or guilt. This exercise is not about changing them, but freeing yourself from the suppressed emotion that is affecting you.

Consider the following definition of *truth* from June Bletzer's *Encyclopedic Psychic Dictionary:*

> **TRUTH:** 1. an individual REALITY (not universal); all individuals have their own Truth within themselves, truth must be found within one's self; no one can teach another a Truth.[5]

Therefore, share your truth from *your point of view,* whether or not you feel your abuser will validate your experience. It is okay and very common to differ in points of view, especially taking into consideration that someone who has hurt you may not be able to honestly own it.

The following themes are suggestions for a free-flowing letter from your point of view (you will have the opportunity to evaluate the recipient's point of view after this exercise). Other themes may suggest themselves to you. Speak your truth to yourself in your letter and create emotional healing for your inner self.

Write a letter to anyone who violated you: Be very specific about how they have harmed you physically, emotionally (feelings), mentally (thoughts, attitudes, beliefs), and spiritually (your truth, reality, ideals, values). What did you experience the moment you were violated, and how has this impacted your sense of self, your relationships, your preparation for parenthood, your life?

Write a letter to both parents: Many self-help and recovery groups recognize the inner child or wounded child that resides within the personality identity of an adult. This is the part of your ego-self that may still feel the wounds of your past as if they are occurring in present time. Your inner child may be affecting your adult sense of self and your way of relating and communicating in present time so that some of your childhood feelings and thoughts dominate your behavior. Many reactive patterns are aspects of your inner child that are seeking attention, and that need to find more mature ways to be expressed. In this exercise allow the authentic feelings and thoughts of your wounded inner child to be expressed freely. What age do you feel as you write about the past to your parents? Perhaps this exercise will reveal to you a time in your past experience with your parents that needs to be healed within you, whether you ever share it with them or not. Give your inner child permission to have his or her own experience.

Imagine if your parents were in the room with you now, and it were safe to tell them anything and everything you have never told them, or any feelings and thoughts you shared but they never acknowledged or honored. (Looking at a picture of them may stimulate a flood of feelings.) Write your truth and be very specific. You are the only one empowered to speak the truth about your experience. Be aware of any temptation to sidestep painful realities, denying your truth to protect them or yourself. Write about such temptations as well.

Write a letter to the wounded child within you from your adult self: Go into your heart and sense whether you treat yourself in any abusive and neglectful ways that are similar to the ways your parents or anyone in your childhood treated you. Write a letter to your inner child admitting the truth. After you have clarified these patterns, focus on solutions and resolutions that will assist your wounded self to understand that you are going to try to find more loving ways to be with yourself. Since many of these patterns are unconsciously adopted through experiencing unhealthy role models when you were younger, you can consider forgiving yourself. The past can be resolved by acknowledging the truth, knowing you did the best you could with the limited awareness you had at the time, and making an effort to behave in more healthy ways in the present and future. If you continue to be self-abusive and experience no change toward expanding your awareness, you may want to seek professional help. When no alternative behavior has been established, sometimes you can be so habitually reactive to harmful patterns that you keep on harming yourself, even though you see what you are doing. In being truthful about your relationship to yourself, you should also consider how this might influence your relationship with your future child, and his relationship with you.

Write a letter to your partner about any unresolved experiences that you want to heal: If you are withholding any feelings or thoughts from your partner about how he or she has hurt you in any way—physically, mentally, or spiritually—now is the time to speak your truth. By holding on to resentments, you only harm yourself. When you resist communicating your hurt to your partner, resentments and mistrust can build up, keeping you from the full expression of love and intimacy.

If your wound is older than this relationship, it may be appropriate for you to clarify how your partner reminds you of someone from your past, and to consciously own it. You may be projecting your unresolved past onto your partner, or your past may cause you to exaggerate a new pain. However, your partner is responsible for his or her present actions. How willing are you to forgive your partner for hurting you? What will it take for you to forgive? Perhaps share this in the letter.

What do you need to own about how you have been harmful or neglectful to your partner (physically, emotionally, mentally, spiritually)? Tell your partner your truth. It is not important that he or she agrees with you for you to trust your own experience. Sometimes you may be misinterpreting a behavior. The purpose of this letter is to create self-understanding, to say what you actually felt, not to either blame your partner or reach agreement. You must hear your feelings in order to clarify issues that need to be healed with your partner, whether the pattern is within you or the other. Imagine if your parents had strengthened their mutual understanding and love before you were born. This is another gift you can give your future child.

Write a letter from the other's point of view: You can creatively open up to the other person's perception without involving him or her. Place a chair directly across from you. Imagine the person sitting there or actually set a picture of them on the chair. You can even say aloud, "I request the presence of *[name]* to please sit in this chair. Please listen to my feelings and thoughts *from my point of view*. We may not agree in our perception of what happened in the past, or how this is affecting our present relationship. All I need is for you to hear my truth. It heals me to be honest with myself and with you." Or say your own words from your own heart.

Then, giving yourself permission to speak the truth, read the letter you wrote in the previous exercise to the other person out loud, as if she or he were physically there.

Once you have expressed your truth verbally, close your eyes and imagine what the other person might say in response, *trying to perceive his or her point of view*. Then open your eyes and allow yourself to write a letter from that person to you. What might be said if he or she actually did sit in the chair and heard your feelings and thoughts? Trust your imagination and intuition. After you have finished this exercise, read aloud the letter to you, and sense whether you really opened up to the other's point of view. Of course, this point of view is not directly from its owner, so it still is experienced through your perception. But caring for and including the other side of the story is an important part of healing between two people. Being willing to speak your truth and then hear the other's reality opens up a lot of new possibilities.

After completing this exercise, consider that it may be healing to share this process with the person to whom you wrote your letter. You can share just your letter. Or share the person's imagined response (telling him or her that you are aware that it is still through your point of view; this is how you imagine he or she may feel). Or share both letters. It is important for you both to remember that you are sharing not to blame them but to create more understanding to heal the past wounds between you. If you are exploring your letters with your partner, then he or she may want to do these exercises, too. Expressing your willingness to hear his or her truth may allow your partner to be more open to you.

Your efforts now can make a significant difference in the psychological health of your parenting experience and your child's life.

Your Child's Psychological Inheritance

Within most family systems, specific personality patterns are passed on unconsciously from generation to generation. You may have discovered that issues surrounding food, sex, drugs, alcohol, or dysfunctional relationship dynamics were modeled to you by your parents or other family members. Whatever pattern you may have inherited from a family member, positive or negative, *someone taught it to this family member.* By creating a detailed genogram you can trace your genealogy, revealing your unique, tangible family legacy. This technique is very useful in understanding how unhealthy patterns such as abuse, addictions, and codependency are passed on between family members, as well as in highlighting your family strengths. Reviewing your family lineage will make you aware of your place in your family's evolution through many generations.

A frequent concern of prospective parents, conscious or unconscious, is that they will repeat unhealthy and reactive patterns of their parents and family members. It is undeniable that your ancestors do contribute to your physical, emotional, mental, and philosophical life. A genogram can highlight the degree to which you are an expression of your unique family qualities and talents, as well as a product of particular family dysfunctional behaviors. It is a detailed blueprint of the biological, psychological, legal, and geographical patterns among family members. It can be an excellent tool for perceiving the physical, emotional, mental, and spiritual design of the whole family system—past, present, and future. See a sample family genogram on pages 124–125.

Constructing a genogram is often referred to as creating a family tree. Each family member with his or her mates and offspring requires a new branch on the central family tree. When you and your partner decide to have a child, you will combine your family trees, thus "growing" a larger tree to include your newly formed nuclear unit. A comprehensive family tree can indicate the origin of particular problems that are repeating themselves in your budding family system.

Thomas feels that reflecting on his family genogram was enlightening in helping him respond to the stress of parenting his infant twin sons:

> When Gloria and I drew our genograms and compared them, we saw that we and our children were susceptible to continuing a long line of emotional neglect and abuse between parent and child, and husband and wife. On top of that, both sides of my family were alcoholics, as were four generations of the paternal branch of Gloria's family. We knew that we needed to remain aware of how we expressed our temperament and attention to our children, since our role modeling had been so unhealthy. We made a great effort to change our ways immediately. Our commitment to break the family patterns inspired us to remain vigilant whenever we behaved like our parents. Since those family behaviors have been the "norm" for Gloria and me, we'll have to be fully conscious of how we use alcohol and what we teach our children about the use of recreational substances, as well as responsibly expressing our feelings to our kids. Without the genogram to objectify our potential vulnerabilities, we might not have made such an intentional commitment to end the harmful generational patterns with our new family.

The genogram map can also help you identify important intergenerational relationship patterns, personality characteristics that may be shared among family members, inheritable diseases, and family beliefs and attitudes. Relationship patterns among family members are particularly informative. Interpersonal dynamics such as blame, manipulation, control, empowerment, fairness and kindness, crisis response, personal power issues, and decision making are all relevant to your exploration. Try to identify roles that various family members embody. You may find such specific personality identities as the provider, rescuer, victim, protector, or caregiver. It is valuable to note family members who repeatedly separate or divorce, as well as substantial family feuds.

All of these elements illustrate the ways in which your family members relate to each other in either healthy or dysfunctional ways. Noting whether a pattern is chronic or an exception can assist you in evaluating whether you, your partner, and your future child may be more likely to express similar behavior. For example, if both you and your partner have a high number of divorces in your family trees, you may want to be aware of your tendency to choose divorce if your own relationship becomes conflicted. This awareness may inspire you to seek counseling to resolve your stresses, rather than choosing the old family pattern of ending the relationship.

Tamara chose to transform her past by confronting it:

> Ollie and I always would get drunk and pick a fight with each other to get out our feelings. Both of our parents did the same thing, and we thought this behavior was normal. The alcoholism led to domestic violence, so that both of our mothers left our fathers when we were small children. Divorce had occurred through many generations of the family so it was normal for me do the same, rather than work through the conflict. I felt myself moving toward the decision to leave Ollie, since Ollie had come close to hitting me. The day I was filing the divorce papers, I heard a voice within me say, "Break the cycle. Take charge and change your behavior, *no one else can do it for you.*" I went into therapy and joined an AA group. Within several months Ollie joined me because he knew he had to change to keep me committed to the marriage. Four years later, we are happily married, with many skills for dealing with stress. Our son has thanked us for changing our ways, and I am sure we saved him from reliving our struggles.

Your personal convictions greatly contribute to your identity, values, and lifestyle choices, and often dysfunctional behaviors and beliefs have their origin in the family expectations and rules. As you work on your genogram, consider a thorough exploration and inventory of your family beliefs. Any of us could spend a lifetime uncovering these! Every phase of family life involves the existence of core beliefs: for example, beliefs about how to birth a child (home or hospital), how to discipline adolescents, educational or marriage expectations, definitions of success, and spiritual philosophy. Some are conscious; many are subconscious. All can be very influential.

Healing your negative parental conditioning is most effective when you acknowledge how similar your unhealthy reactions and actions are to your parents'. By perceiving how you behave like they did, you will bring to light the multigenerational tendencies you inherited. By not denying the similarities between you and your parents, you can more clearly define your differences.

Ed recalls his own awakening:

> I had been going to the same church services throughout my adult life as I did during my childhood. Then, one day, I realized that the spiritual content of my religion was very fear based and empty. After exploring the churches in our community, I found one much more in tune with my values and beliefs. My parents were appalled that I had left the family church, but my wife and kids were happy that we had found a more positive and life-affirming congregation and minister. Had I been more aware, I would have made this change as soon as I began living alone, thirteen years earlier.

I encourage you to expand your exploration to include how you, your partner, and your future child wish to exist within the larger context of society. Explore your political viewpoints, environmental concerns, religious alignments, and moral principles with each other. Review how your families and you contribute to the community, and how the community responds to your family. Clarify for yourselves what you want your child to experience in her relationship with the larger world.

In collecting data for your genogram, I suggest that both partners request information from family members about both negative and positive emotional patterns, discovering how each person feels about the self, others, and life. The temperaments of family members can vary dramatically, from cheerfulness and optimism to depression, phobias, tempers, and violence. Significant details of medical and psychological histories such as alcoholism, organ disorders, arthritis, stress reactions, and compulsions should be acknowledged. Because you are preparing for parenthood, explore family beliefs about children, career, and parenting. Specify multigenerational patterns with infertility, miscarriages, abortions, and stillbirths. What are your family attitudes and experiences regarding conception, pregnancy, and giving birth?

In creating a family tree, you'll want to speak with as many family members as possible, even those with whom you have not been in close contact before. Occasionally, surprising hidden truths about your lineage may be uncovered. Jack remembers when he learned a family secret from a relative:

> I was shocked to discover from my great-aunt that my father had three illegitimate children with another woman after my sister was born and before I entered the family scene. To think I actually have three siblings out there in the world I have never met, and have never even known existed! Now I know why I never trusted my parents; I could tell they were hiding a big secret. It was subtle, but now it all makes sense. My brother and I both have children with women we are not married to. This transgenerational stuff is potent—even unspoken family patterns still appeared downstream in our lives.

Sometimes the existence of past abusive behavior between family members can be threatening for a relative to reveal, especially if the family member being interviewed behaved abusively toward other family members. In such cases, if you fear for your psychological or physical safety in exploring any theme, I suggest you not put yourself in danger.

Creating a genogram is a time-consuming task, and you may find that a brief list of family tendencies suits your purposes. If you choose not to construct a full genogram, please turn to page 128.

Constructing a Genogram

You can construct a family genogram in one of two basic ways. To choose which is most appropriate for you, begin by defining your purpose. To identify a single issue, such as inheritable health concerns or recurrent family addictions, a bare-bones approach is all you need. In your map you will indicate yourself, your partner, and family members, along with only those identifiers that fall within this category. When you're planning for your future child, though, I recommend the more inclusive holistic process described above, which will reveal a world of valuable information.

Once you have decided what type of genogram you need, begin to gather your data. (See a sample genogram on pages 124–125.)

- Across the top of a piece of paper, list all your family members for at least three generations; you may need to use more than one page for larger families.
- Down the left side, list the various types of information you would like to have about family members. You may include such items as intelligence, health anomalies, baldness, obesity, personality traits, giftedness, profession, hobbies, smoking, drinking, disposition toward children and pets, interpersonal dynamics, and much more. Leave enough space to thoroughly detail each item.

  Alternately, you can simply gather all the information possible on each family member and then distill up to ten separate recurrent themes to list on your genogram afterward.
- Then begin to fill in what you know about each family member. Start in your own home, where your immediate family history surrounds you. As part of your process, make a list with your partner of any negative attributes that either of you embody that could affect the way you parent your child. Be willing to face patterns that are harmful for any child to be exposed to. Then clarify the positive qualities you can offer your child. If you already have one or more children, consider how your relationship with them is reflecting unresolved experiences from your own childhood. Can you guarantee your children reliable physical and emotional security? If not, why not?
- After accumulating as much family data as you can from self-inquiry, your partner, and previous children, begin to consider reaching out to other family members. First, choose relatives who you sense are most willing to share the truth—from family ideals and values to the unhealthy dynamics that either existed or still exist. Tell your relatives the true purpose of the life history interview: You are consciously preparing for parenthood and want to evaluate your life patterns so that you can be aware of strengths and weaknesses your future children may inherit. Older family members such as your parents, aunts, uncles, and grandparents may enjoy telling their life stories to preserve personal

and family histories. Take advantage of this to enroll them in your project.

When you are ready to talk with your family members, it is best to meet with each person in his or her own home, where they have access to pictures and memorabilia. You can take handwritten notes or use an audiotape or video recorder to tape interviews. An extended phone call can be very effective if you feel secure in your communication skills; you can also write a letter explaining your intent and enclose a list of specific questions to be answered in writing or by phone.

You may have to do some sleuthing in your research. If you are an only child or your immediate family does not want to help you, you can still try to contact friends of your parents, grandparents, aunts, and uncles. Perhaps your parents' childhood friends or their college roommates are available. Or you may find out where they have worked and talk with their colleagues. You can even hire a genealogy research service.

If you or your relatives are from stepfamilies or have been adopted, work on just one branch of the family at a time. Intimate involvement with a stepfamily, foster family, or adoptive family will still strongly influence the psychological patterns of your childhood family system. Drug, food, or alcohol addictions or personality patterns of the family that raised you can be internalized and embodied, as can their beliefs, values, and lifestyle, but you will not be vulnerable to their genetic inheritance. On the other hand, if you are adopting a child, information about his biological family tree will be very helpful in determining his genetic tendencies. Like stepchildren, adopted children have a blended influence from both adopted and genetic family trees.

If you do not want to create an extensive genogram, spend a few hours developing a simple sketch of the family patterns as you remember them through three generations, beginning with yourself and siblings, then your parents, and moving finally to your grandparents from both your mom's and dad's side. When each partner has created an individual tree, compare the two. Your combined trees growing together is the most comprehensive overview of potential influences that your child may inherit. It is extremely insightful to evaluate mutual weaknesses and strengths that you and your children may experience from each side of the family.

- After you have gathered the data from each family member and logged the information in the correct subject category under each name, you will transfer it to a family genogram map.

To create your own genogram map, use a circle to designate female family members and a square for males. With a large sheet of drawing paper positioned horizontally, draw your own symbol at the bottom of the page, with your partner's beside you. Draw a horizontal line between your two symbols, and draw symbols for any children either of you have, descending from that line. A future child can be designated with a question mark in its symbol. This is your nuclear family, the center or trunk of your family tree.

Next, extend a line up from your own symbol (and that of your partner) and make a horizontal line on which you will place a square symbol for your father on the left and a circle for your mother on the right. Draw lines descending from this line and add appropriate symbols for any siblings you may have. Then, as you did for yourself, draw lines upward for each of your parents to add symbols for *their* parents (your grandparents) and their siblings (your aunts and uncles). If you know or can find out even more about your ancestors, continue to add lines and symbols for as many generations as you can access information for.

If a person in the family is no longer living, place an *X* over their symbol. Record birth dates to the left of the symbol, dates of death to the right. The person's age at death can be written inside the symbol. When you are unsure about dates, approximate dates can be used, followed by a question mark. Since miscarriages, stillbirths, and induced abortions are considered important in preparing for parenthood, especially if there is a recurrent personal or family history of them, they can be included using the death symbol. Fertility and infertility patterns in the family history are of great value for those preparing to conceive a child.

In a genogram the lines that connect family members will indicate biological and legal (marriage) relationships. Horizontal lines symbolize marriage (an m followed by the date marks the wedding date). A marriage that has changed to a separation or divorce is indicated on the marriage line by making a single slash for separation, and two slashes for divorce (use *S* and *D* to indicate the date that disruptions in the marriage occurred).

A SAMPLE FAMILY GENOGRAM

Due to space limitations, children of siblings, aunts, and uncles are missing in this genogram. Your children are represented on the first horizontal line at the bottom of the page.

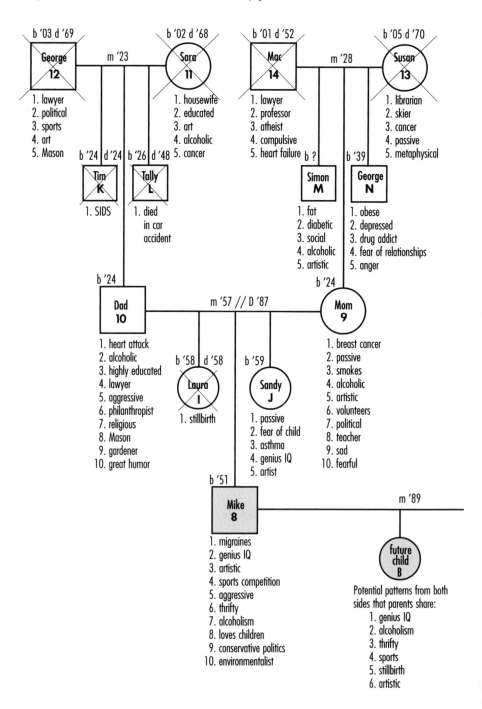

Those with more than two children (and their subsequent family members) in any particular generation will need more space. For comprehensive genograms with many family members, I recommend taping paper together or using large drawing paper.

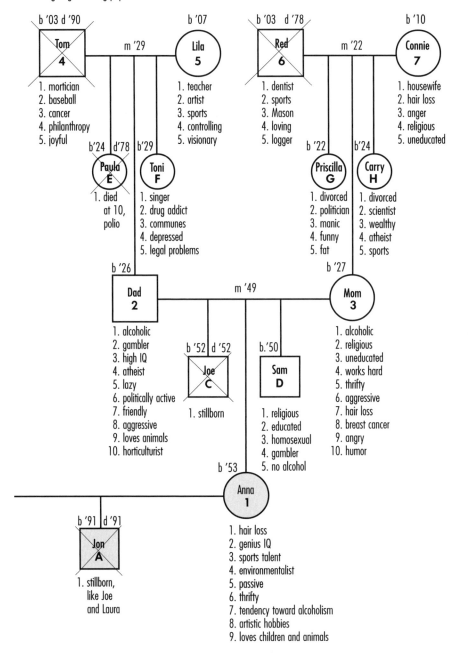

Multiple marriages are more challenging to depict. The different marriages follow in reverse chronology from left to right. When each spouse has had multiple marriages, the most recent relationship is often placed in the center next to the present partner, with the former spouses off to the side. If a couple is living together but not legally married, their relationship is shown by using a broken line.

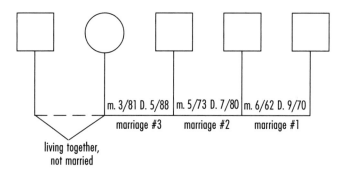

If a couple has children, each child's symbol hangs down vertically from the line that connects the couple. Children are indicated oldest to youngest, left to right. A foster or adopted child is illustrated by using a broken line to the parent's line. With twins, converging lines to the parent's line are used, and if they are identical, they are connected with a short horizontal line or bar.

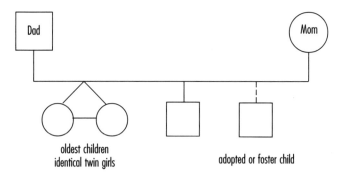

Once you have drawn this basic map, number all family members so that relationships that stand out as special can be described more fully on a separate page if you run out of room. List yourself as number 1, your father as number 2, your mother as number 3, your paternal grandfather as number 4, your paternal grandmother as number 5, your maternal grandfather as 6, your maternal grandfather as 7, and so on. For your mate and your mate's family, continue the numbers. For children, siblings, cousins, aunts, and uncles, use letters of the alphabet. Use uppercase for significant relatives, lowercase for more distant relations. Using the numbers and letters allows you to immediately refer to your list's description of a particular family member.

Dotted lines or colored markers can be used to encircle family members living in a given household, which is very useful for remarried families where stepchildren are shared. The numerous divorces, separations, and multiple marriages of many families create very complex relationships in family structures. Yet this complexity is worth depicting because it is often the reason for challenging interpersonal relationships within the family. For example:

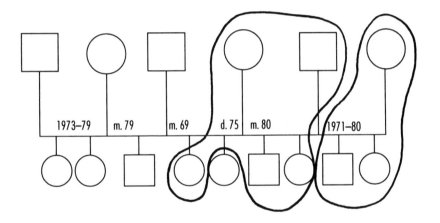

Begin with these basic symbols for mapping biological and legal dynamics among family members, or create other symbols that are meaningful to you. After you have drawn this skeletal genogram, you can begin to record the medical, psychological, and behavioral information you have collected. All of the critical life events and personality characteristics can be added to this basic diagram next to each individual's symbol.

Different lines can be used to symbolize the various relationships among family members. Three parallel lines between two people can be used to represent a very close bond. A zigzag can represent a poor or conflicted relationship. A break in the line may symbolize a broken bond or estrangement, and a dotted line can be used to represent a distant relationship.

As you track many major family patterns, you may be surprised to find that all the cousins on one side of the family have a certain artistic or scientific talent, or all the aunts on the other side have breast cancer, or all the grandparents were alcoholics with children who inherited this tendency. This is what you call a *transgenerational pattern,* a pattern that repeats from one generation to another. Remain aware of these recurrences as you compare your own family tree to your partner's. If there are any patterns of addiction in your family tree—even if you do not personally embody them—be aware of how insidious these can be in the family system. Your child may be regularly exposed to a family member who still exhibits addictive behavior. I have worked with many clients who had very traumatic experiences when they were left as children with a family member for baby-sitting or during family events. Seeing grandparents drunk, for instance, or being ignored by parents because they are intoxicated can be devastating for a child, especially if it is a regular occurrence. As you design your genogram, you'll be able to more objectively discern patterns you and your child are vulnerable to inheriting, and to use this information in preparing for parenthood.

Your Attitude toward Having a Child

The feelings your future child receives concerning your attitudes about parenthood can begin to shape her self-esteem and expectations about herself. Beginning with life in the womb, the subconscious and conscious messages she experiences from you can support or undermine her tender personality. Now is the perfect time for you to explore your attitudes to consciously determine whether you feel prepared for parenthood.

Do You Have Fears or Ambivalences?

It is not uncommon for potential new parents—even those who deeply desire and feel they have prepared for their child—to also feel some ambivalence about conceiving and giving birth to a new life. Having a baby requires major shifts in your lifestyle and relationships, as your priorities will be forced to change. Once you become pregnant, you may experience a wide range of conflicting emotions.

There is a difference between healthy ambivalence and chronic ambivalence about becoming a mom or dad. Healthy ambivalence includes the natural tendency to have fleeting fears or doubts about yourself, your partner, or your future child. Chronic ambivalence is characterized by a *persistent pattern* of reluctance to becoming a loving parent. Continual hesitation about your readiness to handle the challenges of parenthood can profoundly affect your ability to bond with your future child, thus leaving yourself and your baby vulnerable to significant emotional pain. Prospective fathers are also vulnerable to emotional upheavals as they adjust to their future relationship to the new child, along with profound changes in their partner.

It is important that you both invest some time clarifying whether your anxieties about having a child are motivated by a true unreadiness to bond with your little one. During the earliest stages of a prenate's life, a profound connection can be instilled between you and your child. Psychological and biological studies show that a first-trimester fetus possesses enough self-awareness to sense chronic rejection from an ambivalent mother. Dr. Thomas Verny states that "a mother's anxiety-provoking hormones" can flood her baby's system, "making him worried and fearful."[6] The developmental significance of emotional dependency between mother and child beginning in utero suggests that postnatal bonding is a continuum of security that, if missed, can cause a lifelong primal wound.

Irregular doubts and many of the common concerns about balancing career and parenthood, financial challenges, or feeling unprepared to be a parent are appropriate if these feelings are not overwhelming. According to T. Berry Brazelton, M.D., the emotional turmoil that commonly occurs during pregnancy mobilizes a mother to adjust to the demands of mothering. Prebirth anxiety is "a method of freeing her circuits of a kind of sensitivity to the infant and his individual requirements."[7]

Persistent anxiety about becoming pregnant is a sign that you may need some counseling. Distinguish between concerns that are a healthy sign of caring from those that make you feel out of control. If you feel that your emotional stress may prevent you from bonding with your baby or partner, or may leave you feeling consistently afraid that you will not be able to provide your child with love, seek a sensitive friend or counselor who can assist you in feeling more confident.

Sandy and Tim transformed their ambivalence into a reliable sense of certainty:

> We always wanted to have children, yet it was terrifying to actually become pregnant because I was afraid of losing my freedom. One day, after postponing parenthood for more than six years, I sat down and

made a list of all the reasons I was hesitating. Tim did the same exercise and we realized we had similar fears, although mine was about losing financial freedom and Tim's was about losing his free time to pursue recreational pleasures. We realized that our reluctance to sacrifice could be blocking our ability to conceive, and we needed to make a real effort to create practical solutions. We focused on making a list of ways we were self-assured to become parents, and the ambivalence melted away into the truth that we were ready to take the plunge and surrender our childish need for freedom.

Now is the time to consider your feelings of readiness to nurture a child. Find time to talk with your partner about how each of you is feeling. Evaluate your attitudes about conceiving and giving birth to your baby:

- What are your specific fears about becoming a parent?
- In what ways are you ambivalent about having a baby with (or without) your partner?
- Do you need to talk with anyone about your concerns? If so, who?
- Do your concerns feel healthy and appropriate for being a first-time parent? If so, why? If not, what feeling seems out of proportion? Do you need some support from someone?

What Do You Look Forward To?

There is a tendency for those seeking to optimize their prebirth preparation to focus on the ways they are not ready and minimize their confident feelings about becoming a parent. As Sarah observes:

> I am tired of looking at my readiness to be a mom like a cup half empty; in truth, my eagerness to have my baby makes my cup well over half full!

Now is the time to affirm those attitudes that are life enhancing, such as joyful anticipation and the loving desire to bond with and contribute to the child's whole health before he is conceived or born. Focusing on your hopes and dreams can create a warm and emotionally enriching experience for you and your partner. With the knowledge that women and men can actively bond with their child while he is in the womb, you can use your optimism and self-confidence to create a more meaningful relationship with your child from the beginning of his life.

Parenthood can be one of the most profound spiritual experiences of your life. Embracing the idea that having a baby is a spiritual journey, you can begin to realize that not only does the baby need you, but you need your baby to develop yourself as well. You are not only conceiving your child but re-creating and rebirthing yourself as you expand your consciousness for the miraculous events that will occur within you and your partner as you prepare to conceive your child.

Becoming a parent can be a blossoming spiritual revelation about love, wholeness, beauty, and wisdom. Your inner growth is fostered by the continual positive influence of loving your wondrous child. You can use all of the challenges of parenthood to attain a spiritual depth that brings out the best in you. My own journal reflects my personal awakening:

> I cannot overestimate the invaluable perspective of preparing for parenthood as a dynamic force in my self-realization. As a result of committing to be an emotionally and spiritually conscious parent, I have been able to deepen my foundation of self-love, deepen my love for my husband, and open my heart to my daughter in ways I never imagined. Through love, my family has become the most important relationship in my life.

Parenthood can deepen your understanding of how your own loving nature can shape your child's whole self.

Take some time now to clarify:

- In what ways are you feeling confident to become a parent?
- What about your partner's personality and your own makes you feel like you're ready to have a baby together?
- What do you have to look forward to in creating a family?

Communication with Your Partner

Relationships thrive when communication reflects a ready acceptance and respect of people's innate differences.

John Gray

No matter how prepared you may feel for parenthood, having a baby will change you and your partner in many unexpected and significant ways. Fulfilling the constant needs of your child can offer you both opportunities to develop numerous virtuous qualities. You will learn to be selfless, loving, patient, and persevering in ways that you had not imagined. Your mutual ability to communicate your feelings and thoughts to one another will influence the quality of your parenting experience.

As your role as a new parent and your baby's needs become more defined, the familiar patterns of your relationship with your partner will be challenged. There will be many new responsibilities to share as your little one demands around-the-clock attention. Jennifer's story sounds amazing but it is really true:

> Trying to have a shower before evening rolls around is the big challenge of the day. It was a bit mind boggling when I eventually discovered that I had been up since dawn feeding my baby and the next thing I realized, it was sunset, and I was still in my pajamas. This happened week after week after my baby was born; I still occasionally have these timeless days, and my baby is six months old.

Your ability to express your concerns and listen to those of your mate will make adjusting to parenthood easier. The daily sharing of routine tasks requires continuous communication with your partner, as well as with any other children in the home. Even if you and your partner already have a healthy communication dynamic, the time and energy requirements of a newborn will affect all areas of your personal and professional life. If your self-expression has been repressed, expect a crash course in communicating your feelings. If you do not listen to your partner's or child's needs, an uncomfortable tension and potential conflict in these relationships will be the result.

What are some of the most common adjustments that couples must make during this dramatic life change? At times your baby will need you when you feel you have nothing left to give, and your partner may need you simultaneously. Your partner will need to understand that, most of the time, he or she must wait. Also, you can expect that your baby will call for you in the middle of your deepest dream cycle. Heads or tails? Who gets out of bed during these wee hours of the morn? Sometimes, having had no time to eat all day, you will just be sitting down to dinner when your child will need an immediate diaper change; someone is going to have to stop eating and attend to the baby. And night after night, who is going to wash the pile of dishes in the kitchen when everyone is exhausted and needs to go to sleep? Healthy communication between partners will determine a positive conclusion for each of these situations.

If you have never been a parent, you may feel that there are easy solutions to the division of duties, but their frequency will challenge even the healthiest relationships, especially if one or both partners are sleep deprived and stressed from trying to fulfill home *and* work responsibilities. If you have difficulty communicating with your partner before you conceive a child, the natural stresses of having a baby will exacerbate this problem.

Sally remembers:

> Simon would return home from work and could not understand why the laundry was not folded, the dishes unwashed, the garbage overflowing. He had the nerve to say to me the first week after Ira was born, "In the past these tasks have been easily handled. What is the problem now? You have all day to do these things while the baby sleeps." I was livid. Couldn't he see that the baby was nursing for forty-five minutes every hour and a half, all day and night? After changing the ten diapers a day and trying to feed myself and shower, there was no time left. Of course, this eased up after the baby started sleeping more and eating less often, but this took a number of months. Simon and I had many arguments about the messy house—until he spent half a day baby-sitting for Ezra. All of the counseling sessions in the world could not have better illustrated what he learned taking care of Ira for a concentrated period of time. He finally stopped hounding me about completing chores and suggested we hire a person to clean. I wish I'd known how to communicate my needs to him before we had so much stress with our baby.

Most couples feel the demands of their newborn consuming their sexual lives as well. Sleep deprivation has an uncanny way of depleting your life force, and often sex is the last thought to grab a new parent's attention. For women who choose to breast-feed, the constant physical contact with their baby often makes them disinterested in intimacy with their partner. There is simply little energy left for their lover after they have been nursing every several hours throughout the day.

Many couples grow closer emotionally as they are fulfilled by the love and joy that they share with their child. But the bonding with a child should not replace sexual intimacy between partners. Because the demands of a newborn often delay fulfillment of sexual needs for one or both partners, it is essential for couples to communicate about how to care for each other during these times. You will want to know it is safe to tell your partner that your temporary disinterest in sex does not mean that you are not interested in him or her. Do not be surprised if this becomes an issue between the two of you. Couples whose sexual life thrives during the first months after having a child are the exception.

If there is more than one child, quality communication becomes even more essential, because each child must be fed, bathed, clothed, played with, and educated each day—week after week, year after year. Add the requirements of maintaining a household (laundry, cleaning, food shopping, telephones ringing) and the responsibilities of one or both partners working, and presto!—there are a *lot* of task details that need to be clarified. Clear communication creates an atmosphere of harmony when deciding who is to do each chore. How will you and your partner deal with those days when your child's illness means that one of you has to stay home from work unexpectedly? Imagine that you are lying in bed after midnight and suddenly realize that you're out of diapers. Who gets dressed to find an open store and buy a pack on a cold, rainy night? Will each of you be able to communicate your needs and make considerate choices without creating unnecessary conflict?

Cecil and Sharon had to adjust their communication style:

> Sharon and I both had full-time jobs. When our first son, Damian, was born, Sharon would always stay home when he was sick. When our second son came along two years later, she demanded that it was my turn to sacrifice my workday to care for the boys if they were ill. There was never any discussion. She would justify this by saying that she took care of Damian the first two years, and that now it was my turn. After realizing our fights were starting to have an impact on our sons' emotional stability when they were sick, we went to counseling to uncover why there was so much tension between us. I learned that Sharon felt a tremendous amount of resentment that I had assumed she was the primary caretaker in the relationship, and because she was the mother she had to stay home from work. *And* even after she communicated that, I had agreed to coparent our children but only at the times that were convenient for me. I started to realize my selfish choices and began to be more available. We try now to express our upsets at the time they occur, each of us acknowledging when we are selfish and focusing on

creative ways to assist one another. Effective communication has brought harmony back to our family. It's especially important during the holiday season when there is so much more to be done.

Your Child Is Listening: Do You Sound Like Your Parents?

You and your mate will be continuously asked to communicate new ways of handling parenting responsibilities as your child grows. Each of her developmental needs will require new responses and commitments from both parents. And as your child's intelligence develops, your way of communicating will need to adapt as well. If you are having conflicts communicating with your partner, consider that the same patterns may appear between you and your child as she grows older. Mary complains:

> Riley never acknowledges me when I ask him for help. I have to yell at him to get his attention. I noticed our two daughters have adopted the same behavior. They ignore me like their dad, and they yell at me, like I do to everyone else, when they want me to do something for them. I know the girls learned their responses from both of us. And this is the way my parents and I behaved, too.

It's so important that partners who are parents become aware of their conversation style. How similar is your relationship with your partner to the way that you experienced your parents relating? What are the differences? Most important, reflect on how your communication style supports positive role modeling for your future child. Milly says:

> My husband and I both were listened to as children, and honored for our unique viewpoints. I know our ability to hear and honor each other is helping our eight-year-old daughter, Lila, mature socially. Many of her friends come to us for advice because we care about hearing their frustrations, and they ask Lila to help them work through their struggles with their parents. She knows how to listen, and they see how well we get along as a family and they want to learn how we do it.

If you and your partner have consistent conflict and lack the ability to resolve issues and concerns with mutual understanding, then your communication dynamic is an unhealthy one. If you disrespect, verbally or physically abuse, or do not acknowledge your partner's perspective (even if you disagree with it), your way of communicating needs to change. If you frequently respond to each other with anger or judgment on important issues, your child will not learn about compassionate communication. In essence, if your words or attitude disempower or devalue the other, you are choosing destructive interactions. If you feel that you and your partner seem to be speaking two different languages that leave you feeling perplexed and frustrated, you need help.

If you're unhappy with your communication patterns, try to engage your partner in co-creating new ways to talk with each other. Find some books on the subject, or seek professional support. There is always an alternative to reactive dynamics if you are willing to admit the need to change your habitual ways. Peggy recalls:

> George and I used to argue over most of the parenting chores. He would tell me that I nagged him like his mother, and since I knew he did not like her, I always felt he did not like me. Until we went to relationship counseling, he never just sat down and listened to me when I was overwhelmed and needed support. He would just demean my character by telling me I was a chronic complainer. He finally learned that when I was stressed, hugging me and appreciating me for taking care of our sons would restore me to a positive state quicker than anything else. Now when there is tension between us, we know that's a sign that we need to make a conscious effort to communicate to each other. Now George loves to have "date nights" whenever we have a major decision to make about the boys. The rule is that first one, then the other, shares all of their concerns while the other has to listen without interrupting. Then we make a written list of solutions and prioritize them. We don't go home until there is an action plan established and a feeling of love between us.

When a relationship is mutually supportive, each partner values the other's perspective and needs. There is a spirit of respect and appreciation, even if one of you does not agree with the other's opinion or is unable to fulfill those needs. Being a good listener who constantly strives to embody warmth, empathy, kindness, attentiveness, equality, and understanding reflects a healthy communication dynamic between a couple, as well as between parent and child. Genuine interest in and participation with your partner's perspective strengthens the trust that is essential for mature love to be expressed, because your partner can depend on having his or her reality honored and shared.

You will be your child's first teacher. He will learn by your example. Try to embody qualities of love and understanding when you communicate with all of your family members. Specific issues and concerns that will occur between you and your partner and child cannot be foretold, but you can be sure that there will be many problems and challenges that will need resolution. The ability to communicate effectively and compassionately within your family will increase the likelihood that each of your genuine feelings, thoughts, and needs are respected and appropriately fulfilled. When you demonstrate to your partner and child that you care to listen, and all of you consistently honor one another's viewpoints, you are teaching that communication is an active way of expressing wisdom and love.

Creative Exercise:
Preparing Your Mind for Conception

1. What specific feelings from your heart and thoughts from your mind do you consider healthy to express with your future child? What feelings and thoughts are unhealthy?
2. What is the value of meditation in your life? What is the next step you can take to use this tool for psychological and spiritual well-being?
3. What did you learn from your parents about how adults express their feelings and thoughts to children?
4. What inspires you to make a simple or comprehensive genogram, with or without your partner? Specify your resistance to constructing one as well.
5. How can you deliberately use the genogram process to create optimal health conditions for your future child?
6. From which family members do you sense you have inherited unhealthy characteristics, and what are the undesirable behaviors that you express?
7. Which family members have been positive role models for your self-esteem, talents, and abilities, and life choices? Specify what they taught you.
8. In what ways are you ready to be a parent? In what ways do you not feel prepared?

9. What does healthy communication mean to you? What do you consider to be unhealthy?
10. List three or more important concerns you need to communicate to your partner to prepare for parenthood.
11. What do you need to heal or change in your communication style to be the best role model you can be for your child?

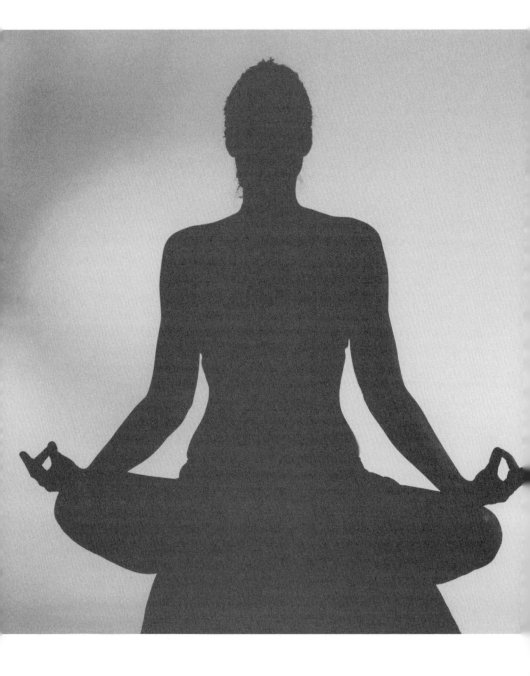

5

Preparing Your Spirit
for Conception

Our Father, who art in Heaven with me,
Thy name be hallowed within my child.
Thy Kingdom come into my womb,
Thy Will be done in my child's growth,
As it is done in Thy angelic heaven.
Give my child its daily spiritual food,
Forgive today its Soul's past trespasses,
And lead its Soul to forgive those who
   trespassed against it on other planes.
And deliver it safely into our world.

Anonymous

There are many ways to nurture a child. To nourish her *spirit* means to care for the Divine Self within her and also within *yourself*. Certain principles and ideals can assist you in preparing to spiritually parent your future child. The conception and birth of your baby will initiate you as a teacher of spirit, for you will have endless opportunities to express your inner wisdom and loving nature in cultivating the true self of each family member. Parenting then becomes a spiritual discipline for you, and a spiritual lesson for your child.

In his book *The Seven Spiritual Laws of Parents* Deepak Chopra shares: "Without being perfect parents, and of course by slipping many times from our ideals, my wife and I found a way to raise our children by

141

inspiration. Showing how to be 'in spirit' is what the word 'inspired' actually means, that is, to 'breathe in the breath of God.' And such modeling also shows what it means to have enthusiasm, which comes from the Greek works, *en theos*, meaning 'in God.'"[1]

Like Chopra and his wife, all parents will experience the ups and downs of trial and error in honing their parenting skills. But beginning with a spiritual perspective will provide you with one of the best foundations possible.

Having an understanding of the law of karma was a reminder to me that my child is an ancient soul who would be born with a spiritual consciousness already unfolding. By allowing myself to care for, and thus psychically bond with, this ethereal presence before conception, my heart and mind opened to the divine plan of my daughter's incarnating soul. By embracing the universal archetype of the immaculate conception, I was honoring the fact that my child was to be conceived and nourished as a sacred life with a divine design. And by consciously identifying with and expressing my highest virtues, I discovered practical ways to sustain a spiritual perspective amid the adversities and challenges that have arisen in parenting my child.

The Law of Karma

All souls incarnate and reincarnate under the Law of Rebirth—
hence each life is not only a recapitulation *of life experiences, but an*
assuming of ancient obligations, a recovery *of old relations, and oppor-*
tunity for the paying of old indebtedness, a chance to make restitution
and progress, an awakening of deep-seated qualities, the recognition of
old friends and enemies, the solution of revolting injustices, and the
explanation of that which conditions a man *and makes him what*
he is. Such is the law which is crying out for Universal recognition.

Djwhal Kuhl

The ageless law of karma is a universal key to holistic parenting. It is often referred to as the law of cause and effect and suggests that your future child will choose his global location, lifestyle, intelligence, physical condition, and relatives—including you as his parent—based on the incarnating soul's entire accumulated activities, thoughts, and emotions throughout all previous lifetimes (or incarnations). In essence, karmic law demonstrates that by our causative actions in one life, we merit certain resulting circumstances in the same or a later life. This is captured in St. Paul's famous words, "Whatsoever a man soweth, that shall he reap. And, if not in this life, then in a life that follows after."

Your future child will incarnate with karmic characteristics that are consequences of actions set into motion in previous lives and that will affect the soul's physical, emotional, and mental patterns for this life as well as future ones. As your child matures and her personality is shaped by family and social influences, her karmic patterns can be transformed through intentional deeds and changes in attitude. The incarnating soul's karma will determine many aspects of her prenatal and birth circumstances as well as her lifelong experiences. Your awareness of the principles of karma can assist your child in unfolding her most magnificent soul expression this lifetime.

According to many of the ageless teachings and Theosophical texts, all human beings are vulnerable to karmic law, so your child may have modest abilities as well as exceptional talents from previous lives. In addition, however, an incarnating soul may have to reckon with moderate or extraordinary limitations during a particular lifetime. As an essential dynamic of reincarnation, karmic forces determine how the family members will potentially relate to each other, and will affect how your future child responds to your consciousness, behaviors, and parenting style.

Reincarnation and karmic law can account for differences among family members and explain why, despite shared genes, each family member may have such different attributes, capacities, faculties, innate wisdom, talents, life purposes, and interests. Genetic explanations that don't include the metaphysical dynamics of spiritual evolution are incomplete. What many call "gifts" or "genius" may be a result of powers and tendencies we mastered in earlier lives.

It is useful to develop a conscious sensitivity to the ways our past and present intentions are responsible for generating our life experiences. In his book *The Seat of the Soul* Gary Zukav writes: "Without knowledge of its soul, reincarnation and karma, it is not always possible for a personality to understand the significance or the meaning of the events of its life, or to understand the effects of its responses to them."[2] Taking responsibility for the fruits of our intentions is an empowering option. This principle can affect how parents prepare for and care for their children. As a parent, practice awareness of how your reactions to your child may affect future interactive patterns between you.

Rabbi Berg discusses the *tikune* process, which correlates with the fundamental principles of karma. *Tikune* is considered the "process of correction made by the soul" through which the "superior metaphysical intelligence of the soul structures the environmental as well as the biological process of evolvement and development." He continues: "From a Kabbalistic standpoint, all forms of pain, suffering, illness and injury have their origins in *tikune* and are there to promote spiritual growth, but *tikune* itself must not be fatalistically interpreted. We cannot escape the results of past actions, but we may change the results by what we do now. If the soul becomes aware of its defects and brings itself into alignment with the forces of the universe . . . the cosmic truths of unity, pain and suffering can be modified."[3]

Those who dislike the idea of karma often feel as if it is "fatefully imposed" by an external source. Rather than a reward or punishment, however, karma is an opportunity for personal and spiritual growth. Its purpose is to refine consciousness and develop positive character attributes. Those who perceive the law of karma as having a positive intent (to grow in self-awareness) realize that they have a chance to use their free will to determine their lives.

Karma goes hand in hand with the principle of free will, which lets us choose how we respond to our circumstances, but free will does not mean that all choices are equal. We are not without inner guidelines and universal laws that determine that certain courses of action are better than others. Whatever we accept or reject, create or destroy, we do not escape the consequences of our choices. In *Serving Humanity* Djwhal Kuhl reminds us: "As to *Karma*, what a man has made, he can unmake. This is oft forgotten. Karma is not a hard and fast rule. It is changeable, according to man's attitude and desire. It is the presenting of the opportunity to change; this grows out of past activities, and these rightly met and correctly handled, lay the foundation for future happiness and progress."[4] Karmic lessons have a very positive purpose. They offer us opportunities to use the feedback from our life experiences, to continue to grow in self-awareness. Sandra recognizes that she had karmic links with her husband:

> I intuitively knew my chronic mistrust of Jake was not based on present experiences of this lifetime. There was nothing in my conscious personal history that justified my fear of his hurting me. He is an exceptionally loving and gracious person who never harmed

me in any way. In a past-life regression session, I became aware of a series of lifetimes where my soul and that of my present husband shared as human lovers before. During each of these lives, we were in a highly reactive relationship where one of us abused and victimized the other. When I learned about the past-life pattern between us, I realized that we had come together this life to heal our karma with each other, using our present-time conflicts to consciously develop the qualities of compassion, empowerment, and selflessness with each other. When we intentionally committed to focusing on these qualities in our communication dynamics, the irrational fear I had of Jake completely disappeared. We transcended our karma by choosing more mature ways of relating.

Karmic Relationships

Souls incarnate in groups to achieve harmonious relations with their fellow humans. The first group we belong to is our family, and as we grow we are attracted to religious, social, political, educational, and professional groups to work out our life lessons and adjust our karmic commitments to other incarnated souls.

According to the ageless wisdom teachings, every physical, emotional, mental, and spiritual characteristic that comprises a personality is perfectly suited to its soul purpose. Within the law of karma, human beings that are brought together are often directed by the soul's need to heal through a new relationship that is either similar to or different from one in a previous life. The act of reincarnating through particular relationships and circumstances is each soul's attempt to make itself whole through the human experience.

You and your future child may be joining together to balance or fulfill karmic needs. To discover whether this is the case, you may begin by inquiring meditatively, "Is there karma with this soul who is choosing me as its parent this lifetime?" Listen for the answer intuitively. Even before conception parents can aspire to minimize conflict with their incoming child, thereby maximizing *positive cause and effects* for themselves and the child.

As I've discussed in earlier chapters, the consciousness of the soul's new personality is imprinted before birth, and its emotional and mental bodies are patterned by the mother's emotional life as well as the father's attitude toward the mother. You cannot fully comprehend the incarnating soul's agenda for this lifetime. A soul coming into incarnation brings with it causes that have been generated and often unresolved in former lives. Many of your child's life lessons have nothing to do with you. Yet you can teach him how to resolve conflicts and challenges, as well as how to develop a positive temperament. By practicing the expression of virtues that will minimize karmic reactions even in the womb, thereby exposing the child to qualities of being that will present a harmonious life experience from conception onward, you can support the spiritual evolution of your child.

Usually, but not always, incarnating souls are attracted to one or both parents through karmic ties from past lives. Karen Schultz points out in her book *A Theosophical Guide for Parents* that the choice of parents "involves the perpetuation of personal or [soul] links from former lives, for nearly always there are links of love between the [souls] of children and those of their parents . . . [yet] sometimes there is a bond of discord, and even dislike, and that also can draw people together and children into a family."[5] Understanding this allows prospective parents to remain aware of subtle, unexpectedly discordant, and, possibly, overtly repelling feelings toward the child. Equally, strong love ties, a familiarity with the child's nature, and a magnetic love attraction can evidence a karmic relationship between parent and child and deepen the bond among family members.

Unresolved psychological conflicts can also draw souls together from previous lives to resolve their issues in present time as family members. In Alice Bailey's *Esoteric Psychology II* Djwhal Kuhl explains that hereditary diseases are "characteristic of some particular family and inherited by the member of this family as part of his chosen karma. Souls come into certain families because of this opportunity."[6] In many varied ways karmic forces may lie behind a particular soul coming to you as your child.

In each incarnation a soul chooses not only its parents and health karma, but also the racial and national conditions to fulfill its destiny. Prior to incarnation, the best geographical conditions for fulfilling the soul's next evolutionary steps are considered. The country is carefully selected, as are the city and the neighborhood, due to the unique growth circumstances required. As you can see, the conception of a child is a highly sophisticated plan on the part of the soul who joins the parents, and not, as many parents think, a chance or "fateful" occurrence. According to the ageless wisdom teachings, nothing is left to chance.

As Schultz describes, karmic factors even "include within fairly wide and flexible limits, the possibility or likelihood of cruelty, as in corporal punishment at home and in school, and the experience of harshness or lack of understanding."[7] John found that embracing this perspective enlightening to his healing process:

> There is no doubt in my mind that my soul chose my parents because of a need for its consciousness to experience the absolute inappropriateness of abusing anyone. As a child, I was always beaten for misbehaving, and I know in my heart of hearts that it was the end of a long past-life pattern between my parents and me, and that in other lifetimes I had been their abuser. It is not that I feel I deserved this pain from my own parents, nor are my parents to be unaccountable for their horrible behavior. But I know that from a soul perspective, I needed to experience the flip side of the karmic patterns that I inflicted on others. So when my human emotions completed feeling their rage and grief, I was able to perceive that my soul had intentionally chosen this family to evolve and transform its own consciousness—to learn that love, not abuse, is true power. Understanding my soul's developmental needs has assisted me in feeling significantly less victimized by my childhood horrors, even though I still hold my parents responsible for their violent behavior toward me.

Remember that your karma, and that of your family members, can be neutralized. How you respond to your reactive patterns impacts the outcomes of your karmic lessons. Penetrating the cause of your behavioral imbalances can reveal a path to transformation. Every misfortune then becomes an opportunity for wisdom to be distilled. Clearly, physical karma that has manifested as a major disability will not be completely alterable in this lifetime, but the state of consciousness with which we live this tough physical condition may be freely chosen.

As a soul works through and liberates itself from its karma, it may choose to reincarnate to serve a plan beyond itself to the benefit of humanity. According to numerous sources, many of these advanced souls are presently incarnating in great numbers in response to the quickening of consciousness in humanity's New Age. An advanced soul may enter this lifetime knowing its life mission and the qualities and faculties it wants to develop. Parents of a spiritually awakened soul have a great responsibility, for they can support or harm its potential life expressions and purpose. Usually, the mature soul is often more advanced than its parents, suggesting that in such cases the parents may be challenged to adopt an attitude of humbleness toward their child. Yet all souls, whether they are advanced or not, must be empowered by their parents to unfold their attributes, talents, and unique self-expression.

Love: Transforming Karma

As I suggested earlier, the universal law that supports you in transcending any past, present, or future karma with the child, partner, or anyone else is the ability to create and maintain harmony and love as a prevailing presence in the bond. This idea can assist in solving many problems between parents and children, and in dispelling apprehension and fear. Parents can use karma's educational opportunities to harmonize and embody their virtuous nature. In *Rays and Initiations* Djwhal Kuhl says, "An incarnation is a definitely determined period (from the angle of the soul) wherein Experiment, Experience, and Expression are the keynotes in each incarnation. Each successive incarnation continues the experiment, deepens the experience, and relates the expression more closely to the latent unfolding divinity."[8]

A common question about the law of cause and effect is: how can you learn to benefit from a predicament that was created in a previous life, especially if there is no ability to remember that life? Most people are living out their karma unaware of why their life circumstances are appearing in a particular way. The soul, however, knows that it needs to evolve and will create the conditions to grow, although often the personality is unaware of who is determining the life conditions. As a parent, it is your lifelong responsibility to assist your child in learning how to recognize the need and will of her soul aspect, and the conditions for karmic fulfillment. How the personality develops for the benefit of the soul can be greatly affected by your openness in asking, "What is my obligation to the soul who has chosen me as its first caretaker as it rebuilds itself into human flesh, depending on me to care for it until it can care for itself?" Lydia and Jonathan used this perspective upon learning they were pregnant:

> When our twins were conceived and we found out we had *two* souls who had chosen us to be their parents this lifetime, we began to consider why they decided to incarnate at the same time. We knew their choice to have us as parents was not a haphazard occurrence

either. We knew that we had to remain acutely aware of their karmic bond with each other, and we knew it was essential that we offer them the best physical and psychological reality to unfold their mutual destiny as twins. As their early-life guardians, we dedicated ourselves to maintaining a conscious perception of their unique traits, as well as their similarities. We sensed that over time, they would show us why they were conceived and born together.

Certainly, all human babies share the same personality needs to be well fed, loved, protected, and provided for. Some karmic influences will cause certain newborns to arrive into a family or cultural conditions where some of these basic needs are not easily available. There are resilient souls who can flourish amid the most adverse circumstances. Parents are not expected to know their child's karma, but rather to be aware of the universal reality that their child is arriving in their life to develop his potentials as a soul-infused personality balancing out his karma.

Offering your future child a loving and safe home life is a dependable intent to start with. Asking yourself whether you and your child may have a karmic dance between you can be helpful in understanding how to serve each other. Simply embodying love is the best first step to a healthy rapport. In *Serving Humanity* Djwahl Kuhl says, "When the heart is full of love and the head is full of wisdom, nothing then is ever done that can cause distress to others in the long run. . . . The man who is fearless, wise and loving can do anything and the effects will be harmless and good producing."[9]

It is a universal principle that a genuine expression of love will draw forth what is best in a child and a parent. The best way to offer your child the wisdom of being loving and harmless is for you to do the best you can to embody and model compassionate presence yourself. As a parent, you can in this way help your child unwind any past, as well as prevent future, karma. You are also creating bonds that evoke the Divine in one another.

All parents will have moments and days when they are reactive with their children or other family members. Changing our patterns can be a lifetime process, especially because some of our reactions originate in the unconscious. But parents will benefit themselves and their child by working toward consciousness and accountability. On the days that emotional stress cannot be avoided, parents can take responsibility to create some peace and harmony after the upset. Love is the great redeemer with karma. You, as the prospective parent, are also alive to experience the progressive development of your own spiritual perfection and intelligent perception. Thus, any challenge relating to your child is an opportunity to cultivate more life-giving, love-enhancing qualities in your own being.

Although the process of perfecting ourselves as divine beings in human form can be slow and painful, we are what we have created ourselves to be, and our circumstances are a result of our actions from many lives on earth as well as our present choices.

As prospective parents, we can choose to eliminate our weaknesses or strengthen our virtues by exercising our free will. By taking responsibility for the conditions of our lives and assisting the incoming generation in understanding these laws of life, there will be no need for us to feel victimized by life's challenges. We can use the principles of reincarnation and karma to our advantage as we learn to be aware of the feedback from our daily interactions in all our relationships. We can progress spiritually as we focus our free will in positive ways, enriching our qualities of consciousness as we become more sensitive to understanding how to evolve our inner and outer worlds.

In essence, reincarnation is the means by which karma is worked out—not as reward and punishment, but as cause and effect—to unfold our divine potentials. This awareness of your future child's motivation for rebirth becomes a vital element in preparing to conceive an incarnating soul. To practically apply the principle of this spiritual law increases the likelihood that your child will be supported in a family atmosphere where patterns of limitation, from the past or the present, can be transformed into freedom, health, faith, and an ever-increasing expectancy that the inner life and the world are good and positive. Goodwill, selflessness, reason, and love prevail. Your responsibility will be to teach your child about healthy relations, intelligent speech, constructive thought, and benevolent action. In this way your child will be given greater opportunity to transform previous life patterns from the old quality to the new, without unnecessary suffering in this lifetime.

> *I hold that when a person dies,*
> *His soul returns again to earth;*
> *Arrayed in some new flesh-disguise*
> *Another mother gives him birth.*
> *With sturdier limbs and brighter brain*
> *The old soul takes the road again.*
>
> John Masefield

Preconception Bonding with Your Child's Soul

Every family is a communion of souls. What we have in common isn't
where we live, what schools we go to, or what we do for a living. We are
sailing the seas of immortality together—that is the real bond.

Deepak Chopra

When Does Bonding Begin?

The bonding process between a parent and child is complex and unique, filled with great mystery and opportunity to develop your loving attributes. In their book *Bonding* Marshall Klaus, M.D., Phyllis H. Klaus, Ph.D., and John H. Kennell, M.D., offer decades of research about the critical bonding experience that occurs during pregnancy, birth, and postnatal periods. This process is not an "isolated occurrence," they tell us, "but takes place on a continuum of experience."[10]

The importance of building secure attachments between parent and child as a foundation for the evolving child's self-esteem and well-being has been addressed for a long time. But when can the bonding between you and your future child *begin?* It is evident to anyone witnessing the extraordinary moments of new parents meeting their babies for the first time that the bonding process is innate for most but can be awkward for others. Those whose parents were detached and inexpressive with them as children sometimes feel helpless and inadequate in their ability to awaken their bonding instinct with their own baby.

Most of the research that has been done on bonding has focused on expressed affection between parent and child, such as feeding, hugging, kissing and cuddling, talking, gazing, or singing. But some begin developing their relationship with their baby during pregnancy, before they can even physically touch her. The concept of prenatal bonding suggests that a dynamic relationship can actually begin with the child in utero before she is born.

The moment a pregnancy is confirmed often initiates a great transformation for parents as they begin to make the internal and external changes needed to adapt to this extraordinary lifestyle change. Efforts to create the optimal health conditions for the prenate's well-being offer the new mother and father the chance to deepen their attachment to the newborn. With the widespread use of ultrasound these days, many couples can see the little fetus by the first trimester and begin to feel a conscious relationship forming between them and their child-to-be.

Others are inspired to connect with their baby when they feel the first fetal movement or "kicking," which occurs during the midsecond trimester. Research shows that even fathers can bond with the child in utero: the prenate begins to recognize his father's voice by the fourth month, when his auditory system is formed.

Yet there are those who feel they are able to form a relationship with the spirit of their child even before conception. Many of my clients report having prebirth contact with a "presence" before their child's physical existence. Even I began to have interactive dialogues during my meditations and journal writing with a presence that identified itself as my future daughter:

> Momma, please relax with your concerns about when to conceive me. Every day I can offer you specific things you can do to prepare and heal yourself so that when the time comes, we will both feel ready. I am a gentle spirit who only has goodness to offer you. Do not indulge in financial fears, for they are irrelevant to my arrival. You will be provided for and I will not burden you with problems you cannot easily solve. I am your daughter. Dad is feeling me and will know his own truth. Today, relax more, take in the essence of nature, and feel my love for you.

I had heard about prebirth communication before, but I was experiencing something very profound, something that I began to call preconception bonding. This was a far cry from what I had learned about the bonding relationship in the 1970s when I was a psychology major at Harvard. At that time there was tremendous excitement about the discovery that bonding *began at the bedside* of a mom and her newborn baby. These first few moments and hours after the baby's birth were considered essential for establishing a healthy long-term attachment between mother and child. Then in the 1980s, as I gathered information for my master's thesis, there were exciting new findings about the contact parents were making with their prenate using ultrasound; Mom and Dad could hear the heartbeat and actually view the fetus in the womb. Prenatal bonding became an accepted reality.

Preconception bonding, too, is literal, and some of my clients report having actual sensations of their baby's spirit hovering around them or communicating through intuitive impressions, or sometimes a voice, dictating ways to prepare for conception. For me this experience was more than prebirth contact; it was the beginning of bonding with my future child.

Upon reviewing the journal I had started the day that I intentionally began my preconception preparation, I found numerous letters I had written to myself, my partner, and to the spiritual presence I began to intuitively feel with consistent familiarity. Her presence appeared as a particular personality with a definite soul quality. Was this real communication, or was it a projection of my desires and imagination? Whichever, I feel both that I experienced direct guidance from my daughter's soul and that the emotional and spiritual desire for my child evolved into a loving attachment. Thus, preconception bonding is not dependent upon you having intimate interactions with the soul of your child-to-be, but upon you developing emotionally and spiritually to care for its well-being. As you mobilize your feelings and thoughts to get ready for the arrival of your baby, the bonding process begins.

Fathers, too, even if they do not perceive the presence of a spirit around them, can begin to bond with an image of the future child and the feelings of becoming a dad. Both parents can give themselves permission to feel love for their child even before they are sure she physically exists. Wondering whether I was pregnant or not, I passionately wrote in my journal to the spirit of my child-to-be:

> Am I pregnant? Am I not pregnant? The vessel of my body has been preparing for you. I see you flashing before my inner vision, sending waves of sensation through my emotional body. The bond between us explodes like lightning on a tropical evening, as you propel me with maternal instincts, reminding me that your conception is occurring, has occurred, will occur? Where are you residing now? Within the nest of my uterus? Or only in the comfort of my imaginary world of desires? It is time to surrender to the truth that whatever form you exist in—body, mind, Spirit—I am your mother, simply by the fact that I am loving you and my whole being wants to care for your magnificent unfolding potential.

Telepathy, Impressions, and Intuition

It is not uncommon for either women or men to dream about their unborn child, to contemplate images and feelings of the dream, to interpret their meaning. Some even feel the presence of a spirit when they are in a deep state of relaxation. Those who want to develop their ability to make conscious contact with the soul of the child must be open to using their imagination and intuition, since it is rare for a precise telepathic communication to occur.

Some describe their prebirth contact as a silent internal conversation that is a mixture of thoughts and feelings. Others hear words out loud or see images or symbols. Some parents describe an undeniable kinesthetic sensation that is felt only when intentionally involving the soul for communion. Some of these conversations with the unborn child, whether literal or abstract, are highly detailed, with both the mother and father asking questions and receiving answers.

Telepathy is a slowly developed sense that requires you as the receiver to be highly sensitive to perceiving what comes to your abstract intuitive mind. For true telepathy to occur, you must learn to be responsive to clear impressions coming from the intuitive world of soul. Because our five senses have not been trained for telepathy, most people only occasionally register accurate contacts from the soul plane, and these are usually mixed with personality reactions. As in all things, practice will bring improvement:

- First, in order to develop your intuitive relationship with your own soul and that of your future child, you must desire to experience this divine connection.
- Quiet the thoughts of your mind so that the spiritual contact can flow directly from the higher planes of consciousness without distortion.
- Focus your conscious intent on being receptive, inviting the soul to impress your consciousness with its message, perhaps telling you what it needs in order for you to prepare for its arrival.
- You may have a specific question that you wish to ask; if so, you can either hold your question in your conscious mind, or even say it quietly to yourself. You may ask the soul, "Do you have a message for me?" Or, "What do I need to do today to prepare for your arrival?" Or even such detailed questions as, "What do you need for me to do to optimize the health of your future physical body? Your emotional body? Your mental body? Your spiritual body?" Remain as detached and indifferent as possible to the question you are asking or the situation you are considering.

- Without censoring, register any impressions you receive. You may wish to write these down in your journal so that you can refer back to them.
- Interpret the impressions you have received intuitively. Try to be aware of your own needs and desires and, as much as possible, keep these separate from any messages you receive from the soul plane. If more than one interpretation seems likely, write both of them down. Developing an intuitive relationship with your child's soul will be a process of open experimentation. As you increase your sensitivity and deepen your communication, its true wishes will become increasingly clear to you.

In your journey of exploring the intuitive realm of spirit, realize that a vision, a message, or a presence may or may not be the authentic expression of the incarnating soul. Yet if the impression feels like it can only be beneficial and will create greater well-being for all concerned, it is useful to experiment with integrating the insight, over time witnessing the effect of your efforts. If acting on the impression can be harmful to yourself or anyone else, it is usually an illusion of your personality, because the soul aspect is universal love and is harmless by nature.

Kara talks about her intuitive link with her future daughter:

All my life I wondered whether to trust my intuition. My rational mind had served me well, and I liked to feel in control of my reality. One night I was lying in bed waiting for my husband to come home. I felt a presence at the foot of the bed, while simultaneously a warm light flooded my whole body. My heart expanded with a feeling of compassion for an image of a small baby who smiled at me. We had a silent understanding that we would be parent and child, and then a series of insights was unleashed about who this being was, when she wanted to be conceived, and what she wanted to be named. But most alarming was that she imparted to me an undeniable sense that my husband, Jerry, was not the father, and that it would be two and a half years before the conditions would be aligned for her arrival into my life. I asked why Jerry was not her dad, and she impressed upon me a vision of my future with another man. Through inner dialogue, the soul reassured me. I felt the loving intent of her message as a way to prepare me for the many changes that would occur in my life. Sure enough, almost two and a half years to the day later, Sasha was born into the arms of her father, my new husband of three months. This initial meeting with my daughter initiated our loving connection before she was conceived, so bonding with her at her birth was as natural as the sun rising.

Prayer and Mediation for Conceiving a Soul

Preparing for parenthood is greatly enhanced when you include the practice of prayer. As you commune with a divine source, you are building faith in divine guidance and protection and strengthening the bond between yourself and your source of spiritual inspiration. Meditation can increase self-awareness so that you may bathe your concerns with positive intent. Both prayer and meditation practices will support you in relaxing and in caring for your innermost feelings and thoughts.

Through prayer you can create an intimate relationship with the Source of Life; you can offer your parenting journey to the will of God, placing your life and that of your family into God's hands. Your prayers may be offered to the Divine Mother, the Divine Father, archangels, saints, masters, or any other divine being whom you feel a devoted connection with and receive assistance from. Regular spiritual practice will deepen your direct experience that there is divine presence in all the phases of parenting you will undergo. You can use prayer and meditation to strengthen yourself when you feel vulnerable to the numerous transformations that the incarnating soul will initiate as it becomes your child.

Prayer and meditation are also opportunities for the bond with your future child to grow. You can use meditation to receive impressions, visions, and messages from the soul. Perceive its nature. Try to understand its purpose for incarnation. Ask what name it wants for this coming incarnation. Use visualization to contemplate images that transmit loving energy and light to the soul. If you find that your attention wanders so that you cannot focus to pray or meditate, find spiritually inspiring books and read them aloud or to yourself, or listen to spiritually uplifting music.

Creating an Altar for Your Unborn Child

In your efforts to develop an intuitive relationship with the incarnating soul who has chosen you as its parents, you may find it difficult to relate to a presence that has no physical form, that you can't see or touch. Giving yourself a visual focal point to acknowledge his presence in your daily life may help make your child more real to you. When I was preparing to conceive my daughter, I built an altar in my room that I thought of as "her place."

My altar was made with a simple wooden table covered with a special cloth. Everything I placed on it was symbolic of my love for her soul and a reflection of my devotion to her divine nature. I chose objects that affirmed our relationship as mother and child and offered gifts of gratitude, symbols of my hopes for our reunion. The altar was a living testimony of my personality, saying, "Yes, soul of my unborn child, you do exist, and I am preparing the way to celebrate your arrival. Bear witness to my desire for you." My husband also added art that he painted for our little one, using his creative expression to acknowledge his emerging fatherhood. Our altar was a specific place where we could objectify our deep subjective feelings of longing for our child, and a way that we could nurture a sacred relationship with the soul.

To create your own altar you can use any special object—something from nature, works of art that you buy or make, pictures of your childhood or of spiritual beings, images from magazines that reflect your dreams, words of affirmation or prayers of gratitude, baby clothes, or anything else that gives you the opportunity to affirm the soul's existence to you.

Art and Music: Food for the Incarnating Soul

Since we know the soul is nourished by the thoughts and feelings of the mother and father who are intentionally preparing for a conscious conception, you can surround yourself with illuminating art and music as a way to develop your prebirth bond with your future child. Find music that is heart opening, life giving, and filled with reverence. Musical selections such as the *Messiah*, "Ave Maria," New Age ambient music, easy-listening jazz, or Bach, Mozart, Beethoven, or other classical musicians are all good choices. Explore classical art, such as the beautiful and sacred images of the Italian Renaissance masters. Surround yourself with art and music that reflect noble qualities, pure colors, beneficent expressions, natural beauty, uplifting sounds, and feelings of rapture.

Your Own Immaculate Conception:
A Useful Ideal

As your mother's egg and father's sperm fused to create the original cell that created your physical existence, a genetic blueprint was born in that first cell, in the image of which all subsequent cells replicated. When egg and sperm fertilize to create the original cell that will replicate trillions of times to become your child, you will want conditions to be ideal. The immaculate conception is an inspirational metaphor you can use to prepare your spiritual awareness for conceiving the body of your child. Choosing to consciously prepare and purify yourself for conception is a natural activity if you are living a holistic lifestyle. Embracing a holistic approach to preconception preparation, a couple is invited to do the best they can—not to be "perfect" and chaste but to create healthy conditions for a child.

The illumined culture of the Essenes lived in private communities in Egypt and Israel from about 150 b.c. to a.d. 68. They cultivated an acceptance of the spiritual significance of the immaculate conception. Their teachings were a part of their temple work, but they also strove to integrate their spiritual lessons into their daily lives. To the Essenes, the immaculate conception signified the highest attainment for a woman preparing for her future child. It is written in the mythologies that Mary was an earthly woman who so purified her whole nature that she was able to hold this state of perfection and purity throughout the conception, pregnancy, and birth of Jesus. She was devoted to these principles of purity and perfection, which are the essence of any condition of optimal health, peace, and immortality.

Many of the teachings of the Essenes can be practically applied to those parents who want to create a conscious conception, but let me clarify: I am not suggesting that parents aspire to an actual immaculate conception like that of Christian and Essene mythology, the conception of Jesus. Jesus was a high spiritual initiate; his parents had to master exquisite conditions of chastity and purity, in conscious cooperation with the angelic ministry and the instruction of illumined beings. It is said that both parents took a vow of perpetual virginity.

I am, rather, offering the immaculate conception as a metaphor for an ideal. Its universal applications do not require a belief in Christianity or any particular religion. Use this metaphor for inspiration as you hold a concentrated image and feeling of your child's divine self. You can contemplate the incarnating soul's perfect form in your heart and mind. Slowly, this thought-form will become energized through your consistent release of love to it, and you will feel the spiritual qualities of your child more authentically. This practice of intentionally nourishing the divine image of your child's soul will deepen your ability to unconditionally love and positively perceive your child-to-be. "When prospective parents prepare themselves through prayer and holy aspiration without thought of self-gratification, the resulting Sacrament of Conception will be immaculate."[11]

By holding this idea in mind, parents-to-be can undergo a spiritualization of consciousness. The immaculate conception becomes a mental focus for positive thoughts about your future child to permeate the physical act of conceiving her. Inspired thoughts of mature love as well as a deep desire for unfolding your child's highest potential are aspects you can cultivate.

It is suggested in the Essene teachings that the redemption of the human race can be found in the essence of the immaculate conception archetype. It involves the sacrifice of something old in order to create perfection. Embracing the idea of immaculate conception means that you let go of any old patterns in your life that may be harmful to a child. Consider the ways in which the archetype of the immaculate conception can be useful in your efforts to be the best possible parents to your future child:

- If you have polluted your body with impure substances (drugs, chemicals, toxins), make the effort to cleanse your body of these substances before they interfere with your child's health.
- Rather than emulate Mary's and Joseph's vow of "perpetual virginity," you might try taking a vow of purity in your emotions and thoughts.
- Paracelsus pointed out that "the imagination of a pregnant woman is so active, that in conceiving seed into her body, she can transmute the foetus in different ways."[12] The conscious conception of the child, held in the heart and mind of the mother, is a significant factor in molding the incarnating soul's form within her body. I suggest that both parents use the image-building faculty of their imaginations to mentally hold a divine image of their child-to-be. Perhaps thinking of the soul as a "child of God" or "in God's image" will help you to achieve this.
- To the very best of your ability, diminish or end discord that can disturb the very sensitive vibratory action of the incarnating soul's consciousness.
- Together, you and your partner can discuss any limiting beliefs about yourselves as parents and release any images that are disempowering either to you as parents or to the soul as

your child, and that keep you from holding an immaculate concept of the soul.

- Learn to magnify your own good nature and that of the soul, and integrate this reality into all your daily activities as you prepare to conceive your child.

These practices are a pretty tall order for even an advanced spiritual aspirant, but that is the nature of an ideal. I suggest that you be content with the process of doing the best you can, and that you use the image of the immaculate conception as a reminder of your child's divinity.

If you find the idea of immaculate conception too idealistic, you may give it a more practical bent. Think instead of a healthy, conscious conception and what that means to you. Your consciousness is always looking for creative ways in which to express itself. But remember one of the great secrets of creation: When you plant corn, you get corn. In other words, the variety and quality of the seeds of consciousness that you plant will determine the kind and quality of fruits that are yielded. The same principle influences the creation and growth of your human child and you, as parents, hold the key. As Edgar Cayce said, "Within the nucleus at conception IS the pattern of all that is possible. And, remember, the soul of man, the body of man, the mind of man is nearer to limitless than anything in creation. Hence, those who consider the manner of being channels [parents] through which souls may enter are taking hold upon the God-force itself."

Embodying Spiritual Virtues

Virtue is the beauty of a person. It is what makes them lovely and unusual.
It is the color, form, shape of the personality. It is the way they do things; the
way they move, speak and dress. They may have no money, but if a person
has virtue, they will always seem rich, for everything that is close to them
will be filled with quality. Virtue shines outwards into everything; into the
body, into the environment and ultimately into the fiber of the planet itself.
It fills what is empty, heals what is sick, settles what is troubled.

Anthea Church

Soul consciousness is developed through the mindfulness and expression of virtuous qualities. If you aspire to actualize your soul presence, as well as encourage the soul expression of your partner and child, you can enhance this endeavor by exploring specific virtues. Virtues are beneficial qualities that exemplify the positive attributes of a person's character. Your soul and your child's soul are made up of these virtuous qualities, often referred to in the ageless wisdom texts as "soul qualities." There are specific virtues that can enhance your ability to spiritually parent your child. The more you intentionally practice personalizing these essences, the greater the likelihood that your child will develop his soul qualities from the beginning of his life.

Perry was inspired by his childhood pain to develop himself before becoming a father:

> My parents were so conditionally loving and impatient. My childhood memories are filled with incidents of my parents reprimanding me for not submitting to their beliefs, never giving me time to express myself, or listening to me attentively. I was determined to be different from them, yet when I honestly evaluate the irritation I feel toward my young nephew, I realize my own child will also be vulnerable to my impatience because I internalized my parents' selfish ways. Now when I notice myself quickly reacting to my partner when she is feeling stressed, I intentionally invoke a feeling of patience and compassion, and I find it is becoming easier to respond to her kindly. During my meditations each morning, as I contemplate myself parenting our unborn child, I imagine relating lovingly to her as a newborn and toddler. I am trying to integrate a new image and identity within myself, so that once she is born, it's a natural tendency to be open to her needs and feelings. Even though my parents did not have these virtues, I can develop them within myself.

Only by your deliberate efforts can you and your partner provide an atmosphere wherein specific qualities can emerge and flourish. It is never too early to prepare for the challenges of parenthood as you learn to handle difficulties in an enlightened way. Perceive your family as a union of souls who have come together to support each other's spiritual evolution. Consider the virtues that are innately a part of your character and those that are lacking in your self-identity. When you practice the conscious expression of your divine attributes, your virtues will, in time, become a part of your personality. Let me discuss some of the foundational virtues to cultivate for parenthood.

Harmlessness: A Spiritual Practice for Parents

Practicing harmlessness embraces the idea that you will never intentionally hurt or wound your child or any family member . . . or any person. Practice this virtue constantly before as well as throughout the pregnancy and thereafter, so that the prenate does not suffer unnecessary pain. A child in utero is a thinking and feeling being and therefore vulnerable to your states of consciousness.

The cultivation of harmlessness means the elimination of criticism of yourself, your partner, and your child, and a conviction to seek loving understanding in all circumstances. It means using your spiritual awareness to shield your family members from harmful words, thoughts, and deeds. Remain mindful of doing the best that you can to arrest each unloving action and devote yourself to being loving and kind to all beings.

Patience: Peace with Time

To practice patience is to remain receptive to the unknown, and to allow a moment-to-moment state of awareness to guide you to consciously respond to the reality that is presenting itself in the now. Patience is an effort to calmly understand something or someone over time. Thus, in preparing for parenthood, you can learn to allow the time necessary to care for your child's long-term well-being. Once you have conceived, patience means remaining aware of the normal and natural pace a child needs to develop and learn. Begin your pregnancy trusting the innate timing of your child's biological and spiritual impulses to unfold and express their true nature in accordance with the needs of her personality and soul. Once your child is born, a patient response to her many needs and inquiries means allowing time to be present for each of them, while other present distractions are ignored.

Purity: Your Child's Essence

Innocence is the state of consciousness in which you can perceive your child as an immortal soul with infinite wisdom and an innately positive nature. It is the beauty of a child whose body has not yet stored the challenges and tensions of life. The incarnating soul depends on you to remember that it is returning to human existence to perfect its divine nature. During the conception and pregnancy, and thereafter, dedicate yourself to protecting your child's purity.

Honor: The Soul

When a soul begins its life with you, a space within its consciousness is already filled with lifetimes of wisdom and spiritual treasures. This precious state must be respected and praised. You are invited to sustain a sense of lightness and optimism. When honoring yourself and your child as heavenly beings, you are honoring the divine presence within each of you. To value your child's beauty and purity means you are honoring his supreme being.

Truth: Be True to Your Self

Your future child is a divine being already. This universal truth can be intuitively perceived. When the soul incarnates, it is up to you as the child's spiritual guardian to nurture the true self expression within her personality. You will have many opportunities throughout life to tell your child that she is really a spiritual being expressing her divine qualities through her body and mind. It is your challenge to express your spiritual awareness in effective ways that awaken the child to herself.

Cultivate an atmosphere of truth so your child can develop the consciousness that she is living light. Your child will innately have the ability to embody her soul. She will depend on you to teach her the spiritual foundation of truth that she is an immortal spirit.

Love: The Building Block

Love is not what you do but who you are. As a soul, your existence is love. Love is the coherent healing force that makes all things whole. Love comes from an original source of compassion and communion that exists deep within your true self. It offers your body and mind suppleness to express kindness amid all inner and outer adversity. Love gives you the energy to build your child's benevolent nature. Love is far-seeing wisdom that supports your child in feeling confidence in you and respect for you. When your heart is full of love and your head is full of wisdom, you cannot do anything that distresses your child's world. True love is noncritical, steadfast, and all-encompassing.

Commit to giving the utmost you have to give, and intentionally release selfish and harmful behavior. Love for your child's whole health will allow you to put your personal needs aside when he needs you to care for him.

Love perceives the eternally perfect qualities in your child even when he is unable to embody his perfection. Cultivate your loving nature and that of your family members, and apply it to all of life's conditions.

Soul Shaping: Virtuous Qualities

The following list of virtuous soul qualities can be used to inspire you to embody more of your spiritual consciousness in preparation for parenthood. Make your own list of all the qualities that you feel are well integrated into your personality. Then make a list of those that you are partially able to express but need more effort to master. Finally, create a list of those qualities that you need to focus on—those that you understand will enhance your parenting abilities, although you have not developed them. Use the creative exercises at the end of this chapter to further explore this list of virtues to become a more soul-infused parent.

Virtuous qualities can be divided into four major categories:

1. Love-wisdom
2. Active intelligence
3. Will
4. Cosmic

These four categories list those virtues that are highly complementary when expressed together. Naturally, many of these virtues could be classified under other categories, but where they appear here may be considered their primary influence.

If you have any question about the virtuousness of some of the following qualities, remember that it's the *positive meaning* or *positive use* of the quality that is to be contemplated or experienced. (For example, think of the virtue "detachment" in terms of letting go of that which is not healthy, rather than as refraining from bonding with your child.) You can also consult a dictionary for clarification.

Have fun with this list, and enjoy expressing more of your soul nature with your whole family.

Love-Wisdom Qualities

acceptance
appreciation
aspiration
association
attachment
attraction
beauty
bliss
brilliance
calmness
caring
cohesiveness
compassion
contentment
cooperation
courtesy
decentralization
devotion
ecstasy
empathy
enthusiasm
faith
faithfulness
flow
forgiveness
friendship

fusion
gentleness
glory
gracefulness
gratitude
harmlessness
health
hope
humbleness
humility
identification
inclusiveness
interdependence
intuition
joy
lightness
love
loyalty
magnetism
mercy
omniscience
openness
patience
peace
purity
receptivity

relationship
respect
reverence
self-acceptance
selflessness
self-love
self-realization
self-respect
sensitivity
serenity
service
sincerity
softness
stillness
surrender
sympathy
tenderness
tolerance
tranquillity
transformation
understanding
unity
universality
vitality
warmth
wisdom

Active Intelligence Qualities

accuracy
action
active intelligence
adaptability
artistic ability
caution
ceremony
change
clarity
comprehension
concentration
concreteness
continuity
creativity
curiosity
decisiveness
detail
discernment
discrimination
dispassion
economy

generosity
groundedness
harmony
honesty
humor
idealism
identity
individuality
insight
intelligence
keenness
knowledge
memory
mindfulness
movement
observation
omnipresence
order
organization
perception
planning

precision
realization
regularity
repetition
resourcefulness
revelation
scientific
   mindedness
self-realization
single-
   mindedness
specificity
spontaneity
synchronicity
thoughtfulness
timing
transmutation
trust
truth
watchfulness

Will Qualities

abstraction
action
alignment
assertiveness
balance
beingness
centeredness
centralization
commitment
confidence
confrontation
control
courage
daring
dedication
detachment
determination
direction
divine indifference
drive
dynamism
endurance
expandedness
fearlessness
focus

fortitude
freedom
goodness
goodwill
illumination
impersonality
independence
initiative
inspiration
integration
integrity
intensity
intent
liberation
mastery
nobility
obedience
omnipotence
oneness
power
promptness
pure being
purity
purpose
radiance

renunciation
resoluteness
responsibility
restraint
rhythm
righteousness
sacrifice
self-control
self-forgetfulness
self-forgiveness
self-reliance
self-sacrifice
seriousness
simplicity
speed
stability
stamina
steadfastness
steadiness
strength
synthesis
transfiguration
wholeness
wide mindedness
will

Cosmic Qualities

abstractness	grace	reality
abundance	infinity	spirit
awareness	omnipotence	timelessness
consciousness	omnipresence	unity
cosmic bliss	omniscience	universality
cosmic mindedness	oneness	vastness
eternity	play	

Creative Exercise:
Preparing Your Spirit for Conception

1. How can the ideas of karmic law described in this chapter assist you in preparing to parent a soul who will chose you as its future mother or father?
2. List three relationships you sense are karmic for you in this lifetime. What is the dynamic between you and the other person that feels karmic? What are the lessons for you to learn through each relationship?
3. How can you prevent creating unhealthy karma with your future child?
4. When do you feel bonding with your future child can begin for you, and for your partner?
5. What are specific ways you want to experience bonding with your child before and after conception?
6. How can you use the metaphor of immaculate conception to inspire you as you prepare for your child?
7. Use your imagination to create ways to use the soul-quality list to prepare for parenthood or to enhance your parenting abilities. Some examples are provided below:
   - List specific qualities that can enhance the conception of your child.
   - List specific qualities that can enhance your pregnancy.
   - List specific qualities that can enhance your relationship with yourself.

- List specific qualities that can enhance your relationship with your partner.
- Each day, choose a specific quality to embody that will enhance your ability to parent.
- Choose a quality each day to embody with your partner in order to enhance your relationship.
- Choose a quality to intuitively send to the child in utero. Surround yourself and the fetus with the feeling of this quality.
- List the virtues you want to embody once the child is born. What efforts will it take to make this a reality?
- List the qualities you imagine your future child will need from you. How able and willing are you to embody these qualities?
- List the qualities you imagine your child will embody as a new human life. How can you support its ability to integrate and develop these characteristics?
- Affirm your existing strengths by putting a check mark next to all the qualities you have already developed.
- Contemplate: "Love is the cause, and love is its own effect." What other qualities can be both cause and the same effect?

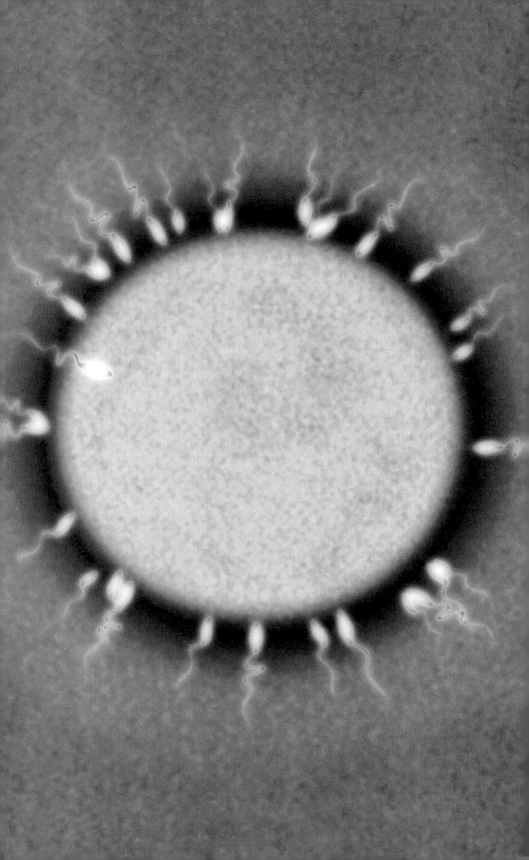

6

The Time of Physical Conception

Mutual aspiration and harmony between the parents lays the ground-work for an auspicious conception—along with love for a being as yet unknown to ordinary waking consciousness.

Karen Schultz

Cellular Consciousness

The idea that during gestation the fetus can experience emotional states and remember them is coming to be widely accepted. But a more recent addition to developmental models of human growth is the idea that emotions also can be experienced during conception and implantation. These primary emotional encounters, which can have an effect on core aspects of personality development, are often referred to in prenatal literature as cellular consciousness.

Graham Farrant, M.D., an internationally prominent psychiatrist, describes cellular memory as a "preverbal memory . . . a body memory, a memory within our cells, of our experiences as a sperm and of our experiences as an egg." Researchers of cellular consciousness use primal therapy, hypnosis, visualization techniques, rebirthing, and bodywork to access these deep early memories. "If you really spend enough time exploring your own psyche," states Farrant, "the experiences seem to naturally progress to dealing with cellular memories of your own conception."[1] In his therapeutical work with thousands of people, Farrant recognized that clinical change occurred after the deep "psycho-physiologic re-experience of conception." Over a fifteen-year period he witnessed a series of "symptoms and conditions that are referable to specific points of trauma in the ten days from pre-conception to implantation," and he has "come to trust the biological reality of conception memories in therapy."[2] Farrant's patients' experiences are memories, not metaphors, he avers.

Over the last decade, as books on prenatal psychology have become more widely available, it is becoming more commonly accepted that individual consciousness exists within the embryo. In addition, significant research is revealing the probability that consciousness is even present in the unfertilized and fertilized ovum, as well as in the spermatozoon. If this is true, then it is likely that primal feelings held within the eggs, and the attraction between the egg and sperm at conception, can influence the blueprint of your child's personality characteristics. In addition to the significance of the biochemical health of the two sex cells, egg and sperm, their life qualities and power of consciousness appear to be very meaningful. David Chamberlain, Ph.D., past president of the Association for Prenatal and Perinatal Psychology and Health, has said, "I do not think consciousness ever ends. Being born is just one phase of life." In the past, Chamberlain explained, memory before birth was rejected by medicine and science because consciousness was associated with the brain. Since brain matter is not developed at conception, it was believed impossible for any conscious activity to be taking place. "It is all there," says Chamberlain. "Consciousness doesn't grow in cells in the body and get bigger and bigger. It's on, period. Medicine and psychology did not teach us this. They are in a different frame of reference."[3]

Thomas Verny, M.D., author of *The Secret Life of the Unborn Child*, also believes that cellular memory exists at conception. He writes: "Since sympathetic messages, like messages along the central and autonomic nervous systems, must also lead somewhere and be encoded somewhere, I hypothesize that they are laid down in individual cells; I call memory so derived 'organismic memory.' This would allow even a single cell such as an ovum or a sperm to carry 'memories.'" Echoing Chamberlain, he continues: "The only thing that I can say is that consciousness is there from the beginning. . . . It is not like a computer with an on and off switch. . . we have moved away from the idea of consciousness being dependent on neurological development, to the idea that the moment you have a living cell, you have consciousness."[4]

In her book *Primal Connections* Elizabeth Noble offers extensive personal and professional research about the experience of conception. She writes: "Rarely is there a perfectly balanced and harmonious union of sperm and egg components. Therefore, it is not uncommon that one gamete feels victimized by the other, was engulfed or invaded by the sperm, or recalls a struggle of reluctance or outright resistance from the egg. There may be an experience of parental ambivalence concerning conception, the man having perhaps second thoughts as he ejaculates and so the sperm shoot forth to their goal but carry seeds of doubt."[5] She continues to cite numerous case histories of adults remembering, while in a deeply relaxed state, the interaction of the sperm and egg during their conception. The original cell is deeply influenced by the pattern of egg and sperm uniting, since this is its first experience of life as a physical entity. If it is true that consciousness exists in this original cell, then the experience of fertilization will become a foundation of the incarnating soul's psyche and body memory.

This notion is supported by some of Noble's case histories. She refers to these initial imprints as "primal life scripts . . . memory matrices that are impressed onto the unconscious mind."[6] Noble has discovered that unplanned conceptions can create a feeling that the person has no right to exist, or they are unwanted.

She writes about her own innate patterns: "I see that throughout my life I have fluctuated between the terrified egg and the ambivalent sperm."[7] Noble then details how her "conception script" actually impacted her ability to conceive her own child. Noble and others have researched correlations between women with apparent infertility and their own unresolved conception traumas. In contrast, I and others have reported our conceptions as being a burst of ecstatic light and blissful feelings. Paula had a very powerful realization when she was regressed into a state of recalling her conception:

> There I was, my soul presence hovering over my parents while they joined in a holy connection to conceive me. Like a tornado of white light I poured into their fused bodies, activating the sperm and egg with my divinity. Like two magnetic radars, the sperm and egg seemed to lust for each other, and I could feel my parents' desire for me become the very fabric of my body and mind. I would forever feel wanted by them.

As prospective parents you can consciously prepare for the conception of your child so that you are flooding the sperm and egg with feelings of love, peace, joy, your desire, and the pure love of your union. Perhaps such positive imprinting can create an important impact on your future child's primary life script. Rather than conception being a haphazard array of semiconscious feelings, you can be aware of conceiving on a day when you feel loving with each other, and avoid days where there is emotional stress or ambivalence about consciously conceiving your child in love. You can also spend some time connecting to the feelings that you have about the sperm and egg—infusing them with positive feelings before you conceive. You and your partner can imagine your egg and sperm uniting in ecstasy as you co-create your future child's "primal script" with all of the other natural and celestial forces present at conception.

The perspective that the consciousness of egg and sperm create an initial imprint, a first cellular memory, has profound implications for those becoming pregnant using reproductive technologies. The potential complexities of these methods are considerable when you take the psychic dimensions of conception into account.

Recently, I attended an in vitro procedure of a client of mine who could not conceive without medical assistance. She prepared herself so that while she was receiving the implantation of the zygote, she was bathing her womb with passionate loving desire for the embryo. Then for many days she focused on flooding the growing fetus with positive feelings. Although the conception itself occurred in a sterile high-tech environment, she had plenty of opportunities to positively imprint the zygote because its primitive consciousness was very mutable and responsive to her loving feelings.

Assisted reproductive technologies (ART) have not been around long enough for psychologists to study the long-term psychological patterns of beginning human life this way. I know many beautiful children who were conceived with medical assistance. Because of the tremendous effort and great expense of conceiving a child in this way, I know these children are very wanted by their parents. My belief is that a zygote conceived in artificial conditions, yet deeply desired by the parents and growing in the mother's womb with constant love, would be healthier than a naturally conceived zygote of ambivalent parents.

What Is Conscious Conception?

*Not having a conscious conception is like
missing the beginning of a movie.*

Sundar

If you accept the idea of cellular consciousness, it follows that you can actually choose to create either a conscious or an unconscious conception. A conscious conception implies that you and your partner are embarking upon your sexual union with full awareness of entering a sacred dance with the incoming soul. As the parents you can actually play with the psycho-spiritual quality of the sperm and egg coming together. A harmonious aspiration on the part of both parents to support cellular consciousness will offer the best conditions for building the personality bodies of the soul. Since conception usually occurs five or six hours after intercourse—if intercourse coincides with ovulation—you and your partner can, through attentiveness, maximize positive feelings for the sperm, egg, soul of the child, and each other in the hours following ejaculation. Give yourself permission to unleash the magnetic feelings of deep desire for your child—flooding your body, heart, and mind with your love. Some people are aware of that miraculous moment when conception does occur, although most women do not sense they are pregnant until they feel physical symptoms. Either way, you can remain mindful of the hours and days following your conception dance as a special time for you and your future child.

Cassandra remembers her excitement at realizing that she was feeling the fertilization of her egg:

> It was a Sunday morning when we made love to conceive our little one. I had been lying in bed all day, basking in the warm glow Mac and I had generated between us. All of a sudden I felt a shock of energy pulsate through my womb. I felt the soul I had been communing with for so many months descend into my body like a lightning rod of moist essence. I knew I was pregnant.

The renowned Theosophist Geoffrey Hodson sums up the opportunities for parents who cultivate a conscious conception. Describing the moment of conception, he says, "When organs of opposite polarity are united, a descent of power occurs. The measure and quality of that power depends upon the level of consciousness at which unity has been achieved. In man the descent of power produces the same measure as that in which the union has been spiritual rather than physical in its nature and motive. In order that the greatest possible advantage may be taken of this fact, the consciousness must be directed away from the physical plane toward the spiritual. The highest level of power will then be released, the greatest possible expansion of consciousness will be attained, and the best conditions provided for the building of the bodies for the [soul] coming into incarnation. At the moment of fertilization, a flash of light descends from the highest spiritual level of the [soul] into the spermatozoon [giving] it its creative power and energy."[8]

As we enter the new millennium, there is a steady stream of souls incarnating with accelerated spiritual needs. It is time to expand our understanding of how these souls are conceived. There is no formula for preparing for a child or raising an evolved soul. What is essential is that the parent be committed to the consistent care for the soul's true self needs. Prospective parents can prepare the soil (their bodies and minds) and offer the healthiest seed (the sperm and egg) so that the innate divine and human qualities, faculties, and powers may develop and grow to healthy fruition. The seed that will unfold into human form can be intentionally nurtured to express its authentic human and soul nature. The attitude of the parents toward their seed can affect the quality of the flower that blossoms.

Creating Sacred Ritual

Conscious conception offers you the opportunity to create a sacred union between you and your partner, filled with love for yourself, each other, and the incarnating soul. At the moment of conception karmic patterns are being established that have long-term implications for the returning soul. Although the soul has come with its own specific lessons that the parents cannot fully understand, "a man and woman [who have mated] together in purest love and altruism . . . will have set up for him an influence at the very beginning of his new life which will aid him enormously in his development, no matter what karmic conditions, good or bad, will be met with in this life."[9]

You may want to imagine yourself coming into incarnation. If you could have told your parents how to create a conscious conception for you, what would you have requested? Feel your mother's waiting egg and your father's dynamic sperm. When the egg and sperm unite, how would you like the energy and the light to feel? What colors and sounds are resonant with your essence? Is your conception a potent and dynamic force or a peaceful or passive feeling? Now imagine the conception of your future child and visualize the sperm and egg that will become your baby. Feel the infinite potential in your genetic offering. Envision the environment you and your partner want to offer to this being. What physical, emotional, and spiritual atmosphere would you like the soul to experience as it creates the original cell that will become the blueprint for all the other cells of its physical form?

As you anticipate the conception of your child, imagine embodying your highest spiritual nature. With your partner design a ritual that invokes divine consciousness between you. Create an ambience of light and music that evokes the divine love between you. Use your environment to lift up your spirit so that you can feel your union as a meeting of soul to soul, as your divine love patterns the physical vehicle of the incarnating soul that will choose you to be its earthly parents. The egg and sperm, each half of the new being, will become united to grow into your child. Feel the loving emotions floating between you and your partner as you join together to consciously conceive.

The First Cell Contains the Master Plan

The body of a woman who is to conceive is being chosen as a channel for the expression of divinity into materiality. Although ovulation is a law of nature, conception is a law of God.

Edgar Cayce

In the world today there are more than six billion living human beings, with ninety million babies born worldwide each year.[10] Yet few of the parents who conceive these human beings realize that there is a lot more occurring at the moment of conception than the union of two "gene pools." There is a growing body of scientific and metaphysical information that suggests that the way parents conceive their children, along with their attitudes, emotions, and health prior to conception, can have a significant influence on the whole health of the child and ultimately society. In a dramatic moment of manifestation, the egg of a woman and the sperm of a man fuse into the first cell that unfolds a human life. The moment you conceive your child you and your partner will be among many intrinsic forces that are contributing to the whole health of his soul.

There is a definite alchemy that occurs at the moment of conception between the biochemical, psychological, and spiritual dimensions of life. Hilda contrasts the conceptions of her two children with her partner, Joseph:

> Our first child was intentionally conceived in a moment of passion on Valentine's Day. As soon as we found out we were pregnant, we looked at Joseph's medical texts to track the development of our child each week. Our perception of our baby was purely biological, and I never even thought of his emotional or spiritual development during pregnancy. I was bonding with an anatomical image. Our second child was intentionally conceived four years later, after we had awakened to the reality of reincarnation and the soul. During this conception, we were consciously honoring the many invisible forces that were co-creating life with us, and we nurtured our relationship with the body, mind, and soul of our child throughout pregnancy. This greatly enriched our experience of our child once she was born, for we had been caring for her whole being from the moment she was conceived.

In addition to the known biochemical activity of conception, psychological patterns may be forming as well. Just consider psychologist R. D. Laing's delineation of his own life into three primary phases: conception to implantation; implantation to birth; and, finally, all of his postnatal life. This suggests that Laing sensed that two-thirds of the major influences of his life occurred in the womb, a full third of these at conception. His perspective certainly places great importance on this fertile moment of life.

We know that when the ovum is fertilized by the sperm, it divides as it travels down the fallopian tubes into the uterus. By the second day the original cell has become 4 to 8 cells; by the fifth day it has become a blastocyst of about 150 cells. Remarkably, when the egg and sperm unify to create the original cell, a complete miniature blueprint of the future human being has already been drawn.

All of the biological complexities of a human life are within this one original cell that combines elements of both parents. The genetic codes that reside in the nucleus of the first cell spawn every other cell that comprises a human body. This faithful code continues to construct every cell out of the prior cell through a process called mitosis. The nucleus of the first single cell provides one continuum of cells differentiating from one to the next. One microscopic fertilized cell grows into a six-trillion-celled human being by the time it is born. When you and your partner optimize the whole health of the original cell, all the cells that subsequently will be duplicated—uncountable trillions of times—stand a better chance of being healthy, too.

An Extraordinary Moment of Multidimensional Activity

From the spiritual planes of boundless freedom, the soul, with angelic assistance, descends into the minute first cell, etherically impressing it with the perfect instruction for this incarnation. This moment of conception—which you and every other human being has experienced—is a multidimensional merging of heaven with earth, containing vast probabilities of unexpressed human potential. Before, during, and after the egg and sperm fuse, complex networks of events are simultaneously occurring on the many transcendental planes of consciousness for the incarnating soul. Corrine Heline, an occult anatomist, states: "An ovum gives no sign of life until it is awakened by fusion with the masculine sperm. In this fusion of male and female life essences . . . the miracle of miracles occurs. The forces of heaven and earth are blended. An immortal Spirit descends to resume physical embodiment."[11]

As invisible agents from the etheric and soul realms mingle with DNA to produce the human body, specific potentialities are created and released. From a metaphysical perspective, divine or vital principles interact with the physical substance of the cell to create a human being in the image of the Divine. Both the ovum and sperm carry the wisdom and qualities of the "universal architect"—the original cell, a microcosm of the potential human self. Your future child's first cell will carry the essence of her soul as well as the design of her human form.

This single fertilized cell is extraordinary in its capacity to duplicate itself to create a human body. Of the forty-five generations of cell-growth divisions needed to create the trillions of cells that evolve into an adult body, eight, or nearly one-fifth, have occurred by the time the embryo is implanted in the uterus; thirty generations, or two-thirds, have occurred by the time your future child is eight weeks old in the womb; thirty-nine by its twenty-eighth week of gestation; and forty-one by the time it is born. The remaining leisurely four generations of cell division occupy the whole of childhood and adolescence. Then there are no more.[12]

Since many couples do not even know they are pregnant until two to four weeks after conception, when about half of these divisions have already occurred, it is vitally important that a woman remains aware of her physical, psychological, and spiritual diet during this precarious and precious period of her cycle.

Some perspectives consider impregnation primarily a spiritual process. Numerous esoteric texts tell of innumerable invisible beings and forces assisting in the creation of the incarnating soul's new life on the physical plane. The Kabbalistic text The Zohar speaks of the "Heavenly Man" who impresses himself upon the aura of the incarnating soul and that of the parents: "At connubial intercourse on earth, the Holy One . . . sends a human form which bears the impress of the divine stamp. This form is present at intercourse, and if we were permitted to see it we should perceive over our heads an image resembling the human face; and it is in this image that we are formed. [If] this image is not sent by God and does not descend and hover over our heads, there can be no conception. This image receives us when we enter the world, it develops us when we grow, and accompanies us when we depart this life." Once conception has occurred and during the prenatal period, the soul "spins threads between itself and the evolving germ" to disperse its divine qualities throughout the embryonic body. The consciousness of the soul does not enter the zygote at conception; rather, it "envelops the embryo as an 'atmosphere' pouring its forces upon the little form as the stars focus their rays upon the earth." The consciousness of the soul increases its contact with the embryo/fetus "as the increasing complexity of development demands the presence of an intellectual force."[13]

The Gnostic doctrine Pistis Sophia describes how the builders or workmen of the higher spiritual realms descend into the original cell of the fertilized ovum: "And forthwith the three hundred and sixty-five workmen of the Rulers enter into her [the mother], to take up their abode in her. The workmen of the two parts [the sperm and ovum] are all there together."[14] Other ageless wisdom teachings such as the Vedic and Buddhist texts describe similar etheric and spiritual phenomena occurring during the human conception as well.

The Chakras: The Soul's Design for Human Form

I have thoroughly explored how the original cell serves as the blueprint for your future child's physical anatomy. There is also a subtle energy anatomy that can be included in your preconception and prenatal health care understanding. The development of the incarnating soul's physical body is preceded by the development of its etheric body. While your child's physical body consists of rapidly dividing cells smaller than a pinhead, her etheric body has already developed a sophisticated structure (see appendix D, From Soul to Cell, for a more detailed discussion). This is actually accomplished through two major stages of differentiation: the chakra system and the meridian system used in acupuncture.

First, according to ancient Hindu texts, the energetic biofield of the future embryo arranges itself into seven vortices of concentrated energy arranged from the base of the spine to the crown of the head, commonly referred to as the seven major chakras. Once the chakra system is established, all incoming informational energy is qualified and categorized by the chakras. Each chakra is itself an energy center on the surface of the etheric body where many strands of energy meet and pass each other, just like major railway junctures. These circular wheels of force swirl etheric, astral, and mental matter into dynamic activity.

The seven chakras correspond to five specific areas along the spinal canal and two locations in the head. They receive and transmit energy, serving as "electric sockets into which a physical gland is plugged" and converting cosmic energy into bodily energy. Chakras draw in the spirit from the air and distribute it to the physical glands in the body, where it is transmuted into physical substance and flows throughout the bloodstream and nervous system. The more evolved the soul, the more spirit the chakra will assimilate.[15]

The function and activity of these energy centers vary according to the evolutionary stage of the soul. Some centers are more awakened than others; less evolved souls function through the lower centers along the spine, with the head and heart centers often remaining dormant. In shamanic and esoteric cosmology, the first three chakras represent the lower worlds, the human condition and psyche. These lower three centers govern the physical life of the material form and the lower psychic faculties and experiences. The upper four centers—the heart, throat, third eye or brow (also called the *ajna* center), and crown—relate to intellectual and spiritual consciousness. Once you've gained a comfortable and grounded instinctual nature, you've refined and integrated your lower three energy centers. The two head chakras are the last to activate, preceded by the throat center. Throughout your pregnancy, you can help ensure the health of your child's chakras as you meditate or reflect on their function.

The Function of the Seven Chakras

The seven chakras are the interface between the soul and the physical-etheric, emotional, and mental bodies. Through these energy vortices you can consciously travel into the spiritual worlds. The chakras are energy and information centers that assist us in knowing and understanding our true essential nature as a spiritual consciousness in human form. Having awareness of the chakra system of the incarnating soul allows you to understand the subtler levels within the developing physical body of your child. Since each energy center has a specific function, the cause of any physical discomfort in a newborn can actually be located in the chakras. You can refer to the chart Your Child's Seven Chakras on page 185.

The first chakra is located at the sacrum or base of the spine. Here is where instinctual and genetic information about survival issues and fears are stored, along with ancestral and archetypal memories. An individual concern for materialistic matters and the lowest parts of human consciousness are perceived at this vortex of energy. This is also the seat of kundalini energy—a concentrated form of intelligent, cosmic energy that is vital to life. It rests in the base of the human spine as a soul begins to evolve during its first incarnation. Kundalini is fed by the chakras along the spine and by cosmic energy entering the feet from the earth. As wisdom is earned in each incarnation, the very potent electromagnetic energy moves slowly up the spine to fill each chakra. In esoteric healing the first chakra is usually associated with the color red. Common issues stored in this chakra are traumas around physical or financial survival. To support the well-being of the first chakra for a fetus, newborn, and child, the consistent experience of physical safety and security is essential.

The second chakra is located just below the navel and is commonly referred to as the sacral center. Its functions are primarily the dynamics of sexuality, reproduction and fertility, primal emotions, and raw creative impulses. The color orange is associated with this chakra. Healing of sexual abuse in childhood, adolescence, or past lives enhances the vitality of this chakra. When the second chakra of a fetus or newborn is cared for, sexual and creative vitality and health are stabilized. Trauma to this center can cause abdominal and sexual health problems, often manifesting significantly in later life.

The third chakra is called the solar plexus and is associated with the color yellow. It is located midway between the belly button and the heart. This energy center is associated with action and assertion. It monitors the energy distribution of the whole body. Issues about misuse of will and power from the present or previous lives are stored here. Encouraging a child to express his creative power and will in a useful, productive, and harmless way is a positive use of this chakra. For adults, a healthy expression of the third chakra is embodying leadership abilities, using creative power to empower others to express their divine nature. If the parents are physically, emotionally, or mentally abusive to the prenate or newborn, this chakra is significantly harmed.

The fourth chakra is located in the heart and chest area. Eastern traditions use green to represent this chakra; Western traditions use pink. This chakra is associated with emotion, affection, intimacy, and self-esteem. Grief and abandonment are often stored here. If a fetus experiences the feeling of rejection in the womb, the health of its heart chakra can be seriously affected. If a child has an openhearted nature and is continuously rejected, this center can easily become damaged. Honoring a prenate's or newborn's emotional nature and embodying a safe, compassionate presence for the new life will enhance the well-being of this chakra. Expressing love and affection can harmonize it as well. Most metaphysical teachings emphasize healthy maintenance of this chakra because it is the balancer and transformer of the three lower and three upper chakras. The three chakras above the heart correspond to the cosmology of the upper worlds or higher planes of consciousness. The heart is the bridge that unites the upper and lower realms.

The fifth chakra is located at the center of the throat below the larynx, superimposed upon the thyroid gland. It is associated with the color blue. This is the center of creativity—when the raw creative energies of the second chakra mature, they are expressed through the fifth chakra. It also mediates vocal expression and is related to telepathic communication and the hearing of your inner truth. When a child's communication and self-expression are invalidated or denied, this chakra can be harmed. If feelings or creativity are suppressed, or a child's truth is judged, this chakra will be blocked. Parents can empower this chakra by caring about a child's emotional, mental, and creative impulses, and by caring about the child's expressive needs.

The sixth chakra is located at the brow between the eyes and above the nose. It is associated with the color purple. This energy center is commonly called the third eye. It is related to *clairvoyance* (clear seeing), *clairaudience* (clear hearing), and *clairsentience* (clear feeling). The pineal gland is an imaging faculty that presides over the nerve center between the eyes. As the focal point of the mind, it transmutes cosmic information into electrical energy so that the brain and whole personality can use it. This is the center where intuition is cultivated. When children are not supported in accessing and trusting their intuitive knowings and inner sight, this chakra is harmed. When this chakra is healthy, your child can perceive visions, intuitions, and inner truth.

The seventh chakra is located at the top of the head and is often referred to as the crown chakra. In some shamanic and esoteric traditions this chakra is where the spirit enters at birth and leaves at death. The color associated with this chakra is violet, white, or gold. Each of the lower chakras unfolds energy into this chakra by graduated steps, giving it the power and intelligence it needs for fusion with the soul nature. Therefore, if any of the lower chakras is damaged or blocked, this chakra cannot fully develop.

The continuity of consciousness from the soul realms into the personality is dependent on the healthy functioning of all seven chakras. You as a prospective parent can greatly support the well-being of your child's seven major chakra centers as they are forming in utero and thereafter. The chakra system is affected by your thoughts and personality. Trauma to any of the soul's personality bodies will affect the health and vitality of the chakras as well, directly influencing the quality and quantity of refined spiritual intelligence, will, and consciousness that the incoming soul will be able to embody as a human personality.

The chakras are activated based on the development of the individual; they affect the various activities of the personality vehicle of the incarnating soul. In fact, clairvoyant individuals can perceive the evolutionary growth of the soul and its karmic debts and assets simply by analyzing the quality of energy of the whole chakra system. When the chakras and glands are in alignment, they offer clear channels for the soul to express its energies. This is rare indeed, but it can be the aspiration of anyone seeking to be physically healthy, emotionally stable, and mentally controlled.

YOUR CHILD'S SEVEN CHAKRAS

Considering that the continuity of consciousness from the soul realms into the personality is dependent upon the healthy functioning of all seven chakras, it is crucial that prospective parents appreciate the importance of enhancing, or at least supporting, the well-being of the seven major chakra centers as they are forming in utero and thereafter. Trauma to the physical, emotional, and mental bodies will affect the health and vitality of the chakras, which in turn directly influences the quality and quantity of refined spiritual intelligence, will, and consciousness that the incoming soul will be able to experience and embody as a human personality.

The lower three centers—the base, sacral, and solar plexus chakras—govern the physical life of the material form and the lower psychic faculties and experience. The upper four centers—the heart, throat, third eye, and crown chakras—relate to intellectual and spiritual consciousness.

First Chakra

Referred to as: Base chakra
Location: Base of spine
Color: Red
Function: Physical safety and security
Traumas: Physical survival

Second Chakra

Referred to as: Sacral center
Location: Just below navel
Color: Orange
Function: Sexuality, reproduction, primal emotions, raw creative impulses
Traumas: Abdominal and sexual abuse

Third Chakra

Referred to as: Solar plexus
Location: Midway between belly button and area of chest where heart is located
Color: Yellow
Function: Action, assertion, energy for physical body, self-expression, personal willpower; expression of creative power and personal will
Traumas: Suppressed self-expression

Fourth Chakra

Referred to as: Heart chakra
Location: In the heart and chest area
Color: Green, pink
Function: Emotion, affection, intimacy, self-esteem, love—unites upper and lower chakras
Traumas: Grief, abandonment, rejection

Fifth Chakra

Referred to as: Throat chakra
Location: Center of the throat below the larynx, superimposed upon the thyroid gland
Color: Blue
Function: Creativity, mediates vocal expression of feelings and thoughts, communication of inner truth
Traumas: Invalidation or denial of self-expression

Sixth Chakra

Referred to as: Third eye or *ajna* center
Location: Slightly above brow between the eyes and above the nose
Color: Purple
Function: Clairvoyance, clairaudience, clairsentience, intuition, inner insights and perceptions, vision
Traumas: No support for intuitive development

Seventh Chakra

Referred to as: Crown chakra
Location: Top of head
Color: Violet, white, gold
Function: Fusion of lower chakras with the soul—where spirit enters at birth and leaves at death
Traumas: Separation from cosmic consciousness

The Formation of the Meridian System
(Acupuncture Channels and Points)

In addition to the seven major chakras, smaller chakras exist through-out the body, probably corresponding to the acupuncture points of Chinese medicine. At the next developmental stage the seven chakras begin to interrelate as seven distinct qualities of energy. As these rela-tionships stabilize, more etheric energy constructively enters the etheric body and the acupuncture channels begin to develop.

The acupuncture channels are hundreds of thousands of threads of bioelectric energy, ordered in precise patterns, circulating in increasingly organized forms. The acupuncture points are "tiny, invisible, concen-trated centers of energy and intellect located in the nervous system (electrical system) of the body . . . seven hundred forty-one [acupunc-ture] points in the body act as transformers and transmitters" of bio-electrical energy.[16] As these vortices increase in strength, they eventually resonate in sympathetic vibration with the finest forms of physical matter. A common holistic health hypothesis is that the physical matter created is DNA.

I once heard a wonderful analogy from an acupuncturist colleague who described how the soul affects physical matter, DNA, through these etheric vortices: "In the same way the crystal chip inside a radio reads subtle energetic signals and frequencies and translates them into music, DNA is the masterful liquid crystal biochip that reads etheric energies and translates them into physical life."[17] Each organ and tissue that will be formed in the physical body is created by a different rate of vibration. The acupuncture points accept the rate of vibrational frequency that comes into them and focus the frequency to form the various parts of the body. This complex network of life energy is guiding the physical formation of your child—before and after conception. By the time the miracle of physical conception occurs, so much has already happened to prepare for the soul's embodiment.

You may find that meditating on your child's chakras evokes images that reflect the subtle energy pathways of the body. An entry in my preconception journal reads:

> I see the living presence of my soon-to-be child as an interdimensional
> tapestry of consciousness . . . streams of light patterns weaving the
> essence of Life into perfect form—directed by natural and heavenly
> forces, produced by her Soul.

Genes: Interdimensional Doorways

In traditional medical models the parents' genetic pools—formed out of their DNA—are considered the primary influence on the health of their child-to-be. The holistic approach, on the other hand, views the parents' genetic contribution as archetypal patterns that are focal points for the incoming soul. When the sperm and egg join to create the original cell, the incarnating soul sets "these primary vortices in motion with its own peculiar rate of vibration [imposing] its will and purpose"[18] upon the new life-form. The *genetic potential* of the new human life is used by the soul based on the soul's evolutionary needs. Therefore, traditional pre-birth genetic counseling that does not include the soul plan and its karmic lessons of the present incarnation is incomplete.

Both you and your partner carry traits in your genes that are not manifesting in you. Your future child is also a repository of traits from the soul as well as influences from universal consciousness. These spiritual traits are carried in the DNA chain in the hereditary patterns—it is more than just biochemistry that determines the traits that are fixed in the biological blueprint at the moment of conception. Hereditary traits represent potentials; the interaction of consciousness, environment, and the soul's innate pattern governs what is used.

In *Wheels of a Soul*, Rabbi Berg concurs with this notion. He states: "The ancient Kabbalistic position is that human beings consist of the mystical compound of physical matter and intangible spirit. . . . Drawing from The Zohar [the basic source of the Kabbalah] and Rabbi Isaac Luria's *Gates of Reincarnation,* I have come to the conclusion that the individuality of humans is not the result of their unique genetic code, but that the personal DNA structure is the result of the metaphysical, individual immortal soul that becomes manifest through the physical individual." Rabbi Berg continues to describe this same relationship between the seed and the tree. The full potential of the tree exists in the seed before it becomes visible in the leaves and branches.[19]

According to Manly Hall, heredity is viewed as "morality, culture, genius, etc., being reducible to rates of vibrations pervading the [parents'] aura, [as well as these factors exerting] a powerful influence upon the external life."[20] The intellectual, moral, and spiritual natures of the parents color the energy zones that are originally established at "the time of copulation." Reincarnating souls are attracted to these energy zones by the law of attraction. The psychic vortices of the parents must be aligned with the incarnating soul's purpose. According to Hall, it is not so much that talents and characteristics are inherited, but that a soul is attracted to its parents based on their mutual soul tendencies and karmic similarities. On all planes of existence like attracts like, and similarly conception is the manifestation of a potent magnetic attraction between three souls. As parents, you do not choose a soul: you are chosen.

The Power of Thought

Many of the esoteric texts suggest that the parents can constructively modify the chemistry of the embryo's body using the faculties of will and imagination. This is especially true for the mother, who is "marinating" the fetus in her own biochemical environment, the womb. In *De Generatio Hominis* the renowned philosophical ontogenist Paracelsus wrote that "the imagination of the mother exerts a great constructive influence upon the development of the fetus, and upon this fact is based the similarity existing between children and parents. The imagination of the father activates the creative power which is necessary to the generation of a human being, and the imagination of the mother furnishes the materials for the formation and development of this being. The rational principle of the child, however, is separate and distinct from that of the parents, having its own eternal subsistence."[21]

A fundamental metaphysical maxim is "Energy follows thought"—in other words, subjective thoughts influence matter. Since all matter is amenable to the power of thought, this original cell is affected by the force of both the parents' minds and the soul's intent. "The Zohar, a Kabbalistic text, teaches that the thoughts of a man and woman during sexual intercourse are what determines what sort of soul will occupy the body of the baby to be born of their union."[22] I invite you to be aware of how the application of your creative imagination can influence and even modify the physical development of the embryo at conception and thereafter.

Connie and Brent actually conceived their daughter, Cynthia, using the eggs of another woman. Connie had been grieving for months that she would not be the genetic mother of her child, and she felt encouraged to discover that she could have a creative influence over her child's development since she would still be the biological mother, growing her baby in her own womb. Connie shares:

Throughout the pregnancy, Brent and I kept visualizing our child in a womb of loving light. I would send feelings of harmony and beauty into my womb during my morning meditation. When Cynthia was born, everyone commented how beautiful she was, and how she resembled me. I have always wondered whether my intense effort to nurture her with spiritual qualities during the pregnancy were utilized by her soul in the development of her body, and her similarity to me is due to my consciousness impressing her throughout the pregnancy. The fact that she is not my genetic child does not disturb our profound connection.

Whether you are conscious of it or not, celestial and angelic forces are influencing every moment of human life. As prospective parents, when you create a conscious conception with an incoming soul, you activate the highest potential that the incarnating lifestream can use as it blends with many earthly and multidimensional forces. You and your partner can develop an appreciation for the many forces that are being created and activated at the moment of conceiving your child and can increase your efforts to create healthy conditions for a conscious conception.

Hot Tips: The Optimal Time and Space to Conceive

When you and your partner decide it is time to conceive your baby, you will know that making love is not just your two bodies making contact, but rather is a heart-opening connection to create a new life. Knowing when you are fertile each month is essential to becoming pregnant; if you did not explore this when you read chapter 3, Preparing Your Body for Conception, now is the time.

All methods for predicting ovulation are based on the woman's reproductive cycle. Ovulation usually occurs about fourteen days before menstruation begins, so the usual length of the woman's cycle will determine what day you are most likely to conceive. For example, in a twenty-eight-day cycle, you ovulate around day fourteen; if your cycles are thirty days, you ovulate around day sixteen; and if your cycle length is twenty-one days, your ovulation occurs around day seven. But these are only averages; some women ovulate earlier or later. If your cycles are inconsistent, then ovulation will be less predictable, and you may want to use an ovulation test kit. These kits are available at any drugstore without a prescription and can predict ovulation within one or two days using a simple urine test. The test kit will actually show a positive result in advance of true ovulation, which gives you the opportunity to accurately time the man's ejaculation.

A woman also can tell when she is most fertile by recording her basal body temperature (BBT), the body's base temperature upon waking, over the course of several months. A natural birth control book found at your local library or bookstore can instruct you in determining your ovulation time based on your BBT, which requires a special but inexpensive thermometer. Another signal of ovulation is a change in the quality of a woman's cervical mucus to a thin, clear, sticky secretion, reflecting the body's change in pH to respond hospitably to sperm. A woman can check her cervical mucus using her fingers every day throughout her monthly cycle, noting the consistency change around ovulation time. Usually the whole vaginal area is more lubricated and full during your fertile time.

Remember that the egg is capable of being fertilized for only up to twenty-four hours after ovulation; the sperm, with few unique exceptions, can fertilize the egg only from the time of ejaculation up to seventy-two hours afterward. The best way to increase the chance of conceiving is to pinpoint the time of ovulation. According to a landmark ten-year study by the National Institute of Environmental Health Sciences, conception is most likely when intercourse takes place on the day of ovulation or during several days preceding it.[23] The importance of timing cannot be overestimated. Lisa's dynamic with her husband offers a poignant example:

> Rick and I tried conceiving for eleven months before our doctor evaluated our unsuccessful track record. My menstrual cycles have always varied a day or two, and I never knew that this made my ovulation time unpredictable. Checking my calendar, we discovered that six of the eleven months we were attempting to conceive, I was traveling during the actual day of ovulation, so it was only in five of those months that the sperm even had a chance during the critical twenty-four hours. Even when we did try to conceive at the appropriate time, I had not been aware of the twenty-four-hour window of opportunity for introducing the sperm. Once we used the ovulation testing methods to precisely pinpoint our window, it only took one month to conceive.

To optimize the opportunity for conception, generally the most of-ten-recommended lovemaking position is for a woman to lie on her back with the man on top of her during intercourse. Her pelvis should be raised on pillows after ejaculation. The "male and female nectars" can be absorbed into the woman's body as she lies in this receptive position and receives them like a sponge. If possible, she should remain on her back for one to two hours in a relaxed state. If you have difficulty conceiving, your gynecologist should check the position of the uterus, because a woman with a uterus tipped forward should be on top of her male partner when trying to conceive.

Many couples trying to conceive want to know how frequently a man should ejaculate to optimize the chance of conception. Some also have voiced concerns about whether the man should abstain from ejaculating before the ovulation time, guarding his reserves, and if so, for how long. Ideally, a man can cultivate the art of consciously controlling his sexual energy so that he can refrain from ejaculating when he does not want to. (The teachings of Tantric sexuality provide techniques to prevent ejaculating while still experiencing orgasm.) Optimally, a man should abstain from ejaculation for up to a week before trying to conceive so that his sperm count will be concentrated and his sexual vitality strong.

A long-standing perspective is that a man should ejaculate no more frequently than every thirty-six to forty-eight hours between conception attempts because more frequent relations are thought to depress the sperm count, while less frequent can miss the ovulation time. Other research suggests having intercourse the night of the woman's LH surge (detected with a reliable ovulation test kit) and again on the following two days. Since healthy sperm will last up to seventy-two hours in a woman's body, by ejaculating the day before ovulation is expected and again a day or two later it may be possible to "surround" the ovulation time. And then there are those times when spontaneity works best.

According to the principles of traditional Chinese medicine, after ejaculation it is important that both the man and the woman keep their bodies warm and eat and drink something warm to replenish their vital energy. For some, air travel is not recommended just before the time of conception (or during the first trimester) because high altitudes can deplete both the yin energy (female essence) and the immune system at a time when an abundance of both is essential for reproductive health.

Classic Chinese texts also proscribe certain times for conception as unfavorable for the health of the future child. Conceiving at noon, at midnight, during a solar or lunar eclipse, during a thunderstorm, during a rainbow, at the summer or winter solstice, or during the full moon is not recommended. When the climatic or macrocosmic energies are highly polarized during conception, these times of disequilibrium can potentially lead to an energetic imbalance in the child's constitution. In addition, try not to conceive while either partner is suffering from a skin disease, or during or for one hundred days after having a hot or warm disease (a fever condition), because the heat in the blood can create fetal toxins. It is also suggested that you refrain from conceiving when intoxicated or with a full stomach, while in mourning, or while distressed or in shock.[24]

According to Chinese medicine, it is best for the woman to orgasm before the man's ejaculation; her orgasm creates a more receptive environment for the sperm. In Taoism—and also in Sri Lankan fertility texts—it is optimal that the couple experience simultaneous orgasm, because the life energies of the woman and man are at their peak for conceiving. It is written in the ancient science texts as well as in the cultural mythologies that when the energies from the mother and father are given to the forming zygote in equal proportions, the child will embody and "radiate its parents' energy equally."[25] With more than one available perspective, you will want to discuss with your partner whether you want to consciously control the timing of your individual orgasms.

In all of this you will want to bear in mind that although your own personal timing and efforts are important, conception is a multidimensional process, and other factors may also partially determine the moment the soul chooses to be conceived. Try to remain open to intuitively connecting with the consciousness of the incoming soul so that you may receive impressions concerning when it prefers its conception to occur. Integrating your own readiness and the soul's preference based on karmic and celestial conditions is fundamental to your holistic preconception health care.

For example, during the time that I felt relatively prepared to conceive our child, I was simultaneously communing with her soul. Although my husband and I were ready to begin our conception efforts in August, I intuitively sensed that she preferred to be conceived in February due to astrological and other considerations. My eagerness to be pregnant tried to defy her request, and although we did conceive in December, we had an early miscarriage. When we successfully conceived again in February, I could not help but wonder who was really deciding the time of conception. Our daughter had been guiding both my husband and me throughout the preconception period, preparing our whole health for her arrival, and I think she even determined when that would be. I began to appreciate the lifelong dance of harmonizing her needs with my own and those of my husband.

Clearly, there are no hard-and-fast rules for how and when to conceive. You can leave the physical conditions up to fate while remaining mindful that you and the incoming soul are beginning a sacred dance with the mysteries of life.

Determining Your Child's Sex

Numerous sources offer various formulas, based on both medical and metaphysical principles, for determining the sex of your child at conception. I resonate with a Theosophical attitude: "The sex of the body which an incoming Spirit is to inhabit is determined by guardian Angels long before the Soul comes into incarnation. This matter is determined in accordance with 'ripe fate' to be liquidated in the coming life. [Whatever this choice], the Spirit is above and beyond the limitation circumscribed by sex; it is in the pure light of spirit."[26] This perspective aligns with the principles of reincarnation in that a human's physical body is determined by the soul's karma and purpose for incarnating. Thus, from a metaphysical perspective, the sex of your child will be determined long before physical conception.

After the soul has finished its experiences in the inner worlds between incarnations, the soul's divine plan determines the quantity and quality of material to be used in the formation of the new personality bodies, including the physical. Vibrating the specific life substance on the physical-etheric plane, the soul's karmic needs will manifest the form—be it male or female—needed to fulfill its destiny.

Though it is very natural for a parent to prefer a specific sex, this viewpoint suggests that the soul's destiny rather than the desire of the parents determines its human sex in each lifetime. Parents need to remember that the soul is incarnating to fulfill its evolutionary needs, not their personal wishes. Therefore a normal yearning, such as "I prefer a son," can be combined with the feeling that "I am open to unconditionally love whatever form this soul needs to fulfill its purpose this incarnation." You are not being asked to deny your preference for a particular sex, or certain attributes or talents. You simply need to keep these preferences in proportion so that the emphasis is on caring for the soul's true needs.

Creative Exercise:
Creating a Conscious Conception

1. How can you use the concept of cellular consciousness in your prebirth experience with your future child?
2. What does creating a conscious conception mean to you and your partner? Do you want to create a sacred conception ritual with your partner? If so, what would it be like? Is there an optimal time and space to conceive your baby?
3. What is your vision of what the incarnating soul experiences at the moment of conception, and soon after?
4. Use the diagram of the seven chakras to describe how you can care for the developmental needs of each chakra of your future child.
5. How can you use the power of thought during the preconception, conception, and postconception phases of your child's life?

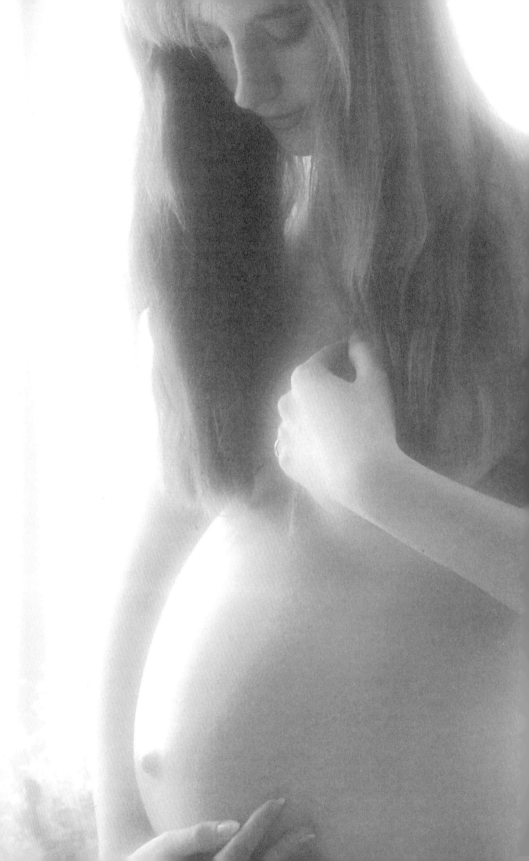

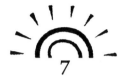

7

The Prenatal
Journey

We can know the future only in the laughter of healthy children.
Ann Wilson Schaef

Throughout this book, I've explored holistic perspectives such as reincarnation, karma, and the conception of your child's mental, emotional, and etheric bodies before physical conception. Perhaps as a result you will choose to explore these ideas and choose to co-create a conscious conception with your child. Once conception has occurred, you will have many other opportunities to further influence the evolution of the incarnating soul who has chosen you as its parents this lifetime.

Pregnancy is a time of profound metamorphosis on every level of your being. But though we all have seen charts of the three trimesters of pregnancy that reflect a miraculous and precise sequence of a baby's biological development, during two decades of research I have yet to see a trimester chart that depicts the simultaneous development of the etheric, emotional, and mental bodies that correspond to the biological phases of growth. Embracing the whole health of an incarnating soul reveals an immediate need to revise the blueprint of how we perceive the stages of human development. Based on a blending of Eastern and Western perspectives, I have developed such a representation. The Holistic Trimester Chart of the Human Personality (see page 198) describes the appearance and interaction of all four personality bodies during

HOLISTIC TRIMESTER CHART OF THE HUMAN PERSONALITY:
A Blueprint of the Development and Integration of the Physical–Etheric, Emotional, and Mental Bodies

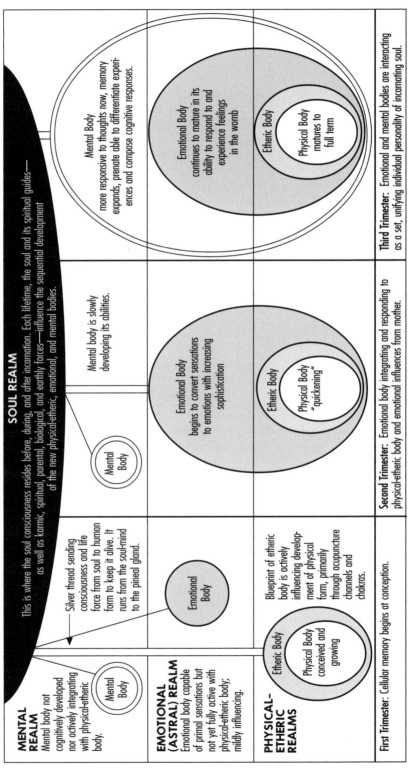

SOUL REALM

This is where the soul consciousness resides before, during, and after incarnation. Each lifetime, the soul and its spiritual guides—as well as karmic, spiritual, parental, biological, and earthly forces—influence the sequential development of the new physical-etheric, emotional, and mental bodies.

Silver thread sending consciousness and life force from soul to human form to keep it alive. It runs from the soul-mind to the pineal gland.

Mental body is slowly developing its abilities.

Mental Body more responsive to thoughts now, memory expands, prenate able to differentiate experiences and compose cognitive responses.

Emotional Body

Emotional Body begins to convert sensations to emotions with increasing sophistication

Emotional Body continues to mature in its ability to respond to and experience feelings in the womb

Etheric Body

Physical Body "quickening"

Etheric Body

Physical Body matures to full term

MENTAL REALM
Mental body not cognitively developed nor actively integrating with physical-etheric body.

Mental Body

EMOTIONAL (ASTRAL) REALM
Emotional body capable of primal sensations but not yet fully active with physical-etheric body; mildly influencing.

Etheric Body

Blueprint of etheric body is actively influencing development of physical form, primarily through acupuncture channels and chakras.

PHYSICAL–ETHERIC REALMS

Physical Body conceived and growing

First Trimester: Cellular memory begins at conception.

Second Trimester: Emotional body integrating and responding to physical-etheric body and emotional influences from mother.

Third Trimester: Emotional and mental bodies are interacting as a set, unifying individual personality of incarnating soul.

pregnancy, and Co-creating Consciousness with Your Child (page 204) suggests practical steps you can take to participate fully in your child's development.

A Holistic Trimester Model of the Incarnating Soul: Development of the Physical, Emotional, Mental, and Spiritual Bodies

First Trimester

In all biological texts and prenatal charts there is a total emphasis on the development of the physical body, the cell divisions and organ development of each progressing week. According to a holistic perspective, while this is going on the fetus literally recapitulates all of human evolution, from a single-celled entity at conception to a miniature human, in the first ninety days in the womb. This awesome fact reflects that during the days and weeks of the first trimester, every child in utero actually experiences millions of years of evolution while the physical body is just forming.

Between day twenty-two and day twenty-eight, for example, this tiny living system metamorphoses from a basic neural tube to a primitive "fish creature," an animal form in just six days. Most pregnant parents are not aware of this first rapid growth phase, which the embryo experiences in less than a week. In fact, the first several months of pregnancy are a delicate time when the developing fetus is highly sensitive to subtle energy influences. So each day of your potential pregnancy, it is important that you be conscious of what substances your child in utero is exposed to. A woman who is not yet aware of her pregnant state may take a drug to care for a common flu and dramatically affect the embryo's growth. The safest approach is to assume you are pregnant until you can confirm it.

Since the emotional body is present at conception, exposing a pregnant mother to a psychologically traumatic experience, such as a death or an emotionally abusive interaction with someone, can affect the subtle energy anatomy of her prenate as well. Although the emotional body is not yet fully active during the first trimester it is mildly influencing the fetus, since primal cellular consciousness already exists.

Clara describes the impact of her brother's illness:

> I was four weeks pregnant when Joey was diagnosed with a terminal
> illness. From the moment I heard the news, I completely withdrew

my attention from the baby growing inside of me. It was as if I felt responsible to fight for Joey's life, rather than protect the one inside me. It was no wonder our little one decided to go from my body less than a month later. She was not being nourished by me anymore, as I rarely felt anything but grief for my brother's pain. When I miscarried, I realized how much I contributed to sustaining the little fetus's will to be released. In retrospect it is clear to me that our baby was encountering more feelings of grief and death from me than feelings of love. I did not feel guilty, yet I knew not to conceive again until my heart was free to welcome and delight in the life growing inside me. When I finally did become pregnant again, I was ready, and my baby got the best of me. Her buoyant personality reminds me daily how important it is to celebrate life.

Emotional stress becomes even more significant during the second trimester, when the emotional body is actively integrating and responding to the physical-etheric influences from the mother.

Honoring the delicate energy needs of the growing prenate can help to ensure a positive outcome. Rather than letting an understanding of the strength of the mind-body connection make her unreasonably fearful, a pregnant woman and her partner can use the first several weeks and months of their child's life as an opportunity to remain vigilant of the biological and psychological nutrients needed for their baby to flourish.

For Sally, knowing that "there was more going on in my belly during the pregnancy than those prenatal charts in my doctor's office" gave her a way to include her husband in the early-pregnancy experience:

> After each office visit, Todd and I would discuss ways we could create the emotional atmosphere to communicate to our unborn child that she was loved. We learned that the child could respond to sounds in the womb. From then on, we were more aware of what we said to each other and made sure we played peaceful music around the baby. Our doctor never told us the importance of being this sensitive. Focusing on the baby's emotional needs in utero really invited Todd to be actively involved in her development, starting in the first trimester. Although he could not connect to the baby physically, he knew he had a lot to give her emotionally and spiritually.

Second Trimester

As you'll discover, the classic medical second-trimester gestation charts are not very illuminating. This is because there is little more that can be graphically represented about the physical development of the child than what is in the first-trimester charts. By the end of the third month of prenatal life, all of the biological systems are formed. During the second trimester these same structures grow. From the beginning to end of the second trimester increasing size is the salient feature of the baby.

The same second trimester of the holistic chart is far more fascinating, illustrating the growth of the subtle bodies that are behind the scenes of the developing physical body. During the beginning of the second trimester, the emotional body makes very direct contact with the fetus as it "takes up residence" with the human personality. Until then, the emotional body has been developing in a primitive way by recording primal cellular impressions in the womb. During the fourth month, the soul begins to experience increasing emotional consciousness through the human personality of the developing child. Modern scientific prenatal research describes the child becoming highly sensitive to the emotions of his mother around this time, as well as having his own independent emotional reactions. During the second trimester, as the brain matures at the cerebral cortex level, the child is learning how to translate maternal messages into emotion. By the sixth month in utero, the fetal consciousness is able to transform a feeling into an emotion and create a response. Verny explains that as the fetus gains awareness "as a distinct 'self' and is able to convert sensations into emotions . . . he begin[s] to be shaped increasingly by the *purely emotional* content of his mother's messages."[1] As a pregnant mom, you can begin now to more actively nurture the emotional well-being of your child. In my journal I wrote:

> As we enter the second trimester, you are feeling my feelings more precisely, and I am responsive to your sensitivity. I like this. It means I get to open my heart more, to be more loving. It means I have to remember to still my mind, to become more peaceful. It means I can make the extra effort to meditate, to feel our spiritual bond. It means I can let go of that which drains me, to choose that which enlivens us. Your arrival in my life inspires me to be aware of choosing that which is life-giving.

The desires and thoughts of the mother have a significant effect on the developing life matrix in utero as the soul hovers nearby. Christian mythology describes Mary spending this time communing with hosts of angels during her pregnancy. The daily stresses of modern civilization may challenge our ability to make contact with angels; still, a woman can create a contemplative time each day to reflect on positive thoughts, walk in the beauty of nature, read an inspiring book, look at sacred art, or listen to peaceful music. There are many ways to create a sacred state of awareness. Even while driving in stressful traffic, a pregnant woman can use audiotapes that are relaxing and soothing.

The father can also contribute directly to the emotional state of the mother, and thus the child. Any action that uplifts the pregnant mother will benefit the child as well; likewise, any behavior that upsets the mother can potentially affect the child, since the prenate is immersed in the mother's psychic reality.

Third Trimester

In the traditional third-trimester prenatal charts you can usually see the body of the fetus with all the essential biological systems that were established in the first trimester growing larger, along with some additional traits and a more mature appearance. In a holistic prenatal chart you can also see the emotional body continuing to mature in its ability to experience and respond to feelings in the womb as well as the beginning of the mental body identifying itself actively with the fetus as it, too, now interacts with the developing personality. As the child's physical-etheric and emotional bodies become more sophisticated, the ability of the mental body begins to differentiate as well. Verny continues to describe the intimate relationship between the personality bodies: "As his memory and experience expand, he gradually acquires the ability to make more discriminating and subtle connections. By birth . . . the infant is mature enough to be able to respond to maternal feelings with great accuracy and compose physical, emotional, and cognitive responses."[2] The prenate is now able to be more responsive to her own primal thoughts as well as those of her parents throughout the pregnancy. In my journal I wrote:

> It is month eight. Welcome, you are descending quickly. You are now a solid blend of heavenly *and* earthly forces. I try to focus my mind on the beauty of life. Yet the tumultuous news in the world

reminds me that I cannot protect you from that which you have come to live amid. As your delicate mind is forming, my idealism would like to cocoon you from the agitation of *my* mind and the collective one. I will do my best, until you have the resources to protect yourself and pierce the illusions of this world so that you can always remember you are Divine.

Theosophical perspectives describe the soul as only dimly conscious through the physical body during the prenatal life. At quickening during the second trimester, when the mother is able to perceive her baby's movements, the nervous system has developed to the point where a small measure of the soul's consciousness can manifest, increasing vitality.[3] Just before birth, the soul receives a vision of the life it is entering. This preview is mentioned by both H. Q. Blavatsky and the Tibetan Book of the Dead as the complement to the "life review" that follows death. The soul is offered an overview of its karmic lessons for this life, the conditions that will be encountered, and appropriate responses to each. There is an awareness of the causes and the justice of the new life circumstances.

At birth, however, the physical and subtle energy bodies are shocked from the warmth and safety of the embryonic life, and a veil seems to separate the soul from this conscious preview stage—suddenly the soul's consciousness is perceived through the limitations of the primitive infant personality, and the soul may wonder where the freedom to express its divine nature has gone. Your loving care can ease this transition for your newborn as he moves from the sublime states of the soul dimension, through the disorienting experience of birth, to face the adjustments of inhabiting a highly sensitive physical, emotional, and mental body. Parents can undermine or enhance this process, depending on their own physical, emotional, mental, and spiritual stability. The soul who has chosen you to be its parents this lifetime knows that you will do the best you can to care for it.

CO-CREATING CONSCIOUSNESS WITH YOUR CHILD

You can focus your consciousness to assist the development of your child's physical-etheric, emotional, and mental bodies. Set aside a quiet time in the morning and evening to commune with your growing child-spirit. You and your partner can also do this as a couple.

	First Trimester	Second Trimester	Third Trimester
Physical-etheric body	Your unborn child will grow from a single-celled being to a miniature human with all of her biological systems formed. Concentrate on all of her physiology being vibrant with light, vitality, and the soul's essence. If you are inspired, pray for or visualize perfect health. Welcome her into your life.	The physiological structures, organs, and systems are forming and developing rapidly. You will feel your baby move between week 16 and 20. By the end of this trimester, he will be more than half the length of his newborn size. Continue to visualize and feel your child's body filled with light and vitality, or any healthy quality you sense is beneficial.	This is the time of the greatest weight gain as your baby's body grows to full term. Send positive images and feelings to your child's whole body. Focus on her organs, structure, and physiological systems flowing and glowing with light and life.
Emotional body	The primal emotional body is able to sense if it is wanted and loved or rejected and neglected by the mother. Allow yourself to bond deeply with your child. You can imagine a psychic cord of light or energy between your hearts—pour your love and desire for her from your heart to hers. Talk to her throughout the day and express your love telepathically or verbally.	As the emotional body develops the ability for greater emotional expression and perception, bathe him in positive feelings. When you are emotionally agitated, surround him in a cocoon of loving light. Or talk to him and reassure him that he is safe and your upset has nothing to do with him.	The emotional body is becoming even more receptive and responsive. Continue to deepen your prenatal bond by sending or infusing feelings of love and joy directly into the body of your child. Let him feel deeply wanted and cared for by talking or singing to him. He already recognizes your voice.
Mental body	The mental body is not very active, yet the soul is drawing on the mental substance of your thoughts. Beginning now and continuing throughout the pregnancy, avoid exposing yourself to negative or violent energies and images.	The mental body is only mildly active. Yet, because the emotional body is so receptive and because your emotions are affected by your thoughts, continue to keep your mental attitudes and attention positive.	The memory is expanding and cognitive responses are awakening. Continue to avoid exposing your unborn child to negative or violent energies. Focus your own mind and heart on uplifting thoughts, feelings, images, and beliefs—send these emotional, mental, and intuitive impressions to your child.

Your Child Embodies Kingdoms:
The Developing Zygote

Even if we propose that a spirit or soul exists apart from matter, the embryo weaves the two entities together as organism and psyche.

Richard Grossinger

Embryogenesis, the science of the biological process of human evolution from the moment of conception, rarely describes the reproductive cells of the mother's egg and the father's sperm as the result of hundreds of billions of years of evolution and transmutation. The ageless wisdom teachings, on the other hand, regard a human being as the epitome of the whole universal order and a reflection of earthly and divine mysteries.

When the sperm and egg unify to create the zygote, the first cell of the human form, billions of years of history are infused into it and are repeated as that cell continues to divide and multiply, becoming a baby. In this process, along with the original blueprint of the DNA, the cells use energetic phenomena such as psychological, spiritual, angelic, astrological, and cosmological forces. As a prospective parent, you can begin to view your child's emerging human body as a temple for his soul, a divine individualized human expression of the "one all-pervading Life."

According to Manly Hall, the "beginnings of the universe are recapitulated in the fertilization and cleavage of the cell. Ages so vast that the human mind cannot invoke even a shadow of their duration in the intellect are summarized in the activities following immediately upon the union of the sperm and ovum."[4]

Hall's contention—that within the memory of each cell is a recapitulation of humanity's condition throughout all the ages of the remote past—concurs with the view of embryologists that you cannot expand on a pattern without *including* the pattern, and therefore all first life-forms must be included within all successive life-forms. In his book *Embryogenesis* Richard Grossinger gives this example: "In a dramatic case that has been recognized from ancient times, the growing butterfly in the cocoon melts down the caterpillar until its integrity disappears within her own."[5]

In the first few weeks and months of your child's prenatal life the human embryo embodies numerous archetypal patterns that took the human race millions of years to evolve. Every human life actually embodies distinctive patterns of the four kingdoms—mineral, plant, animal, and human.

As esoteric anatomy texts describe the first four weeks in utero, the "infinitesimal nucleus of man is composed of the same elements as is the stone [mineral kingdom]."[6] In the next phase the embryo has been described as similar to a plantlike composition of thin layers enclosing a liquid. By the end of the first month, "the embryo has assumed a plant-like appearance; the esophagus, stomach, and intestine look like a vine."[7] During the fifth week, the hands and feet begin to develop, representing a correspondence with the fins of amphibians. Amphibians and reptiles are "partially individuated, and have inklings of personalities."[8] The third month is the recapitulation of the animal state and sexual differentiation. As we evolve in the womb until birth, we develop conscious awareness of words and symbols, thus transcending animal behavior, which has remained primarily unconscious and instinctual. We have become human. Sally describes her revelation when she conceived her child:

> When my son Alan was conceived, I felt as if I was experiencing the formation of an entire planet inside me. Knowing that he was evolving through the four kingdoms before the end of the second trimester inspired in me an awe for the miracle of human creation that was growing in my body. Becoming a mother meant I was a powerful expression of natural intelligence and evolutionary impulses. This was not just a batch of cells growing within me—it was vast kingdoms of life that I powerfully unfolded with my child. My pregnancy became a fascination about the miracle of life that I was to consciously assist.

By the fourth month the fetus takes on a human shape, her face has human features, and her characteristics distinguish her from all other vertebrates. Yet according to Hall, the fifth month of the prenatal epoch is associated with the ape, "as the body is thickly coated with woolly hairs." The apes have established an extensive social blueprint for humans to follow—living in groups, playing, and expressing intense emotions, especially love for their young. Grossinger observes that "ninety-nine percent of our genes are identical to the apes,"[9] yet we have mutated to such a degree that we could not effectively mate with one. This 1 percent difference provides a psychological and spiritual factor that no ape has experienced. As humans we know the difference between past and future. We recognize the presence or absence of virtuous qualities in each other, and we know the importance of spiritual law. And unlike the apes, each human being has the unique reality of an individualized soul. Mike says humorously:

> I was glad to learn that our sons were not just another reenactment of the evolution of the four kingdoms, but that along with all the wisdom of human evolution, they also possess the great consciousness of their minds and evolving souls.

Angelic Influence

This all sounds to you peculiar and too abstract and farfetched to make much sense. I would have you remember that much which is familiar to you today and which constitutes a definite part of the recognized facts of daily life would, a few hundred years ago, have been regarded as unusually peculiar, incomprehensible, and impossible.

Djwhal Kuhl

Along with all of the practical aspects of preparing for your future child, it can be comforting to remember the help you will be receiving from the spiritual realms. The angelic kingdom makes a vital contribution to your child's development down to the most minute detail. Angels have a great responsibility for the evolution of all human beings on earth, and they have a hand in designing the etheric blueprints for every form of nature, including the human kingdom. Consider Georgia's experience:

> I have always had a clear intuition that has guided me well in my life. From the moment my husband and I climaxed, I knew I had conceived twins. I saw two etheric presences over our bed with a very distinctive pink color. They felt totally loving and deliberately present for the incarnating souls. As we lay together, they came toward me and seemed to mingle with my own physical body for about two hours. Then I felt a literal physical sensation in my body that felt like the sperm and egg had connected, and the original etheric beings left my awareness . . . and it felt like new ones had appeared, although the actual feeling was very subtle. Fourteen weeks later, my husband was flabbergasted to learn that the ultrasound had confirmed what I had already told him: we had twins!

Outside our everyday awareness, angels are always present. Their dynamic, intelligent, and loving energies are not detected by the physical senses. The properties they carry are of a spiritual nature. To better understand how you can use this perspective in your preconception and prenatal journey, it is worthwhile to deepen your understanding of angels. Then you can decide whether this is a reality you wish to include in your prebirth health care program.

Angelic Perspectives

Most of the knowledge we have of angels comes from great mystic traditions and from the prophets and sages of different religions. According to these sources, angels operate on various levels, each level having its own properties and responsibilities. Angels are always aware of the source, the divine perfection, and the order of eternal life. Their purpose here is to serve creation and its many forms. Our entire universe is composed of a dance between angelic and human consciousness, on every level, from micro to macro. Our physical, emotional, mental, and spiritual bodies are constantly being influenced by the angels. What is more, according to many spiritual texts our subtle energy bodies and our chakras are actually partially *composed* of angels.

Angels have been depicted in Eastern art for thousands of years as the deities in the chakras. Angelic forms embellish many of the great paintings of Western art, especially those of the Renaissance period. The innumerable renderings of the Madonna and Child nearly always show angels accompanying Mary's aura and Jesus' birth, suggesting the innate presence of these etheric beings around the pregnant woman and newborn. Many cross-cultural myths depict angels as allies to the stories' protagonists; the religious texts of Sufism, Judaism, Christianity, and Hinduism all mention the creative influence on humans of the archangels Michael (leader of the archangels, "Slayer of Evil Intentions"), Gabriel ("Bringer of Good News"), Auriel ("Angel of the Night"), Raphael ("Divine Healer"), Melchizedek ("Eternal Lord of Light"), and Sophia ("Source of Wisdom"), to name just a few.

Theosophical teachings describe the intricacies of the angelic kingdom as it assists the process of reincarnation. Geoffrey Hodson, a great Theosophist of the twentieth century, described a clairvoyant study of the human embryo in his classic book *The Miracle of Birth:* "As a rule, it would appear that at least three members of the angelic hierarchy are present from the time of the opening of the life cycle. One of these operates from the higher level and is in possession of full knowledge concerning the karmic conditions of the Soul about to incarnate; he cooperates with his subordinates at the lower mental and emotional levels and passes on to them sufficient knowledge of the particular aspect and measure of karma which is to be worked out in the forthcoming incarnation."[10]

Angelic Influences in the Womb

According to esoteric theory, one presiding angel oversees the prenatal development process. This angel is guided by its own superiors and determines the balance of positive and negative karma to be experienced in the new incarnation without harming the progress of the soul. The physical, emotional, and mental personality bodies each have their own karmic patterns. Parents, race, nation, era, religion, environment, sex, and type and condition of body are all decided by the presiding angelic intelligences. The presiding angel determines which karmic position will allow the greatest flexibility for the incarnating soul to work them out. As discussed in chapter 5, karma—both positive and negative—is for the purpose of harmonizing, balancing, and learning and so is to be highly valued.

Your future child will have a building angel who is responsible for the development of each personality body until the moment of birth. While any adverse physical tendencies or potential diseases are given the best possible outcomes, the angels cannot ignore the karmic lessons that the personality and soul need to experience for their evolution.

The building angels who fashion the personality vehicle for the incarnating soul are assisted by nature spirits, semi-intelligent beings on the lower level of angelic evolution. Each nature spirit is associated with a specific natural element—air, fire, water, or earth—and they remain present with the soul from conception until death, building, repairing, and regenerating as karmic and physical law allow.

Once the karmic conditions are established by the higher angelic authorities and the lords of karma, the soul initiates its incarnation into human form, focusing its attention away from the soul realms and toward the physical plane of human life. Hodson observed that the foundation of the body is not solid matter but flowing electromagnetic energies. Throughout the pregnancy, the angels weave these energies and forces in response to the vibrational patterns of the incarnating soul. They adjust the seven chakras in the mental, emotional, and etheric bodies, as well as the associated physical nerve centers and glands.

According to Hodson, the various angels extend their auras around the mother and the mental and emotional bodies. Within the determined karmic conditions, they protect the newly forming personality vehicle from outside intrusion or shock. Debra recalls:

> During my fifth month, Ike and I were driving on a windy road and found ourselves sliding on wet leaves into a red clay bank. The car hit hard, but all of a sudden I felt a large white being embrace me— it felt like falling into a featherbed. My head whipped back and then the next thing I knew, I was on my feet outside of the car. My husband had a similar experience. We knew that some spiritual presence had intervened. We had no signs on our bodies of any harm, and yet when the police came, they said it was a miracle we came out unscathed. I knew our child was safe, for I had been cushioned in the bosom of an angel, a presence I had been feeling throughout my pregnancy. This experience confirmed my sense that our child was connected to angels. I had never even entertained the idea until I felt their distinct sensations the first month I became pregnant. I could feel them in the quiet hours of the night, combing my aura. When I would walk in the woods, I could feel them interacting with nature and my subtle energy body. We named our daughter Angelica in honor of their gifts to all of us. Sometimes she looks like an angel in a human body.

In Hodson's clairvoyant investigations of the prenatal life he perceived that during the fourth month, the angel in the soul realm instructs the mental-building angel about people from past lifetimes that the incarnating soul will meet again. Hodson saw these people as tiny figures in the angel's aura, some of them smiling, while others frowned, indicating pleasant or unpleasant associations with the incoming soul. The angel in the soul realm also instructs the mental-building angel about the entire karma that will be explored in the soul's present life. The building angel for the mental body communicates to the emotional body's building angel the essential karmic patterns concerning the emotional disposition of the incarnating soul. Hodson and others witnessed continual creative activity between the different angels and nature spirits during the entire pregnancy. In fact, it is not at all uncommon for a woman to intuitively feel, see, or hear angels while she is pregnant.

Angelic Assistance during and after Birth

According to the Theosophical tradition, all of the angels and nature spirits associated with preconception and prenatal life retreat into their own realm at birth. As the prenatal angels leave the scene of the birth, a great angel called the World Mother creates a thought-form of her image and projects a vivifying presence of her life force, infusing the mother and atmosphere with spiritual qualities of power, love, peace, and reverence. Angelic servants assist her during the birth. Then within eight to ten hours of birth, the life energies of this great angel are withdrawn. Some women report consciously working with the angels while attending births. Pam, a midwife and mother, reveals:

> Every time I am at a birth, the room fills with a light that seems to illuminate the whole space. Sometimes I think it is the incarnating soul filling the human form, other times I wonder if it is a special kind of spiritual entity. But I must admit, there is always an infusion of the Divine Mother qualities that seem to permeate everyone who is open, especially the new mother.

Your child will not be abandoned by the angelic kingdom during those precious moments following his birth. Along with the nature spirits, each incarnating soul also has a guardian angel who is with it from the moment of birth until death. Phoebe Bennet, another renowned Theosophist and clairvoyant, captured this cooperative dance between different angels as she observed their angelic assistance at the birth of an infant: "As far as one could tell, the angels spoke and worked in terms of consciousness rather than through any more concrete medium of expression. A ceremony seemed to be going on, in which the angels attendant upon the doctor, the incarnating ego, and the presiding angel were the chief celebrants. They appeared to be enacting a definite ritual, simple and yet profoundly mystical, which culminated, after the actual birth, in the giving of the infant into the charge of another angel, apparently its guardian angel, who up to this point had been quietly waiting [to] one side."[11]

According to these metaphysical perspectives, the angelic kingdom is not only present but actually essential for the development of your future child's human personality. These subtle energy beings are as responsible for the development of the soul's physical, etheric, emotional, and mental bodies as the atoms, molecules, and biochemicals of your own genes and those of your mate. As your conceived child grows in the womb, know that you will not be alone as you co-create a precious life *with the angels.*

Prenatal Bonding

"How do we learn prenatal bonding?" the newly pregnant couple asks.
Be loving to yourself, each other, and your baby as often as possible—
purposefully caring for the body, mind, and spirit without hesitation.

The Earliest Imprints

When we explored the idea of preconception bonding in chapter 5, you learned that you can intentionally begin loving your child and caring for her whole health before conception. Most people understand that once born, the baby's first cry and first look initiate a lifelong communication between parent and child. In the past decade the concept of prenatal bonding has achieved widespread support as ultrasound imaging, electron microscopes, and other laboratory procedures have allowed us to peek into the life of a child in utero.

Since the early 1980s, when prenatal psychology was publicly introduced through the pioneering work of Thomas Verny, M.D., and the research of many others, especially members of the Association for Prenatal and Perinatal Psychology and Health, we have learned that a baby in the womb has developed the emotional and intuitive sensitivity to experience the mother's inner and outer life. He hears his mother's voice and senses her love. Prenatal research demonstrates that your unborn child will see, hear, remember, taste, and think before and during birth. By the fourth month, he has well-developed senses of vision and touch—he will suck if his lips are stroked and shield his eyes if a bright light shines on the mother's womb. By the fifth month, he will raise his hands to cover his ears if there is a loud sound. Your child will be emotive, capable of communicating his aversion to your behavior.

Prenates clearly respond to the thoughts and feelings of the mother and to the father's style of communicating with her and the baby. This all-important communion can foster a dynamic interaction between you and your baby as she begins forming her personality. You can actually soothe, stimulate, and love your little one from the moment of conception onward. A child who experiences prenatal bonding is often more alert and enters the world with an innate sense that she is loved and wanted.

The Effects of Stress on Your Child in Utero

During the past several decades, many researchers have studied the behavior of babies in the womb by using ultrasound devices to perceive their reactions to certain stimuli. It is now clear that the child in utero is a very sensitive being who responds to overt stimulation from the inner and outer environment of the mother as well as to her interaction with other people, especially the father.

One of the leading pioneers in this research is David Chamberlain, Ph.D. In his book *The Mind of Your Unborn Baby* he describes in great detail the remarkable growth of the "preborn." The prenate's nervous system is already responding within five weeks of conception as his heart muscle is activated. Less than two months after conception the vestibular system—the part of the baby's nervous system that responds to gravity—begins to develop; if you jump about, your baby also jumps about, whether he likes it or not. The brain has measurable electrical activity by six weeks. Four months after conception your baby's "liquid breathing" is influenced by his mother's lifestyle—caffeine, alcohol, drugs, and nicotine can slow down or speed up his breathing, necessitating a stressful effort for him to get the oxygen he needs.[12] Your future child's higher brain centers are also forming in the womb. Many researchers have discovered that babies begin hearing as early as the eighteenth week of pregnancy, and they have distinctive musical preferences. In a London maternity hospital preborns who were four to five months old appeared restless when exposed to the intensity of hard-rock music. Vivaldi and Mozart, however, seemed to calm them.[13]

Measuring brain waves in prenates has shown that no later than the end of the seventh month of pregnancy, the brain responds to stimulation of vision, touch, and hearing. Chamberlain deduces that "this supports the assumption that even in the womb, your baby is capable of responding meaningfully to experience."[14] He firmly believes that preborns do not prefer loud sounds and benefit from more peace and harmony in their world. Chamberlain cites studies that show how important the mother's voice is to her preborn child, since the baby continually bathes in her sounds. He suggests that the "earliest experiences of sound in the womb can [either encourage or discourage] your baby's desire to listen and communicate. In extreme cases where the womb is a noise box, a baby may want to hide from life."[15] Prospective mothers—and fathers—can contribute to their baby's well-being by speaking lovingly and refraining from being excessively angry or chronically emotionally reactive. Your unborn child will like you to sing and hum soothing songs.

The wide-ranging effects that physical changes of pregnancy can have on the emotional state of the pregnant mother can be difficult to control. Deep, fluctuating emotions—including fear, sorrow, and joy—can take even the most conscious woman by surprise. But because the heart rate of the preborn can double when her mother is frightened, for example, you have a responsibility to protect your child from adverse stress and overstimulation. So . . . how will you cope with your authentic emotional experiences, the myriad changing feelings about yourself, your body, your baby, your partner, and your emerging role as a new mother?

My journal entry captures such feelings as I write to the soul during a more stressful month of the third trimester:

> Here I am, a vessel for your arrival onto earth, and I am not a reliable source of peace and joy. We have to move and we have not found a new home. We are having a home birth in less than two months and I have yet to know where your first moments of life will be—certainly in my arms, but where will my body lie as you slide out of it? I sense you feeling my chaos—my late-night worries bathing me. I surround you with white light and love to give you a "sound-proof" room from the static of my mind. I know you do not ask me to be perfect, just to be aware when I am really being anxious. Expressing my worries releases them and thus releases you from them. We are finding our new home together, and as you are feeling my fretting, you are initiated into the challenges of life on earth. You can bring heaven with you, and I will do the best I can to provide you with daily well-being—inside and outside of me. I have learned so much already from you the past year as I dedicate my life to nurturing your magnificent beingness. I have faith that we are together to love and heal each other as we both awaken to our true needs—moment to moment.

Once your child is born, he will thrive on stimulation if it is not excessive. When distressed, he will also be able to communicate by crying, fussing, or going to sleep. However, while he is yet in the womb you will not be able to clearly perceive your baby's needs. Since your preborn is sensitively alert to your voice and that of his father, he has no choice but to absorb any "vibes" that are disharmonious along with those that are harmonious into his sense of self, and his sense of you as a safe or unsafe caretaker. Be self-nurturing. Allow yourself to authentically, and frequently, feel your misgivings about being pregnant so that you can clarify the support that you need. When they arise, acknowledge your disquieting feelings so that when you *do* feel excited about your baby, you can experience that love more freely.

There is no such thing as a perfect way to experience pregnancy. As soon as you discover you are pregnant, you leave one part of your life behind and begin a new one. The momentous news that you are expecting is usually met with a mix of shock, acceptance, and, frequently, rejoicing. Which emotions you experience can vary greatly, depending on how prepared you feel. If the pregnancy is not planned, you may feel more overwhelmed than elated. Conflicting emotions are common, so do not be surprised if joy is mixed with doubt, denial, and fear of entrapment—but realize that your emotions can generate anxiety that will be passed along to your child in either subtle or direct ways.

As we explored in chapter 4, Preparing Your Mind for Conception, if you are feeling chronic ambivalence about being a mother or have any sense that you may become depressed or predominantly disconnected from your child in utero, please seek some professional counseling. It is possible you may just be going through a challenging adjustment that will resolve itself with time. It's appropriate to feel some anxiety, because your whole life is going to change radically; for some women, giving birth feels like a big hurdle. But if you have a sustained period when you are not feeling emotionally positive about being pregnant, or if your psychological state is such that you may be harming the prenate in any way, find someone who is trained to help you.

No matter what your personal history, you do not have to adjust to motherhood alone. New mothers often feel a deep yearning to be mothered themselves. As soon as she became pregnant, Sandy went through an unexpected shift in her relationship with her own mom:

> I never felt close to my mother. She judged me and withheld love when I did not meet her expectations. I have always felt emotionally "motherless." But once I became pregnant, my need to be nurtured and reassured by her became so strong that I called her up hysterically several times. For some reason, my vulnerability opened her heart to me. Our relationship went through a major transformation so that I was able to forgive her for her past neglect. My own impending motherhood felt so exciting yet the unknown was so

scary. My mom was able to offer me comfort because I allowed myself to need it from her. There were times when she still is unable to be physically or emotionally available to care for me. Then I ask for the support I need from my nurturing women friends.

Knowing that there will be times when you will feel overwhelmed, create a clear vision now of how you want to nurture your unborn child—physically and psychologically—in times of personal stress. Rather than getting stressed about being stressed, use this plan to develop a heightened sensitivity to the true needs of your prenate.

When you are agitated, try to create an activity that calms you. For example, try to meditate on peaceful images or sounds, or go somewhere and relax in silence. You can use soothing music to bathe your nervous system. You can use yoga or any form of dance or movement to release bodily tension and quiet your nerves. Sometimes simply expressing your feelings in a constructive way will release pent-up energy. Bella had a creative approach to caring for her unborn child:

> When I was newly pregnant with my first child, I wanted to offer her an idyllic environment, protecting her as much as possible from every harsh stimulus. I refrained from going to movies or watching TV programs with violent images, I listened only to light, relaxing music, and I made every effort not to have prolonged emotional bouts of anger with anyone, especially my husband. This ideal inspired me to try to let go of everything that strained or stressed me. Although the outer-world stimulation was easily controlled, my highly reactive emotional nature was hard to harness. At certain times, and under certain conditions, I just could not quickly transform my agitation.
>
> I discovered within the first month of my pregnancy that even with all my good intentions, I still would become irritated, especially when pregnancy hormones magnified every feeling. Yet I realized I could be more mindful to regulate the volume of my voice and, when I did get emotionally riled up, to release those negative emotions as soon afterward as possible. If, for example, my emotional expression had made my belly contract, tightening my uterus and possibly affecting my baby, I would talk to her, reassuring her that she was safe. I discovered that I could have a simultaneous awareness of my upset state while parts of me were able to consciously and intentionally separate her from me. Sometimes, while

in the throes of upset, I would intentionally surround her in a calming, warm, white light and send her feelings of peace from the part of me that was not aggravated.

At times when I was feeling really inadequate in controlling myself, I would place my hands on my belly and just rub it with a loving warm feeling for her. Thus, I was always free to communicate a sense of love to my unborn baby, even while unable to be loving to myself or another. I began to feel the power of my mothering instinct to protect my vulnerable child, even when I myself was the source of irritation. It gave me greater confidence that I would continue this sensitivity with my little girl for the rest of her life, and that I did not have to be perfect for her to feel trust and my love for her.

Note: Although it is definitely useful for specific medical indications, recently the extensive use of ultrasound has come under challenge as an invasion into your baby's natural world (for more information on the potential risks of ultrasound, see *Immaculate Deception II* by Suzanne Arms). Because of this, I do not advocate exposing your prenate to unnecessary scans in order to verify the information presented here. Rather, use this research of others to inspire you to create a peaceful inner and outer world for you and your child during your pregnancy.

Nurturing Your Child's Personality Nature

There are many things you can do to nurture your child's personality nature and enhance your pregnancy, whether you are emotionally reactive or not. Use your intuition or your imagination as you sense your child's perspective. For example, my pregnancy journal states:

> Today our new home fell through. We are less than two months from my due date and no home on the horizon. Bad enough I cannot nest. I am planning a home birth and have no place to deliver. Okay, Life. I can choose how I respond to this challenge. I am scared. I could get angry, too. When I entertain those feelings, I know that they are reasonable to feel. But do I want to bathe our baby in days of anxiety (for a solution to this may take a while)? How can I give her what she needs from me now while still being authentic to my bubbling fear? [I spent several minutes focused inside myself.]

When I just closed my eyes and felt the fear inside of me, I imagined it like stormy clouds passing through me. I also sensed our little baby needing to feel safe and secure. I filled my womb with a warm golden sun, which is always shining behind the clouds even on the bleakest day. I knew she would prefer this weather, even though other parts of me were feeling rather gray. I was glad I could remember to give her what she needed while being true to my reality. Now I am going to meditate and pray, restoring myself to a feeling of Faith in Life. I have never been abandoned yet, and I want to trust that the perfect home will be there for all three of us soon.

Journaling

You can see in this passage how visualization, meditation, and prayer can be used to calm feelings of distress. Sounds simple. It is. It works. You can also use journal writing to explore your feelings and thoughts about pregnancy as well as communicate your feelings directly to your baby in the womb. A paragraph from my journal reads:

Dear One, I write to you as a magnificent Soul, and as my beloved human child growing symbiotically within me. Today was really a challenge for me. I have soooooo much to do before you are in my arms and I am not nurturing myself enough in the process. I have not had time to meditate in weeks as I try to find us a home with your daddy. Are you noticing my pushing and lack of rest? Yet as I wobble about, there is the daily joy I feel for you, and the years of yearning to kiss your precious face—these fill me with a profound awe that seems to soften the tensest moments into a deep inner peace. I love being able to talk to you directly about my feelings, and know you are listening.

As I described in chapter 1, journaling is also very powerful to use when you are feeling the deeper, darker emotions about being pregnant. You can openly express the full spectrum of your prenatal feelings and thoughts because your journal is a completely nonjudgmental listener. Simone used her journal as a compassionate friend. She wrote:

Dear Journal, I need you to hear my fears again today. I am insecure about becoming a mom. I am insecure about my marriage. I am insecure about giving birth. I feel so relieved just to be honest with someone. To be truthful to you, which means to be truthful to me. Can I find a solution to this emotional roller coaster? I guess I need to listen to my gripping fear and care for it. Should I get some counseling or do I just need a dose of self-love? I think I need some real help as I hear how overwhelmed I feel. Thanks for listening.

Visualization

Using visualization, you can create meaningful images that deepen your rapport with your baby or enhance her well-being. You can imagine your baby in a specific form or as her majestic soul presence, perhaps appearing as an abstract image or symbol. While in a relaxed state, try to imagine meeting your child in a special place of peace. If you cannot see an image, sense her essence, feel her qualities, hear her voice speaking to you. Ask her if she has a message for you. Tell her anything your heart and mind spontaneously want to express. Share your concerns, hopes, dreams, visions. Write down any impressions you receive in your journal.

Music

You can use music to assist you in your relaxation as well as to soothe or stimulate your unborn child. Select calming tunes that open your heart to your baby. You can use the same piece of music each time so that it automatically is associated with the intention to relax, or you can choose a fresh piece to meet the mood of the day. If you do use the same piece of music throughout the pregnancy, do not be surprised when your baby recognizes it once he is born. Tory describes an experience that is common to prenatal stories:

> I had to commute sixty-five miles each way to my job during rush hour throughout my pregnancy. Before I got pregnant, the drive would stress me out. Then when I got morning sickness it became unbearable. Just when I thought that was done, I discovered that because of the baby's weight, my lower back would pound when I had to sit for more than a half hour. I knew it was up to me to keep my consciousness in a relaxed state so that the baby would be at peace. So I chose to listen to a tape of a very heart-expanding song that my friend wrote about a mother's love for her baby. After several weeks I began to enjoy my commute because it was precious time to bond with my baby without interruption. When she was born, we played the tape at her birth. She immediately stopped

crying. Eighteen months later she still responds to this song as if it were my very arms embracing her.

Research has shown that babies in utero prefer slow-paced music that resembles the rhythm of the resting maternal heartbeat. Compositions by such classical composers as Bach, Mozart, Haydn, Handel, Fasch, and Vivaldi are excellent for the pregnant mom. It has been commonly noted that prenates do not like hard-rock music. There is an easy way to decide if the music is a "thumbs up" or a "thumbs down"—if it does not relax you, it is not going to relax your babe.

Don't forget, the father can consider himself as having equal access to your child. He can sing songs and openly express his feelings to your child in utero by putting his mouth up against the mother's belly. Also, when the father frequently expresses his love and appreciation to the mother, her heart will open more to nourish the baby with kind feelings as well.

Sacred Space: An Attitude for the Pregnant Mother

As the pregnant mother you are providing a sanctuary wherein your baby can physically, psychologically, and spiritually thrive. Multiple states of consciousness will flow in and out of you like the tides during a full moon. Some will be subtle, like whispers from your child's soul, reminding you to stay calm and feel the divine life flowing through you. Other times, especially during the first trimester, the undertow of morning sickness—which can last through the day and night—may grab your attention so that the spiritual presence that can permeate your pregnancy is obscured while you cope with nausea. During such challenging, physically uncomfortable times, as well as the days when you may be overcome with irrational anxiety, focusing on the wonder of your pregnancy can be the most soothing, healing balm.

In my journal, I wrote about the challenge of remembering the blessed opportunity of having a soul incarnating from heaven to earth . . . in my body:

> Today I woke up feeling morning sickness and I have had no relief all day. Whenever I mention the discomfort of my pregnancy symptoms, others seem to love to tell me their horror stories about how difficult their pregnancy was, or how the tiredness only gets worse after the baby is born. The common attitude was one of distaste—

as if having morning sickness was like having a bad flu. I never heard anyone describe the absolute joy and awe that make these symptoms are tolerable because we can simultaneously focus on feeling the miracle of life growing inside the womb.

I know that I have the choice, moment to moment. I can feel dominated by the discomfort, or I can feel that my tiredness is a loud voice from my body telling me to relax and quietly celebrate that my little baby needed all of my energy resources to grow her precious spine and organs this week. The emphasis on my exhaustion blinds me from sensing the wonderment of her using *me* to grow and energize her heart—the temple for our love bond. Why don't the prenatal books I'm reading describe my experience as awesome, astonishing, incredible, extraordinary, beautiful, profound, and sacred? Why am I permeated with reverence for the divine essence unleashed within the very hormones that sustain this pregnancy? Together—child and I—we are *Divine Life* realizing *itself.*

Include the Divine

During pregnancy you can consciously remain connected to the spiritual presence of your baby. While lying in bed in the morning or night, or during times of feeling overwhelmed, place your hand on your belly and imagine her literal physical body in its particular stage of development. Then invite the incarnating soul to reveal its essence to you. Sense its attributes—often qualities of love, light, peace, joy—and bathe the little fetal form with these emanations from the soul. When you feel nausea or tiredness, try invoking the eternal life and light of the soul and allow it to pour into your heart and down through your hands, radiating the energy into your womb, warming it with feelings of reverence.

I wrote in my journal:

> Sometimes when I am so tired I cannot imagine going to work, I lie down and empower my hands to massage the unlimited vitality of my Soul into my nerves. With my intent, I can infuse the essential qualities of life into my breath, so that as I move through the stresses of life today, each inhalation and exhalation is imbued with celestial forces. And as I stand here on earth, growing an earthly body with my own, this union with the Divine reminds me that

there is a holy truth to "As above, so below." I pledge to include the Divine in my prenatal perceptions of myself, of my beloved, and of our baby. To honor the beatific qualities of her soul, as well as her emerging body is to embody the fusion of heaven and earth.

Think about how you and your partner can deepen your relationship to your baby while he is growing inside of you. Sometimes my husband would meditate on the soul and use his hands to massage his own inner sensations into the womb or other parts of my body. (There is nothing like a good back massage from your partner when his heart is filled with loving feelings for you and your baby!) Sometimes your partner may need to be reminded that he is free to develop his own relationship with the incarnating soul, and then translate that through his touch or voice into your body, where his child is housed.

This is a time to be shared fully with your partner. Meditate together on the soul qualities of your child and talk about your perceptions. A bouquet of flowers is a wonderful way to celebrate the miracle of your co-creation with your partner. You can draw pictures of your experiences to capture the subtleties that words cannot describe. The journal I shared with my husband is filled with entries from us both about our inner explorations. My husband wrote to our baby:

> What will emerge from the void of silence? Do you live in a light of a dream I know so well? Is your hair like the stream of golden sparks showering my meditations? Will you breathe on the belly of your mama and awaken us into your dream?

If you are reading this while pregnant, go ahead now. Delight in discovering ways to sustain a spiritual inner world for your baby. If you have yet to conceive, prepare yourself for the soul's arrival. Its first moments of human life, and thereafter, can be infused with your efforts to personify the divine.

Creative Exercise:
Optimizing Your Child's Prenatal Life

1. Understanding that your child-to-be is a multidimensional being who has specific needs each trimester to actualize the soul in human form, what do you want to do to assist this development?

   First trimester
   To enhance the baby's physical health, I choose to . . .
   To enhance the baby's emotional health, I choose to . . .
   To enhance the baby's mental health, I choose to . . .
   To enhance the baby's spiritual health, I choose to . . .

   Second trimester
   To enhance the baby's physical health, I choose to . . .
   To enhance the baby's emotional health, I choose to . . .
   To enhance the baby's mental health, I choose to . . .
   To enhance the baby's spiritual health, I choose to . . .

   Third trimester
   To enhance the baby's physical health, I choose to . . .
   To enhance the baby's emotional health, I choose to . . .
   To enhance the baby's mental health, I choose to . . .
   To enhance the baby's spiritual health, I choose to . . .

2. How can you use the understanding that there is angelic assistance for your baby and you throughout the pregnancy? Be specific.

3. In what ways are you concerned about stress affecting your pregnancy? Make a detailed list of the stressful activities and behaviors that you and your partner can eliminate from your life. What concerns and challenges need to be consciously worked with while you are pregnant? Be specific.

4. How do you want to integrate the limitless ways of prenatal bonding with your baby?

5. If sacred space is one of many attitudes for the pregnant mother and father to maintain throughout the pregnancy, what attitudes do you and your partner want to declare as part of your prenatal experience?

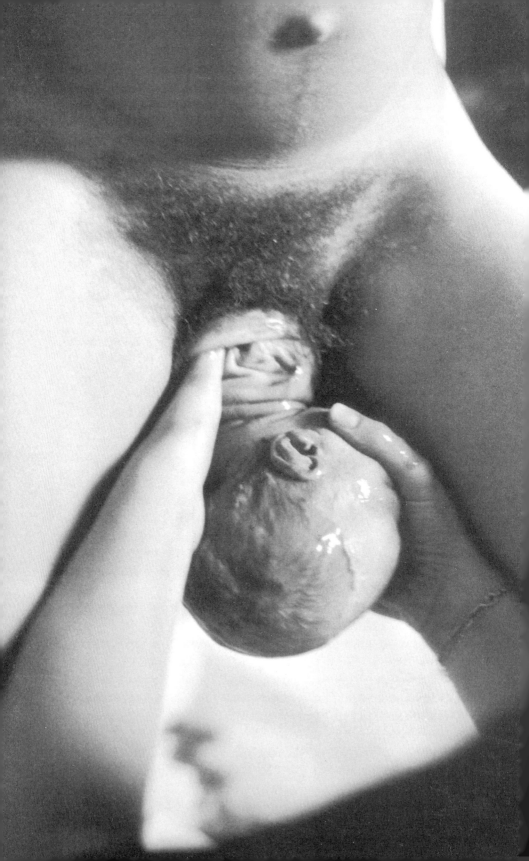

8

Birth and the Beginning of Your Baby's Human Life

The truth is, much of what we have traditionally believed about babies is false. We have misunderstood them and underestimated their abilities. They are not simple beings, but complex and ageless—small creatures with unexpectedly large thoughts.

David Chamberlain, Ph.D.

Birth is a rite of passage for you, your partner, and your baby. The process of birth is designed by nature to be a healthy passage into a natural world. Yet in the Western world during the past several decades, technological advances and interventions have placed most births in hospitals, rather than in a natural setting at home with an attending midwife or doctor present. In this process the emphasis has been focused exclusively on the physical health of the child, obscuring the psychological and spiritual aspects of birth. It is unlikely that anyone was consciously aware of your psyche and soul during your birth. Who, you may wonder, will be conscious of your newborn as an incarnating soul as well as a baby?

Birth is a life initiation of great complexity. Esoteric texts describe a great flurry of spiritual beings actively preparing for the moment of birth. Spiritual forces and beings impress their influences upon the soul as it is born into its earthly form. Descending from the heights of the spiritual world, the incarnating soul loses its perception of itself as divine; its awareness of spiritual states of consciousness fades. Communion with the highest spiritual sources dims, and vivid memories of the spiritual life cease at birth. Birth is often described as a soul leaving the spiritual realms of light through a dark, narrow door to be born into a human body. The loss of spiritual connection in the soul's descent into matter is further compounded by the stressful physical experience of birth.

The Lifelong Imprint of Birth

You have discovered how your child is conscious, with the capacity to develop her senses and memories, even in the womb. Since babies can have memories of their gestation, it is natural to assume that they are aware during their birth. Trauma experienced by your child at birth can produce lifetime ramifications.

In his historic book *The Mind of Your Newborn Baby* David Chamberlain, Ph.D., relates credible cross-cultural scientific evidence that some adults can accurately recall the events surrounding their own birth. Some people report abstract impressions, while others recall detailed descriptions. In Chamberlain's research pairs of mothers and children accurately recalled similar memories when hypnotized, although the mothers had never discussed details of the births with their children. Allowing for minor distortions in the facts, Chamberlain concludes that objectively gathered birth memories are reliable and "genuine recollections of experience."[1]

Other psychologists have reported recall of birth memories with such various psychotherapeutic techniques as hypnosis, psychodrama, psychoanalysis, primal therapy, breathing techniques, water-stimulated rebirthing, and guided imagery. The research of some of Chamberlain's colleagues includes extensive documentation of toddlers who spontaneously describe explicit birth memories without having previously been told of those events. Numerous child therapists are finding correlations between birth trauma and the presence of nightmares and phobias in their clients and troubling physical symptoms related to the head, spinal column, and breathing. Some also relate birth trauma to learning disabilities.

The highly respected primal therapy psychologist Arthur Janov enumerated many connections between the birth experience and psychological trauma in his book *Imprints: The Lifelong Effects of the Birth Experience*. Many prominent prenatal and birth psychologists share the belief that birth can often be trauma producing. Though the birth experience itself is generally brief, it is during this very sensitive time that the child's first experiences of life in the body are being imprinted. The newborn's first experience of human relationship can determine whether he feels love and safety or indifference and abandonment. Many prenatal psychologists have concluded that the inherent trauma of birth is likely to create lifelong personality patterns, a natural conclusion to be shared by those who believe that consciousness already exists at conception and in the womb. Anyone involved in birth, from the parents to the childbirth assistants, midwives, and doctors, can benefit by understanding birth trauma, its causes, and how to treat as well as prevent it.

According to Dr. Raymond Castellino and William Emerson, Ph.D., both pioneers in the identification and healing of prenatal and birth trauma, imprinting that occurs during birth and the period of time immediately following can affect our patterns of relationship and motivation, and how we assimilate nurturing. The way your child is born will leave a unique physical and psychological imprint. Vaginal births, cesarean section births, and surgical interventions, including forceps and vacuum extraction, each can have particular physical and psychological impacts. Anesthesia, epidurals, and any drugs that are used can chemically imprint your baby, including the development of the central nervous system, the psyche, and motor (movement) patterns. Variables such as twin birth, breech, and adoption can also affect personality and character structure in babies, children, and adults. Emerson and Castellino have developed groundbreaking healing techniques for assessing and resolving prenatal and birth trauma imprinting in children as well as adults.

With so much mystery and many uncontrollable forces involved in your baby's birth, even the best-informed parent cannot control all variables. Birth can be traumatic to a greater or lesser degree, and you cannot be expected to prevent all trauma that may occur.

However, with conscious awareness, you may be able to minimize a birth trauma and help effect a positive transition for your child from the womb into the world. Explore the impact of drugs and medical interventions on your child's whole health so you can make informed choices and decline invasive extras if there is no obvious need for medical interference.

Adverse impacts from a baby's birth may be responsible for the baby's inability to nurse and can also impact the bonding process between the baby and parents. Resolving the existing trauma releases the depths of human potential in your baby. The healing of a birth trauma is an opportunity to learn greater emotional expressiveness and empathy between you and your child.

If your child should experience adverse birth imprinting that results in problems with nursing, bonding, attachment, or development, or you are aware of trauma that may have an impact on your baby's well-being such as having the cord wrapped around her neck, loss of oxygen, forceps or vacuum extraction, cesarean birth, or prolonged labor and delivery stress, you will benefit from getting an evaluation by a birth trauma specialist.[2] After resting relatively peacefully in the dark womb with no stimulation from human touch, comforted by her mother's heartbeat, your baby will be thrust into the external world, bombarded by light, noise, and stimulation. Trauma as a result of this great change is not unusual, and the lack of proper postnatal care can cause long-term health challenges.

In preparing for your baby's birth, however, you have an opportunity to provide the most gentle and nurturing conditions for your baby's transition.

Preparing for Your Baby's Birth

Now that you understand the implications of birth trauma, look into some of the ways you can lessen the degree of trauma your baby experiences by learning how you can prevent some of the potential complications of childbirth. Whether you choose a natural or medicated delivery, decreasing your anxiety about birth will increase your ability to respond to the challenging phases of your birth experience. The dilating of the cervix, the uterine contractions, and the pressure of your baby's head as it moves down the birth canal and pushes against the tissues of the vagina and perineum are all healthy, normal sensations and pains. The pain inherent in childbirth is not just physical; it also can be psychological. The body-mind connection that affects preconception and prenatal health continues to play a role with a woman's emotional state and her reproductive system responses during birth. Researchers have found links between unaddressed maternal fear and unhealthy labor patterns.[3]

If you feel a lack of confidence in your ability to give birth and mother your child, now is the time to address your concerns. A holistic approach to childbirth preparation will guide you to extend your commitment to include the physical, emotional, mental, and spiritual aspects of your baby's birth. You, your partner, and your baby all will be profoundly affected by the birth environment and by the people participating in the birth. I encourage you as the mother to choose to make it an empowering experience for yourself. Take charge of your childbirth before it happens. Locate childbirth educators who can teach you skills for coping with labor pain in addition to the mechanics of labor and delivery. Choose someone who embraces your emotional concerns as well. As with the preconception and prenatal phases of parenthood, childbirth is a potent time for personal growth.

During your labor you will be extremely suggestible and will be vulnerable to internalizing the emotions and thoughts of those who attend the birth. If you are in a deep moment of fear and doubt, do you want someone there to offer you medication, or do you want encouragement and reassurance that you can endure the challenge?

Since your doctor or midwife will strongly influence many aspects of your birth experience, do not underestimate the importance of choosing these attendants. You'll want to find someone with whom you can have an open, communicative relationship before and during the birth, rather than an authoritative person who disrespects your feelings and need for support. If you're opting for a hospital birth, learn your doctor's position on drugs, monitors, episiotomies, cesarean section, and father involvement. Make sure your doctor supports natural childbirth, if that is your choice, and will not interfere with normal labor unless there is a real medical need. Educate yourself thoroughly about the side effects drugs may have on you and your baby, as well as the risks of medical intervention. Do not depend on your doctor as your only source of information about the ramifications of medicated childbirth, for many physicians' views are biased based on their medical training or personal beliefs.

Read numerous perspectives. Explore your local library or bookstore as well as the Internet. There are many birth preparation methods, each offering specific breathing and relaxation techniques. Some instructors are true to a single method while others blend techniques from more than one system. I like the comprehensive approach of William Sears, M.D., and his wife, Martha Sears, R.N., authors of *The Birth Book.* Dr. Robert Bradley's *Husband-Coached Childbirth* and Grantly Dick-Read's *Childbirth without Fear* were among the first to popularize methods that challenged the traditional notion of escaping from childbirth pain. These systems emphasize fully experiencing birth sensations. A woman can learn to focus on her inner signals to manage pain during labor. Rather than dissociate from labor pain, she can enroll the support of others who will support her in this. This natural approach to childbirth encourages mother and father to take responsibility in choosing attendants who will align with their desires.

If you do decide to choose a hospital-managed birth, realize you may be signing up for scheduled inductions, Pitocin augmentation, electronic fetal monitoring, and epidural analgesia. While clearly there are cases when this technology is medically appropriate, interventions should not be a routine package deal. In her book *Immaculate Deception II* Suzanne Arms passionately reveals the unhealthy impact of technological and medical interventions on the mother and baby. It is certainly possible to arrange a more satisfactory hospital birthing experience, but it requires perseverence and a supportive medical team.

You should also be aware in a hospital birth that you are allowing the hospital or doctor to determine the first moments of your child's life in the world. Impersonal hospital protocol may become your newborn's first exposure to human touch, sound, and relationship. Because your newborn will also have received any drugs you choose to take, he may need to be medically evaluated before you are allowed to bond with him. You may be separated from him immediately once he comes out of the womb. The Birth Wish List in appendix B can guide you in creating a more positive hospital birth for you and your babe.

In choosing medical birth you will want to choose a doctor and nurses who are highly sensitive and compassionate toward the mother's, father's, and baby's well-being throughout pregnancy and labor. If you are to have an empowering experience of creating your birth journey together, your doctor should encourage you to trust your body—rather than technology or drugs—to deliver your baby. Take as much time as you need to interview doctors, midwives, or birth attendants, and trust your intuition in creating the best possible birth team to assist and comfort you. Be aware, too, that while your own doctor may agree to your requests for a gentle birth, he or she may not be on duty during your labor, and your requests may not be honored by the other personnel. You should discuss this possibility with your doctor well in advance of the birth.

Terry and Joel felt deeply regretful of their decision to leave their child's birth up to their doctor. Terry says:

> When I was in early labor, I called my doctor to tell him my waters had broken. He told me that I could go to the hospital and begin being monitored. He never gave me the impression that he was the least bit interested in supporting me to give birth naturally as he began to rattle off my drug options. He told me it was unlikely I

could do it without medical help because it was my first time. Then he told me he would meet me at the hospital when it was time to push my baby out. I was devastated because I had told him I was afraid and I needed him there to support me. He scolded me and told me doctors are there only for the delivery, not the labor, and that it is standard hospital procedure. He seemed indifferent about my need for him, not even referring me to anyone else at the hospital for support. He said the fetal monitor would protect me from danger. Imagine that. Mother Nature and my own body strength and breath were less important than a darn machine. I wish I had been informed of other options.

Our second child was delivered at home, a striking contrast to our first son's birth. Our midwife honored my fears, and she walked me through each contraction with great patience and love. Most important, she exuded confidence in my ability to trust myself in surrendering to the birth energies—which I discovered was quite easy with her nurturing support. It was so healing to reclaim the power of birth that was always there inside me.

As you take greater responsibility for the birth of your child, remember that the beginning of your child's life profoundly matters. Do whatever it takes to surround yourself with the most loving and wise support you can find.

Home birth with a qualified midwife offers an entirely different alternative to a hospital birth with a doctor, nurses, and technicians. In *Gentle Birth Choices*, Barbara Harper, R.N., cites landmark studies that suggest childbirth can be as safe, if not safer, outside of a hospital setting as long as there is quality prenatal care and the support of a qualified midwife or physician during labor and delivery.[4] Numerous studies also show that the quality of care given by a midwife is often superior to most doctors' care. This is because the midwife usually takes more time to educate and support women during the pregnancy. There is often a greater focus on nutrition and psychological concerns throughout the pregnancy and more enthusiasm, patience, and skill to support you in a natural low-tech birth. During labor the midwife remains with you, whereas many doctors manage your labor over the telephone with the labor and delivery nurse until it is time for you to deliver, or you or your baby become "high risk."

If you are not able to find a qualified midwife or if home birth is illegal in your state, a safe alternative to hospital birth is a freestanding birth center. Most birth centers avoid invasive or restrictive procedures unless medically necessary, and the primary care givers are midwives. Birth center professionals screen potential clients carefully and recommend hospital births for those women who are high risk and need to be cared for by specialists.

If you choose a hospital birth, you may want to arrange for a birth assistant, often called a labor coach or doula. Continual emotional and mechanical support from a birth coach has been shown to significantly reduce the use of oxytocin, pain medication, forceps, and epidurals, as well as decreasing the length of labor, the incidence of cesarean sections, and other birth complications.[5] During your third trimester, ask your childbirth educator or doctor to recommend a coach in your area. Most people who use a midwife do not have a birth coach, since the midwife is present during the entire birth. In most hospital births fathers have little or no experience with the process, so an experienced coach can offer her skill to enhance the mother's natural ability to trust her body. She does not dominate, control, or manage the labor but offers a nurturing presence that empowers the father's involvement and allows the mother to feel confident that all is progressing well. She also has the ability to advocate for the couple if the doctor or nurse recommends medical treatment. This becomes very important if the mother needs emotional support and tranquillity to endure labor pain when there is not yet a clear need for medical intervention. At the same time a seasoned labor assistant will perceive the real need for medical support when the couple may be unaware that mother and baby are entering a risky condition.

Birthing plans (or what I prefer to call a birth wish list, since the mystery of birth cannot be planned or controlled) are commonly brought into the hospital birth experience. This list itemizes the parents' requests so that any nurse or doctor on duty will understand their wishes. Such lists typically include that no medical interventions will be undertaken unless the mother or child is at risk. Other common requests are no episiotomy, no forceps or vacuum extraction, no drugs, and no unnecessary monitoring. Keeping the mother and baby together immediately following birth to promote bonding and breast-feeding is another important item to include, as is, if it is necessary to separate mother and child, permitting the father to be with the baby at all times. A comprehensive birth wish list can be found in appendix B.

Inform yourselves about the use of silver nitrate, vitamin K, and any immunizations, which are often given to your baby only hours after the birth. This is your baby, not the hospital's, so feel free to protect her from routine medical protocols that are not always necessary and can cause harm. In his book *Vaccines: Are They Really Safe and Effective?* Neil Z. Miller explores how mandatory vaccines can trigger developmental disorders and autoimmune diseases that have lifelong implications for a baby's health. Immunizations have become very controversial, so research the most current information.[6] As a parent, you do have freedom of choice in how you safeguard your child.

There are so many ways you can create your birth experience—at home, at the hospital, in a birth center. Some couples choose water birthing because the buoyancy and warmth of the water deeply relax the mother, often shortening labor and alleviating pain. Some couples create their own birth tank, resembling a hot tub, at home; others use a deep bathtub. Michel Odent, M.D., author of *Birth Reborn*, who successfully facilitated underwater births in birth tubs at a general hospital in Pithiviers, France, says, "The right place to give birth would be the right place to make love."[7]

In determining where to give birth I always tell my clients that choosing a place where they feel safe will help them reduce inhibitions and deeply relax. Soft lighting and low noise stimulation are frequently chosen by those who are trying to create a conscious environment in which to give birth. Not only does the mother benefit, but the baby has a more gentle transition into the new world of sensations. Those who are spiritually oriented may want to create an intentional sacred space that can include devotional music, prayer, and flowers. You can invoke the presence of the soul, guardian angels, saints, birthing angels, or any holy being—real or imaginable. Many of these elements can be brought into a hospital birth.

Wherever you choose to create your birth experience, your baby will enter a world where all will appear new and strange. His miraculous entrance into the world can be surrounded with love and safety or fear and insecurity. Now is the time to envision your child's first experience of the world.

My journal entry four hours into giving birth to my daughter at home:

> It is 6:15 A.M. . . . I have been up—oops, here comes a contraction— since 2:30 A.M. with gentle contractions . . . easing slowly into the

Tao of Birth. Primal Instinct moves the waves of energy through my body . . . as I continue breathing into the opening and softening of a warm liquid life that is our baby—oozing through my body. I feel the baby align with me, and I align with Divine Presence. Our baby is on her way and is welcome. There is One Life and we are one with this all-pervading life . . . and I ask this Life to bless us with an ecstatic birth, as I surrender.

It is finally happening—over a decade of waiting to meet you, beloved child. Here comes another contraction . . . open, breathe, yield, flow, go, move, adjust, adapt, blend with it . . . and it pulses through my nervous system. My body knows how to do this—to open to fresh life itself . . . to say *yes!* to motherhood, love, family, and devotion to you, our Divine Child. Welcome.

The Fourth Trimester: Your Child Still Linked to Heaven

Written several days after giving birth, my journal entry reflects my dedication to honoring my daughter's spiritual heritage:

You were born in the beauty and bounty of our home. I knew you were a girl all along, from before conception. Your birth was amazing, transformational. Labor pain: like a cannonball of potent energy . . . my body expanded to accommodate your emerging presence into this world. When your head crowned through the opened gate of my pelvis and you came pouring through and out my body, you were placed on my belly. I will never forget your warm, wet skin sliding against my tummy and chest. Seeing your radiant presence shining through your vulnerable physical body, I realized Daddy and I were your first earthly experience with Divine Love. You are counting on us to sustain your connection to the sublime world of spirit that you descended from into our arms. We will protect you from the harshness of this world during your transition. We are dedicated to providing you with the life conditions that will enable you always to remember your true spiritual birthplace.

The miracle of birth. A soul, your child, has incarnated. Having both contributed your love and energy to the soul's coming, you celebrate this time of elation in wonderment that your baby has arrived. Birth is life's beginning, yet it is a continuation as well. From the soul realms, your child has been on a long journey of evolution and preparation for this lifetime, most of which will be veiled from her awareness unless you help her remember her true origins.

At the time of birth a baby is still totally dependent on his mother for food and protection, as he was in the womb, and interconnected with her psyche and biochemistry as well. Ashley Montagu calls this "fourth trimester," the phase of gestation outside the mother's belly, "a womb with a view." Studies indicate that mothers who lovingly bond with their babies through breast-feeding, constant skin contact, and eye gazing immediately after birth and throughout infancy have children who are more independent and confident in early childhood.[8] The bonding relationship is powerful, and the need for this profound interdependent attachment in both mother and child are undeniable. If bonding has been established before birth, it is simply a natural deepening of an already secure relationship.

After the birth both your partner and you undergo many physical and psychological transformations. The force of your thoughts and feelings imprints upon your child's inner and outer life. Psychically, your love blossoms and enfolds your baby with a soothing tenderness. Esoterically, this outstreaming of a mother's psyche and soul surrounding her newborn is referred to as a Madonna's Cloak. This protective psychic garment radiates into the atmosphere around the child. If the mother's soul consciousness is loving, the cloak is filled with warm colors and radiates light; if her soul life is dull, the quality of the cloak will reflect this. For the newborn, this cloak is a spiritual reality that genuinely envelops her. During her early months, and even through her first three years, your baby is affected by the quality of your psychic soul life. The father also weaves his own qualities into the cloak's texture and tones. When the parents' relationship is full of warmth, peace, light, and love, it imbues the cloak with the forces of heaven that the incarnating soul requires for its optimal evolution in its new human body.

During the critical "fourth trimester," there is a need to protect your child from any threats to her well-being. The sensory stimulation of modern civilization can be stressful even for adults. During her many transitional stages, your baby's soul will require sensitivity. She will be far from mastering any of her personality bodies—physical, emotional, mental, or spiritual. Your newborn is designed by nature to need you totally, to depend on you for all of her security and comfort, to drink deeply from your loving touch, gaze, and voice.

At birth the baby comes from the water element of the womb to the air and earth elements of the world. It can take your baby's nervous system several months to adjust to the external "disturbances"—the new auditory, visual, and tactile stimulation—which can actually create irritation and a feeling of intrusion for your newborn. Up until now, your newborn has only heard the steady, dependable sound of heartbeats. Now television, music, or voices may blare in his ears. Many parents choose to avoid exposing their newborns to harsh mechanical sounds, which can feel jarring to the delicate senses of a budding nervous system. Some people who live in cities or busy suburbs choose to keep their babies indoors as much as possible for the first weeks or months, in a soothing, protective environment.

East Indian birth customs prescribe that for the first three to six days after birth, only chosen relatives are allowed in the room where the child resides. The belief is that the newborn's mind is like a photographic plate, and the first sensory impressions of life affect the foundation of her whole life. The mother, too, is protected from visitors for the first six days because she is hypersensitive to disharmonious energies.[9]

As a newborn, your baby will be sleeping a lot as his consciousness transitions from the spiritual realms to his earthly existence. At around six weeks you will begin to notice a change in his alertness to his surroundings: he will become more responsive to your normal activities and noises. Yet you should still surround him with refined sensory impressions. You can begin to introduce him to nature, soothing music, and gentle, positive interactions with people. While adults can differentiate and reject a sensory stimulation that is unappealing, the infant is not yet able to protect himself from harmful sensory impressions. His state of peace or disharmony is largely dependent upon you.

Breast-Feeding

Rudolph Steiner, founder of Waldorf education, wrote of the close connection between your child's soul life and her senses. According to Steiner, a child has at least ten senses—the usual five, plus rhythm, balance, movement, warmth, and "sense of the other's ego." Although your child has the ability to see and hear from birth, rhythm, warmth, and touch are the most important senses for the child less than six months old.[10] The infant will become more actively conscious of the world of sights and sounds after about six months of age.

Steiner states that a rhythmic pattern to your child's day will be very beneficial for his long-term health. Eating, sleeping, and playing should be on an ordered, yet not fixed, schedule; the latter is not realistic for a newborn feeding on demand. When breast-feeding, the child will be aware of the rhythmic pattern of his mother's heartbeat. The importance of warmth is often underestimated in many newborn care books. According to Steiner, a baby must have a consistently maintained body warmth to perfect his organs and maintain good health. This suggests securely wrapping your baby in a blanket in the early weeks (leaving his arms free to point upward), offering him the enfoldment he experienced in the womb. Later, your baby's gestures will suggest that it's time to simply place a blanket over him. Check throughout the day that your baby's feet, hands, and tummy are warm.

Regarding the awakening of your baby's sense of touch, soft clothes made from natural fabrics are most beneficial for her first kinesthetic experiences. Kissing, cuddling, massaging, and breast-feeding are supreme ways to nourish the primal need for early skin contact. In fact, breast-feeding is the most nurturing way to provide the three primary senses of rhythm, warmth, and touch to your baby throughout the day. Parents of babies who are bottle-fed will need to be creative in finding other ways to provide this sensory development. If you choose to bottle-feed your child, let her rest in your arms in a cozy embrace rather than feeding her in a baby carrier. You can simulate the kind of contact the breast-fed baby enjoys by holding her in a similar position, skin-to-skin and near your heartbeat.

Breast-feeding is one of the great joys of motherhood and an initiation of profound love with your baby. It is very important to thoroughly explore the benefits of breast-feeding. La Leche League's popular book *The Womanly Art of Breastfeeding* is very informative. Suzanne Arms has also written a comprehensive and empowering guide called *Bestfeeding: Getting Breastfeeding Right for You*. Both of these books detail many positive reasons to breast-feed, including enhancing bonding, stimulating constant skin-to-skin contact, and maturing eye and facial development as mother and baby share gazes. Breast milk produces complete nutrition for at least the first six months of your baby's life, and the colostrum produced during the first several days after the birth also provides your baby with antibodies to disease. Also, colostrum coats the digestive tract so that only beneficial bacteria begins to proliferate.

You will probably feel that you and your baby are nourishing one another in a mysterious bond that transcends your physical connection. Karen feels that she and her first daughter missed a fundamental life experience that she was able to share with her second daughter:

> When Susie was born about twenty years ago, there was no information about breast-feeding anywhere. The norm was to feed your newborn with formula. I decided to breast-feed anyway, but my child was having trouble with her sucking reflex, and there was no such thing as a lactation consultant in those days. I finally had to let go of breast-feeding her. I was in so much grief, my body ached for the closeness that a bottle feed could not provide.
>
> When my second daughter, Lynn, was born ten years later, I had the same problem. But a lactation nurse showed me a very simple solution. All I needed to do was hold her in different positions. I realized how a little education and support can make all the difference for so many new mothers struggling with the first few days of breast-feeding. I feel sad that the lifelong benefits of breast-feeding Susie were simply lost due to the lack of aid and understanding. Now whenever I can, I tell pregnant women to make sure that they really understand the great benefits they give up if they choose not to breast-feed. I'll always remember the blissful states of love that would wash through my body as my little one suckled away at my breast.

Circumcision

"To circumcise or not to circumcise"—that is the question for many new parents of a boy. The belief that circumcision is necessary for medical or hygienic reasons has been proven obsolete, and since 1975 the American Academy of Pediatrics has not recommended routine circumcision. Parents should be aware that routine circumcision is not medically necessary and can be harmful to your son. Circumcision surgery is traditionally done with the boy tied down on a restraining board without his parents, and sometimes without anesthesia—using clamping devices and scissors for a five- to ten-minute procedure. During a routine circumcision, it is common for "newborns [to] scream, tremble, choke, wail, hold their breath, vomit and agonize."[11] Now that we know that newborns perceive pain as fully as adults, we must rethink this procedure, especially because it is often performed for social rather than religious reasons. Please devote yourself to the lifelong well-being of your son by researching the latest findings about the physical and psychological traumas that accompany this practice.

Whether or not your religious or family beliefs include circumcision, choosing this procedure means that your baby's first adaptations to his body will be fraught with pain and discomfort. In his book *Say No to Circumcision!* Thomas J. Ritter, M.D., a diplomat of the American Board of Surgery and a general surgeon for more than three decades, reports that the Jewish community is reexamining its position on circumcision and that "Christianity does not require or promote circumcision."[12] A national organization, Jews Against Circumcision, counsels families who are trying to reclaim their religious traditions while honoring their own differing values. In addition, many insurance programs and companies, including some Blue Cross and Blue Shield groups, will not pay for routine circumcision, since the procedure is not medically necessary.

Those who are concerned about their uncircumcised son feeling uncomfortable in the locker room should take heart: the locker rooms of the next millennium will reflect the steady decline in U.S. circumcision rates. If you are a circumcised father who is concerned about your son looking like you, realize that he is entitled to his own identity and appearance. You can always explain to him that medical recommendations changed and that you did not want him to undergo a painful procedure.

Numerous well-known physicians oppose circumcision, including Benjamin Spock, M.D., who wrote, "My own preference, if I had the good fortune to have another son, would be to leave his little penis alone." Ashley Montagu, Ph.D., writes that "circumcision is a very cruel, very painful practice with no benefit whatsoever." Commenting on Ritter's book, Dr. Frederick Leboyer said that "no one is aware of the deep implications and life-lasting effect [of circumcision]. The torture is experienced in a state of total helplessness which makes it even more frightening and unbearable."[13] If the primary dictum in medicine is "First, do no harm," one has to wonder about the wisdom of exposing a newborn to this surgery, usually without even his parents to comfort him.

If you choose to go forward with this procedure, make sure your baby has anesthesia and that you are there to help him with the pain and shock. Carefully choose doctors who will be authentically compassionate toward your baby and you before, during, and after the surgery. Empathically reassuring your son that he can express his fear and anger during circumcision will help him release the tremendous physical and psychological stress that he will incur. Immediately afterward breastfeed him, rock and reassure him with your voice, and surround him with relaxing light and sounds. Remember that your baby is freshly born and is more in heaven than on earth.

Nourishing Your Body, Mind, and Spirit—For Moms

My journal entry describes my first expressed dilemma with my newborn girl:

> It has been a week and I am trying to let go of Time and surrender to your needs—eat, snuggle, diaper, sleep—the daily dance between us—again and again. I am exhausted and challenged to know when you will need me. Changing diapers is a tall order, a major project for a woman who is used to mastering her reality. Confidence is building a little more each day. Yet I fret about my ability to take care of you. I wonder if your diaper is changed enough, is your belly button clean enough, are your clothes washed with the right detergent for your skin, is your body cleaned correctly, are your little nails clipped painlessly, are you well fed? Are you sleeping and playing enough? Am I? *Can I take care of myself? Can I nourish me?* If I run out of energy, who is going to energize you? All day long I have to choose whose needs are more important at any given moment. Ah! So this is motherhood.

As a new parent, the absolute joy and wonder of bonding with your baby will be mixed with many trials—sleepless nights, endless caring for your newborn and other family members, and the never-ending housework. After the birth, the mother will experience many physical and psychological changes. The instinctive tenderness and compassion that will awaken in you toward your baby will sustain and guide you through the challenges of early parenthood. You may experience a loss of identity, a death and rebirth of your life values, a radical shift in your social and professional life, and a grand awakening to a new sense of life purpose and goals. Deep and rich insights will surprise you at the most unexpected times, awakening you to new aspects of your character while changing your baby's diapers at 3 A.M. Who would have believed you could be awoken every few hours throughout the night and still love your child so much? Several weeks after Kylea's birth my journal entry reads:

> Time melts into days of nursing, hour upon hour of melting into loving this gorgeous child and beautiful, sweet Soul. I adore Kylea. The bond. A mystical cord of loving energy that ties us through a feeling of mutual giving, caring, being. Time merges into the endless cries of breast-feeding—weeks have fused into one long instinct to mother my precious girl. Goals have become as simple as getting

a daily shower, sneaking in a walk, or making a phone call. Eating a meal creates a feeling of having a successful day! She cries—my life drops into full service of her needs. My relationship with Jared is strained. Yet I know it is temporary as my exhaustion demands that I conserve my energy to feed and care for Kylea. It is a phase, I trust, and our relationship is strong enough to withstand this grand initiation called "learning to sacrifice my own needs for something greater: unconditional love for my newborn."

Your partner, friends, and relatives can help with essential everyday tasks, allowing time for both parents to bond with the new babe. Yet if the mother is going to be the primary nurturer, she must first be able to nurture herself. Within a day or two of birth a woman's progesterone and estrogen levels will be lower than before pregnancy. Prolactin surges to meet the demands of breast-feeding. Other hormones such as endorphins and oxytocin, as well as huge changes in the thyroid and pituitary glands and massive loss of blood and body fluids from the birth experience, can create major chaos in a woman's body. You will need rest and the relaxation of unstructured activities to help you adjust to the hormonal changes in your body. You'll need to be very gentle with yourself so that you can rebuild and replenish your reserves.

If you are breast-feeding, you will need to devote your energy to nourishing yourself so that you can nourish your baby. To breast-feed your newborn, you will need an average of five hundred extra calories per day.

It can take new moms many months to regain the energy consumed by the birth experience and breast-feeding. Giving birth depletes a woman's vital energy, and she is often left emotionally exhilarated but physically exhausted. Depending upon your prenatal health, you may experience varying degrees of postpartum imbalances. Whether you had a natural delivery or a cesarean section—which is major surgery and requires four to six weeks of bed rest—also will play a role.

Most women need about six months to regain their energy reserves. Certainly during the first days and weeks, a new mother must rest and sleep whenever possible and refrain from any kind of work except caring for her newborn. According to traditional Chinese medicine, exercise should be restricted to walks—no excessive or strenuous activity—to optimize postpartum recuperation. You will have plenty of time to get your normal muscle tone back. Now is the time to nourish yourself and replenish the life force that your baby has used from your body for prenatal development. Gentle Kegel exercises, which are recommended throughout pregnancy in most prenatal exercise books, can begin soon after delivery to strengthen the perineal muscles as well as body tissues and organs.

A doctor trained in traditional Chinese medicine can prescribe a custom-designed herbal remedy to assist you with postpartum recovery. If you experience symptoms such as excessive bleeding, an inability to create breast milk, an overproduction of milk, or inflammation of the breasts during lactation, consider contacting a Chinese medical doctor and herbalist, who can recommend herbs that are healing for you without being harmful for your breast-feeding baby to consume.

Get Some Help

Very few first-time parents have been adequately prepared for caring for their newborn. Many new mothers expect to feel capable of meeting the demands of their baby. Most couples were never taught to expect that they would need guidance and support. If the newborn is breast-feeding, the mother must be available to her child around the clock. As the newborn's needs become inseparable from her own, her abrupt loss of independence can create in her a dependency on someone else. This changes within several months (usually between weeks five and eight) when the mother can pump breast milk and the dad or other caretaker can feed the baby with a bottle. The mother then has a chance to revive herself with a self-nurturing activity. If the father chooses to actively coparent and be available to assist, his daily presence can help immeasurably. Or if a family member, friend, or hired professional assistant is able to "mother the mother," then she is replenished to mother her baby with greater joy and ease.

If all of your basic needs are met by others, you'll easily be able to surrender into the role of round-the-clock loving care for your baby. It is natural for you to desire to spend the first weeks and months melting into divine union with your baby. Free from the stresses of your normal daily responsibilities, you can delight in the timeless cycle of getting to know your baby's personality and needs. For their optimal well-being, this is a holy period of bonding for mother and child. For the first several months after the baby's birth, the father needs to become a reliable presence of support who will nurture and protect the baby and the mother. He can be an intermediary with the outside world, thus sheltering the new mother from anything that would disturb her care of their child. If, perhaps because of work responsibilities, he is unable to provide this unconditional support, he can enlist the help of others in his support network.

Sleep deprivation can affect both you and your partner during the first several months, challenging the best of relationships. It is normal for the dynamic between a new mom and dad to be strained; the more outside help you can rally to cover the daily household chores, the greater your opportunity will be to rest and restore yourselves and your relationship. If you are a single mother, outside support is imperative. Nature never meant for new mothers to be alone.

Sometimes when women feel isolated from their previous life, and they have no time for self-care due to the demands of a newborn, they may experience a mild or more severe case of postpartum depression (PPD). PPD is not uncommon. Usually symptoms appear several days after the birth, but they can appear anytime the first year following birth. Symptoms of PPD include anxiety, depression, restlessness, insomnia, anger, frustration, memory loss, excessive tiredness, crying, hopelessness, and confusion. Some women feel ambivalent about their baby and the responsibilities of motherhood and do not feel an innate bond between themselves and their newborn. Overwhelming fear or aggressive tendencies toward your child require immediate attention from someone who understands the physiological and psychological causes of PPD. According to traditional Chinese medicine, excessive blood loss during delivery can leave the heart empty of vital chi and blood, "leaving no place for the heart spirit to rest."[14] Lily describes the anguish of her fourth-trimester experience with her son, Aaron:

> When Aaron was born I had a very difficult delivery with lots of blood loss. Afterward I had no one to help me but my husband, Stu. His parents and mine were dead, and we had no friends because of a recent move to a new community. Stu had to work overtime to make up for the money I was losing during my maternity leave. I was unable to rest enough to restore my health because our step-daughter needed to be driven to and from school and her many activities throughout the day. After a month, I had to return to work. By this time, I was so tired and I felt so isolated. I went into a severe depression and disconnected from my baby; I could not even keep my own body strong enough to stay awake, much less feed him. Luckily, as I began to despair Stu contacted our local

church, and there were many eager grandmothers ready to fill our house with care and comfort so that I could rest and regain my sanity. As a new mom, I needed to be mothered.

If you experience similar symptoms, do not suffer in silence. Call your doctor and seek a referral for someone who specializes in PPD. If you experience frequent feelings of being overwhelmed or of frustration, assess whether you may be sleep deprived, or whether you feel the need for support. Also, make sure your diet is replenishing you. You will be loving your baby by loving yourself.

Astrological Influences

To deepen your spiritual understanding of the timing of your child's birth, the influences of the stars may offer you a unique perspective. Astrology suggests that when your child is born, he receives in his body an imprint of the position of the stars at the exact moment he takes his first breath. Many new parents are aware of the sun sign of their own horoscope and often also know the astrological sign of their child. Yet very few parents really understand the significance of the birth horoscope.

Your child's familial and childhood conditions are not the only forces that will determine her identity. If you have embraced the idea that your child's earthly life personality coexists with her inner life of soul perceptions, a soul-centered approach to astrology will allow you to attune to the essential energetic qualities embodied in your child's natal chart. This chart suggests potential aspects of her evolving consciousness.

The earth and each of us are affected by gravitational and magnetic forces. We know the gravitational pull of the moon affects both the tides and our psychological moods, so it should not be surprising that other celestial bodies such as the sun and other planets also trigger responses in us. Spiritually, a natal astrological chart is often used to describe the soul's expression on earth. It may shed light on potential life lessons and challenges the soul has selected to experience. Thus understanding your child's chart can help you better understand the physical and psychological aspects of the personality that the soul has chosen this lifetime.

Although a computer program can produce a natal chart that is moderately accurate, I suggest that you have such a chart read or interpreted by a qualified professional. A computerized rote interpretation cannot capture the unique design of your child's consciousness. Avoid any astrologer or interpretation that suggests there is a predetermined future for your child based on his chart. All of us have choices regarding how we use the forces presented in celestial influences. Qualified astrologers will give you a comprehensive perspective that does not predict your child's future or crystallize his personality nature. Rather, they will make you aware of possible karmic predispositions that may or may not manifest in your child's demeanor. If a tendency for an unhealthy behavior is indicated in the birth chart, you will understand that this is a karmic pattern the soul has chosen to experience so that it can, with your guidance, transform that tendency into healthier ways. You will, of course, use your own consciousness as you intentionally guide the unfolding of your child's self-awareness.

The Soul's Celestial Message to You

Although the soul of your child exists prior to her human birth, the moment of birth initiates a different kind of development for her, beyond her soul existence. The astrological influences at birth simply reflect certain forces and influences that exist in potential form. Since throughout her life she will have considerable free will to work with the celestial forces that have become part of her destiny, the birth chart is not a snapshot of a static reality for the newborn but an informational guide for a lifelong developmental process.

Your baby's first breath, his first moment of independence from you, will be his astrological moment of birth. Since natal charts are based on the position of the planets at the exact time and location of birth, it is important that you have someone at your birth responsible for noticing the precise moment of your newborn's first breath. Often in both home and hospital births, no one is aware of this exact time, which then has to be estimated. In an astrological chart, the planets and constellations can change locations within one minute, which can cause an incorrect reading of your child's astrological influences. Whether your baby is born naturally, born by cesarean section, or requires use of life support systems in his birth, the first breath will signify his exact birth time.

Each planet in your child's natal chart will hold physical, psychological, and spiritual meanings that will be colored by its position relative to all other planets. Each planet's placement within the constellations, or signs, is also relevant. Each sign has positive and negative attributes that influence how the qualities of a particular planet placed within it will be expressed. While a complete explanation of astrology and interpretation of your child's natal chart is beyond the scope of this book, I have created a simplified chart called Astrological Archetypes and Affirmations (see facing page) that you can use to understand several primary qualities of each planet and constellation. Although all have many attributes that affect the personality and soul, I have chosen one or several qualities that can be universally applied to the process of getting to know your child based on her birth chart.

Once a natal chart has been created for your newborn, simply knowing the constellation position of three planets—the sun, moon, and rising sign (ascendant)—will give you a strong glimpse of the qualities that the soul has chosen for its personality in this lifetime. This is because the sun sign represents the personality nature of your child in which it seeks to maximize personal potential. The moon influences the quality of the emotional nature of your child, and the rising sign indicates the identity the soul is aspiring to evolve toward this lifetime, which may be very different from the personality sign (the sun sign) it chooses to express during the beginning of its life.

Knowing the significance of other planets—Mercury, Venus, Mars, Jupiter, Saturn, Uranus, Neptune, and Pluto—can deepen your understanding of your child: Mercury and the sign that it is in will reflect the mental nature of your child. Venus indicates your child's values, female qualities, and sense of beauty. Mars reflects the male energies, including the will to pursue personal desires. Jupiter suggests your child's spiritual and educational inclinations, while Saturn illustrates the realm and degree of responsibility and discipline as well as the nature of karmic patterns to be resolved by the soul. Uranus indicates areas of innovation and uniqueness, while Neptune demonstrates the expression of the intuitive nature and spiritual tendencies. Pluto tends to be impulsive and transformative as well as provoking the deep, unconscious karmic patterns of the past and present life.

It is important to understand that each of these planets has strengths and weaknesses. A child with a strong Pluto aspect may be very emotionally volatile in youth but if parented and educated appropriately, this characteristic could mature into an adult personality that is very powerful, with great healing and leadership abilities. Without parents' wise and loving guidance such an individual could be abusive and chronically reactive.

When I reviewed my daughter's natal chart the day after her birth, I understood that there were many ways to interpret it. Yet there were clear patterns and qualities indicated that made me aware of potential

ASTROLOGICAL ARCHETYPES AND AFFIRMATIONS

For each constellation, begin with this invocation followed by the specific qualities described under the affirmation column. "I [We] call upon the essence of [constellation name] and the incarnating soul and invoke the highest expressions of . . . [complete with affirmation]."

Constellation	Positive Potential	Negative Potential	Affirmation
Aries	Independent, assertive, adventurous	Pushy, aggressive	Independence and will
Taurus	Resourceful, playful, loyal	Stubborn, stingy	Persistence and determination
Gemini	Versatile, mentally agile, multidimensional, curious	Undependable, distractable	Intellectual diversity and clear communication
Cancer	Emotional, nurturing, family oriented	Insecure, smothering, needy	Psychic powers and emotional sensitivity
Leo	Magnetic, self-expressive, enthusiastic	Egotistical, selfish	Creative expression and selfless, heart-centered generosity
Virgo	Purity, perfection, and service oriented; discriminating	Critical, judgmental	Ability to manifest the ideal within the real with precision
Libra	Cooperative, loves beauty and harmony; relationship oriented	Indecisive, vain, imbalanced	Peace, truth, beauty, harmony, balance, justice
Scorpio	Intense, emotionally deep, powerful, and passionate	Compulsive, abusive, overly reactive	The soul's ability to focus its psychic powers for positive transformation
Sagittarius	Philosophical, expansive, optimistic, spiritual	Self-indulgent, dogmatic, fundamentalist	The soul's potential to seek truth and expand consciousness
Capricorn	Responsible, ambitious, structured, realistic, practical	Rigid, domineering, controlling	The soul's ability to be disciplined in creating useful forms
Aquarius	Visionary, group and future oriented, inventive, unique	Disruptive, rebellious, quick changing	The soul's ability to interact for the highest good of groups
Pisces	Compassionate, psychic, highly sensitive, healing	Victim oriented, addictive, moody, codependent	Compassion and healing
Planet	**Positive Potential**	**Negative Potential**	**Affirmation**
Sun	Illuminating personal potential, expressing personality	Egotistical and self-centered	The divine design of the soul's personality
Moon	Emotionally expressive	Emotionally reactive	The most beneficial emotional qualities and nature of the soul
Mercury	Positively uses thoughts and ideas, effective communication	Lacking mental clarity	Optimal mental potential
Venus	Healthy values, high ideals, creates harmony and beauty	Vain, undefinedly idealistic	Beauty, harmony, values, and idealism
Mars	Asserts self and personal desires in positive way	Overly aggressive	The purest desires for this soul in alignment with its divine design
Jupiter	Expands and disseminates knowledge, freedom of ideas	Dogmatic, unwilling to learn from others	Possibilities for growth, truth, and freedom
Neptune	Develops intuition, expresses compassion, has faith	Actively deceptive of self or others	The universal qualities of faith, unity, and unconditional love
Saturn	Organizes, disciplines, defines, and creates forms	Domineering and controlling	The discipline to build useful forms for the soul
Uranus	Innovative, creates new ideas and forms for future	Rebellious, impulsive, explosive	Universal awareness and creative opportunities
Pluto	Profound transformation, cycles of death and rebirth	Compulsive, destructive	Its power to positively transform obsolete realities

weaknesses in her character that could be limiting for her as well as positive personality attributes that could be intentionally nurtured. Many aspects suggested that she would be innately sociable, unlikely to be shy. Now at the ripe age of four, Kylea is clearly a natural extrovert who loves any opportunity to socialize with anyone, anywhere, any age. As her parent, I try to create many ways she can express her social interests.

An important lesson is reflected in the interpretation of her friend Joshua's chart. When his mother asked me to explain his birth chart, I saw planetary aspects that reflected the potential of an explosive emotional nature. Joshua's sun was located in the sign Scorpio, whose characteristic is emotional intensity—compulsive and violent in its extreme—in close relationship to his moon, placed in Taurus, whose challenging aspect is potential stubbornness. His Saturn was located in Capricorn, which can create a rigid disposition. This cluster of planets suggested the possibility that Joshua might be emotionally reactive until he learns to channel his feelings in responsible ways. Potentially, such a personality could become an aggressive or impassioned leader as he matures, or a penetrating, practical healer who has a great sensitivity and ability to be psychic as well as resourceful. Joshua's mother, Hava, describes how she integrated her understanding of her son's astrological tendencies:

> Knowing Joshua's propensities from the beginning of his life gave me a special sensitivity to his intensely willful personality. From day one, he was always feisty whenever I changed his diaper or clothes, and always cried whenever anyone else held him. He knew what he wanted and when he wanted it, and this stubborn quality followed him throughout his childhood. Unlike his sister, whose natal chart and personality were completely opposite, I knew not to personalize Josh's determined nature—that he needed my compassion and guidance to help him channel his aggressive temper in creative and useful ways.
>
> I knew that if he learned how to develop his loving nature, his strong will would always serve him in beneficial ways. People always describe him as intensely loving. I know if I had been impatient with him during his formative years when his will was raw, he may have become combative and never learned to use his passionate temper in a constructive way. Astrology helped me to recognize and remain aware of his potential weaknesses. It was up to me and his dad to help him develop his potential weaknesses into personal strengths.

Your child's birth chart will indicate both active and latent celestial forces. The planets are symbols of his future potential and purpose. They reflect certain personality drives and behaviors that can be nurtured or redirected as they manifest. You can use astrology to help your child make the most of his life.

Birth and the beginning of human life offer endless opportunities to perceive your child as an embodiment of the Divine in a delicate human form. Along with celestial forces, the experiences of birth and the fourth trimester contribute to the early imprint of life in the body. Your child will always be linked to heaven. As her parent, it is up to you to remember this universal truth and care for your newborn with this inspired awareness.

Creative Exercise:
Envisioning Your Baby's Birth and Beyond

1. Knowing that your baby is affected by the birth experience, how would you like to assist in a gentle arrival? Make a birth wish list specifying all of your desires and needs for all individuals involved—your baby, you, your partner, your labor assistants, and anyone you want at the birth. (Refer to the birth wish list in appendix B.)

2. Once your child is born, what does the fourth trimester mean to you? How do you want to create this phase of your child's life? Who do you need to include in this awareness?

3. What do you think you need to do in order to nourish your body, mind, and spirit once you have given birth to your baby? Be specific.
   - My body
   - My mind
   - My spirit

4. How can you use astrology as a tool to better understand your child? Do you want to have a natal chart prepared? Will you have your child's chart interpreted by a professional astrologer, or would you like to learn how to do this yourself? How do you sense celestial forces can affect your child's personality?

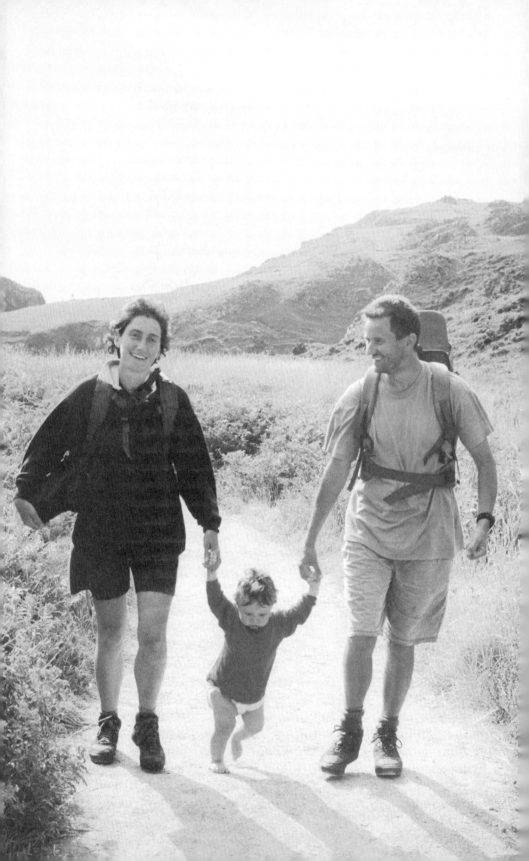

9

Holistic Parenting:
Practical Next Steps

*The greatest gift you can give your child is your self. This means
that part of your work as a parent is to keep growing
in self-knowledge and awareness.*

Myla and Jon Kabat-Zinn

Choosing a holistic parenting style means incorporating your recognition of yourself and all of your family members as incarnated souls, each with specific physical, emotional, and spiritual needs. Implicit in this is a continuing devotion to your child's whole being—body, mind, and soul—whenever you have health care choices to make, and equal respect for the well-being of your partner and yourself.

Being a parent has its own unique set of challenges. Each of you will find it a delicate and daily balancing act to discover ways of being true to yourself while being a reliable source of love for your family, a beloved to your partner, a contributor to your community, and effective in your career.

For many new as well as seasoned parents, balancing parenthood, career, partnership, and self-care is a mighty task that challenges even the most proficient time manager. Just as your child's developmental needs will forever be changing, so will your work commitments, and these will need to be redefined often. A mother may find herself exploring and transforming her own expectations of being a "superwoman" or "supermom." A father may need to heal internal conflicts about being "superdad." Sierra remembers a decision she made when she was young:

> My mom gave up her career when my twin brother and I were born in 1955. For years, our family meetings were sprinkled with little demeaning innuendoes about Mom sacrificing her professional work to take care of me and my brothers. I decided before I was ten that I would never give up my career for my children, so when I had my two girls one year apart, I was determined to keep my work schedule. Suddenly I was not enjoying motherhood or my work. It was all too exhausting, and "supermom" was far from healthy. I had to reevaluate my priorities, because if I couldn't keep myself balanced, my kids would suffer with a depressed mom. I had to redesign my professional life so that it supported my being a mother. I had to build creative strategies to integrate family life and career.

While both jobs require significant skill, time, and experience, parenthood and career hold different meanings and responsibilities for everyone. Some full-time parents have the opposite challenge of being overwhelmed with family life and needing outside creative outlets for their self-expression. Often volunteer or part-time work fills this need. And parents, like everyone else, also have the need sometimes for personal time—without children, partner, or work.

The unique physical and psychological demands inherent to parenthood, combined with rigorous professional expectations, require that parents in the workplace intentionally develop a personal and professional lifestyle that benefits their family life. Your employer's plans for phasing you back into part- or full-time work after maternity or family leave should take into account the developmental needs of your child as well. Your relationship to your work will be a healthy one to the degree that you are able to use your time and energy such that your family responsibilities and interests are not neglected.

Assess your daily challenges, and clarify any support you need to manage the process of change in your life, including the needs of your child. If your current employment is too rigid to support your new needs as a parent, you and your partner may explore work options that provide the flexibility you need:

- Look into whether your company allows the use of personal days for maternity or paternity leave.

- Look into whether your company allows part-time or flextime work for parents returning to work after family leave.
- Try to organize a regular schedule. Unpredictable appearances and disappearances can disorient a young child.
- Even if you work at home, planning is necessary.

Whatever decisions you make concerning how much time you devote to parenthood, your newborn will survive. However, studies clearly indicate that the strongest bonding requires the mother to be available to her baby frequently and with ongoing regularity, day and night, through the first years of life. As the child grows older, the time mother and child spend apart expands, and the child who has been allowed to be dependent naturally grows independent. This may require that you reevaluate your financial responsibilities and lifestyle to minimize activities that keep you from spending the time that you want with your baby and other family members. If commitments or hardship prevent you from providing your child with this experience of security, then be sure that you are completely present during the time you are able to spend with your little one. If the mother and/or father must work, it is important for the child's internal security to provide a *consistent*, loving caregiver with whom the child will have a primary attachment.[1] Holistic planning can help you discern your true physical, emotional, mental, and spiritual needs so that the family will not only survive but really thrive.

Taking Care of Your Physical Needs

Regenerating Your Body

Once a mother gets beyond the birth and early postnatal adjustments, she may feel the urge to rebuild her body from the impact of being pregnant. For some women, the pregnancy and birth will have seriously depleted the body of vital energy reserves. It will be necessary to replenish essential nutrients, vitamins, and minerals that were used by the growing baby or expended in giving birth. Even if a woman considers herself out of shape after giving birth, rather than dieting I recommend finding a good nutritional guide to help you determine the best foods and supplements for restoring your physical well-being. If you are breast-feeding, make sure you take into account the nutrition required to fully nourish yourself and your babe. If you are concerned about your weight, you will discover that breast-feeding is the best way to lose weight naturally without dieting. If you are not breast-feeding, remember, in any case, that your body will need to replenish its supply of all the nutrients the baby used to grow in the womb.

Many women and men feel the need to balance their parenting responsibilities with a regular routine of self-care activities. New moms should wait until all bodily discharges from the birth experience have stopped before resuming dynamic exercise. Gentle movements such as yoga, walking, and swimming are usually recommended in the first months after the birth experience. Typically, interrupted sleep patterns leave new parents with little excess energy to exercise regularly. Don't push yourself. Let the energy level of your body dictate the pace of your exercise. This is a time for regenerating your physical vitality, not further depleting it through overexertion.

Financial Planning for the Family

Many couples or single parents will be further challenged by financial stresses. Money and children: they are inseparable. You can have money without children, but it's hard to have children without money! Your short- and long-term spending habits will undoubtedly have an impact on the quality of your family's lifestyle. Whatever your financial "building and spending" habits were before becoming parents, it is time for you and your partner to consider how your daily and yearly expenses will be affected by having a child. Unlike your investments in material possessions, investing in your child means giving him the opportunity to enjoy good health, expand his natural intelligence, explore his creativity, and nurture his curious and joyful nature.

How Much Is Enough?

Some parents lavish their kids with new and expensive items, while others can afford or even prefer only secondhand clothes, toys, and baby furnishings, hand-me-downs from family members' or friends' children. Mary and Tom had a combined income of only twenty thousand dollars a year but needed very little to feel secure:

> We had two children without any savings. We lived month by month, and our children never suffered for it. Although we lived simply, there was always enough quality food and clothes for the kids. Instead of new toys and furniture, we gathered secondhand articles. We asked friends for hand-me-downs that their children

had outgrown. We went to thrift shops and found wonderful things. We created play activities using inexpensive art supplies and things collected from nature. And although we did not have a lot of money, our kids were secure in our positive attitude that living a simple life is healthy and filled with creative opportunities.

On the other hand, Donna and Perry gave real importance to having financial security before conceiving their child:

> Before our son, Michael, was born, we spent seven years establishing financial assets so that I could be a full-time mother at home without the need for my income. I came from a poor family and I knew how much I wanted my child to have all of the material comforts and educational resources I'd lacked. I wanted to have money for all of the best and newest baby products and furniture available. Creating a large savings was part of my preconception planning experience. It has been healing for me to buy Michael anything that interests me or him for his development. His father continues to work hard to maintain our lifestyle, but this is a choice we both made so I can be the primary child care provider in the family.

Many couples share the financial responsibility of having a child. Both partners may work before or after the birth to provide for financial needs. Some potential parents find it reassuring to build assets before having children, while others create an unstructured financial reserve that develops over time. For most people, the challenges of balancing financial responsibilities continue throughout the child's life. Alice recalls how she resolved her own dilemma:

> When Jed was born, we had minimal savings and we kept our mortgage payments and retirement plans at their lowest rates. Our commitment was to maintain our careers and earn enough money to provide Jed with the best child care once I returned to work. When Jed was six months old we decided we wanted to have at-home day care, a decision that forced us to sacrifice our love of taking expensive vacations. We saved money by eating at home more, buying less of nonessentials, and taking long weekend trips rather than exotic vacations. Our "extra" money went to giving Jed everything he needed. Our material sacrifices were worth it. Our reward was that our son had a life full of wonderful experiences, even though there were real limits to how much we could spend.

As you can see, there are no rules governing how much is enough in financially preparing for having a baby. If you want to clarify your own goals of what and how you want to provide for your child, you will find a financial guideline in appendix C that describes many common expenses for the first four phases of parenthood—preconception, prenatal, birth, and postnatal.

Taking Care of Your Emotional Needs

From your baby's birth, you are her first teacher of understanding and love. Your child's soul virtues will begin to be cultivated during her very early years. A loving emotional temperament is demonstrated through your example. Your child will absorb your and your partner's dispositions, making them part of her personality and soul. Fostering attitudes of self-love will enrich your child's psyche as well as your own.

Self-Love

Your little one will be very sensitive to your emotional states and stresses, soaking them up like a sponge. For your own sake and that of your baby, give yourself permission to compassionately accept the full range of your feelings as you adjust to parenthood. Self-acceptance *is* self-love. Self-acceptance is not a passive state, but a conscious inner orientation that allows you to see things as they are and then explore more life-affirming possibilities.

Any kind of "negative" emotion you experience will be a chance to achieve greater understanding, if you are able to view yourself without judgment. Sometimes expressing your darker feelings in a creative way— such as talking with a sympathetic person—allows you to regain your equilibrium as you harmoniously release pent-up energy and renew your connection to your true nature. As long as your emotional expression is discharged in a healthy manner it will not harm you or your baby. Remember, your child will internalize your outbursts or prolonged states of tension. Not all your emotions will be appropriate to express in front of your child, since he will not be able to self-regulate the stimulation. It is your responsibility as a parent to express your emotions in a productive way that protects your child from being emotionally hurt. Practice consciously feeling and deliberately letting go of disharmonious emotions for the purpose of inner healing and wholeness. Focus intentionally on your loving nature to bring out the best in yourself.

Parenting will involve you in countless emotional interactions with your child. How you perceive yourself will influence your behavior in these. Begin to develop a conscious repertoire of emotional expressions that honor your deepest internal experiences. The more awareness you bring to the feelings that flow through you, the easier it will be to accept the myriad emotions your child will express throughout the years to come. Accepting your own ups and downs with compassion, a willingness to love all parts of your inner self, will be reflected in a willingness to understand, accept, and love all parts of your child. It's an ongoing process to find appropriate and satisfying ways to attend to your feelings and all the subtle messages they evoke. During the third month of parenting, I wrote in my journal:

> I can't believe the waterfall of emotions that pour through me each day. I consciously remind myself to affirm the presence of love that pervades all other feelings. I simply need to honor whatever emotion reveals itself as a part of me needing attention. When I listen within and focus on what I need to feel better, the particular emotion in question always tells me what to do to heal myself. I must remember when I feel agitated to stop for a moment, dialogue with the feeling, and ask it what it needs to be comforted. Invariably, I'm relaxed just by paying attention to my irritation, and then I understand how to care for it. Often, it is simply to accept what's going on; other times some action is required. Loving myself is loving my baby, since she then gets to bathe in my quietude.

Gather Support

In many of the emotional waters you will navigate while parenting your infant, you'll benefit from sharing with others on the parenthood journey. It is not unusual to feel conflicted, anxious, or confused, as well as overwhelmed or frustrated with sleep deprivation and no time to see to personal needs. Conversely, spontaneous states of pure joy, love, and even ecstasy fill many new parents' hearts as they get to know their baby.

Frequently, new parents postpone caring for their own emotional condition because they've made meeting their child's needs a higher priority. Then days or weeks of suppressed emotions explode when unexpectedly provoked. Every parent needs support. It's okay to ask for help. Being a parent is a big deal.

For many new mothers, finding reliable assistance with the constant demands of nursing and infant care is essential for sustaining a harmonious adjustment. You may need to be reassured about your caretaking style, or guided in your mothering methods. Some moms feel the need for a trusted friend or family member to help out with household tasks on a regular basis so that they can depend on a specific window of time to rest and recharge their energies.

Support groups can also offer wisdom and encouragement from other new parents. Your local parenting or community center will likely offer parent and baby classes, at which you can network and share information. Your local park is another place where you can meet mothers and fathers. This is especially helpful if you have given up a job and feel socially isolated.

Most people love to share their personal stories, and other couples who have been through the early-parenthood initiation can be a great support. Even if you do not agree with their overall child care style, don't overlook the gems of wisdom in their stories about their own adjustment to life with a newborn. Clara was upset by her mother's intrusions yet recognized their gift:

> Mom is always telling me what to do with Jason. Her methods are so outdated; she does not understand there has been a drastic change in perspectives since she had me four decades ago. But I realized that every time I disagree with her, I become more clear about my own truth, and what I feel is right for my family. So our differences really just reinforce my own decisions. Also, since I don't feel obliged to disagree with her entire viewpoint, I often can learn a new technique or two.

Upon opening up to support, be prepared to be inundated with advice. There will be those only too glad to advise you how to feed, bathe, and sleep with your new baby, even when such feedback is unsolicited by you. Just remember that it's okay to do things differently from everyone else, including your own mother. Only *you* know your needs and those of your baby and your partner. You'll want to experiment with those suggestions that ring true for you as you and your partner customize your parenting plan. Being a parent is very much trial and error. Don't make perfection your ideal—in parenting, it simply does not exist.

As you've seen in earlier chapters, parenthood can stress the healthiest relationships. A new baby can bring out the best and worst in each of you. Be willing to work through difficulties with your partner, deepening your bond of love for one another. One of you may at times feel emotionally abandoned or neglected because of the time the other is spending with your baby. Make the effort to creatively nurture your relationship while you both adjust to your new responsibilities. Remember that Dad should bond with the baby as much as possible to keep him completely included in the love loop.

Taking Care of Your Mental Needs

Your mental beliefs and principles will be guideposts that help you make the endless choices parenting requires. Awaken to the power of your mind and you can use your thoughts to sustain a positive parenting experience. Strive to remain aware of the ways you reinforce beliefs that enhance conscious parenting, as well as those attitudes that limit higher states of consciousness in caring for your child and perceiving yourself as a parent. Pay attention to those beliefs that support your true nature, and intentionally let go of any that are not a reflection of your values. Holistic parenting asks that you remain conscious of dysfunctional psychological patterns that can hurt you or your child. This will increase your sensitivity to the Divine in yourself, your partner, and your child. Unless your *conscious thoughts* affirm the existence of such realities, you will not be able to perceive the presence of the Divine in yourself and your family.

In their book *Everyday Blessings: The Inner Work of Mindful Parenting* Myla and Jon Kabat-Zinn show how the simple practice of mindfulness honors the present moment and, within it, the inner potential of your child and of yourself. Throughout your child's life you will be given opportunities to discover who you are and who your child is, as well as to understand what particular contributions you can make to her personal growth. "In the process," they write, "we may find that this ongoing moment-to-moment awareness can liberate us from some of our most confining habits of perception and relating, the straitjackets and prisons of the mind that have been passed down to us or that we have somehow constructed for ourselves."[2]

Now is a fruitful time to explore your beliefs and attitudes about yourself and your partner as parents, and the thoughts each of you hold about your child. Consider whether you tend to be critical, limiting, inflexible, or self-righteous in your thinking. Are you open to new points of view, or are you stuck in your childhood belief systems or obsolete social expectations? The primary rule concerning healthy parenting is that you continually seek to understand the guiding principles that empower you and your child to attain your highest potentials. Take a moment to evaluate what beliefs and attitudes you hold that do not support you in being true to your divine nature as a parent. Release those habitual thoughts that undermine your ability to nourish your child's personality and soul needs. Tamara's grandmother always scolded her mother for not disciplining her and her siblings well enough:

> Throughout my childhood my grandma used to tell my mom that she was a lousy mother because she was too easy on us. She would tell me and my two sisters that we would be lousy mothers, too, because our mom was a bad role model. Here I am, nine months pregnant, and terrified that my grandma has cursed my future. I know that I'm free to choose my own methods of educating my child about the rights and wrongs in life. I have to rid myself of my grandma's negative thoughts about my ability to mother and consciously create my own principles that are a reflection of my own essence.

The Perfect Parent: An Illusion

Once more I'll say it: perfect parenting does not exist. This is true for seasoned as well as new parents, yet first-timers often think that there is some secret formula they can learn to meet their baby's needs flawlessly all the time.

You will not be able to fulfill your baby's every whim; learning patience and self-soothing will be important lessons for him so that your occasional slip-ups can become productive growth opportunities for you both. Parenthood is an art form that by its very nature is filled with experimentation—including mistakes—as you address your child's ever-changing developmental requirements.

If you have a personal history of needing to be in control of your world, now is the time to give up this attitude. Your child will begin to internalize your need to be in control and will feel that she is disappointing you if her behavior does not rise to what she perceives as your expectations. If your child feels that she is not fulfilling your image of perfection, she will not feel free to explore her spontaneous expression.

An obsessive or controlling approach to parenting limits everyone's expression of compassion, self-assuredness, and authenticity. Take pleasure in the experience of being a loving and thoughtful parent, rather than a perfect one.

Taking Care of Your Spiritual Needs

When I was preparing for parenthood, I feared the loss of my personal time. I'd heard about the incredible demands of having a baby to care for, and how many of my friends had lost their self-care and spiritual practices to the daily chores of parenthood. I sensed that my ability to meditate would be greatly diminished for years, and my spiritual growth sacrificed. But less than one week after Kylea's birth I wrote to her in my journal about this illusion:

> I never knew the true use of the superlative adjectives *supreme, unrivaled, great.* Until I met you. Though exhaustion can limit my enjoyment of this sacred meeting between us, the sublime love that awakens in me is more blissful than the highest meditation I have ever experienced. The peace is deeper than the most beautiful blessing of nature. The divine communion of our souls (you, me, and Dad) is more holy than the most spiritual state I have ever achieved. The beauty and innocence of your presence is the purest I have ever witnessed. You are my spiritual teacher, my daughter. You are a constant meditation in love, a daily spiritual practice of selfless service. You are a living blessing that has graced my life forever. Thank you.

Parenting Your Child: A Lifelong Spiritual Path

Perceiving your child with devotion is the key to spiritual parenting. It will bring out the best in him and in you. It will encourage the divine self within all family members to prevail. In the four years since my daughter was born I have come to know and experience the essence of love. Of pure joy. Of spirit in matter. Of soul embodied. Of divine union. Of sacrifice and surrender. Of selfless giving. Of teaching virtues. Of being virtuous. Of the miracle of life. Of delight, wonder, awe, gratitude.

I am on a spiritual path with my lovely child. For me, she is the best source of divine inspiration I have found on this planet. In all our daily interactions are chances for me to guide her to the inner awareness that she is a divine spirit in human form. I get to experience that truth of myself and my darling husband, Jared, as well. If I get upset or reactive, I can become love itself—flexible, giving, soft. As her mom, I can help Kylea discover her unique journey with spirit. Every moment is an opportunity to embody a virtue—to exemplify goodness, wellness, wholeness.

The love her dad and I have found for one another is like a succulent garden that she can sink her formative roots into and blossom into her glorious beingness. Jared and I have worked diligently to weed out old patterns that restrict well-being for any of us. Before conceiving Kylea and once she was born, we have been determined to create a home—a safe and beautiful haven—for our daughter to unfold her wings. Our reverence for Kylea has allowed her self-esteem to be founded and grounded in divine love. All of the spiritual texts that I have ever studied are applied to my daily practice of caring for this beloved child of God.

I hope this book has helped inspire your own awakening to the wonders of becoming a conscious mom or dad. Parenting is a sacred activity in which you are able to cherish, cultivate, nourish, empower, uplift, and embrace the divine in each family member, every day—all day long.

Both of you can raise your child with spiritual skills—love, patience, sharing, generosity, prayer, meditation, truth, honesty, goodwill, and reverence for all life—and so bestow her with a lifetime connection to her divine self. This in turn will assist your child in effectively meeting the challenges of life, as well as enhancing the meaningfulness of your relationship together, and all of your child's relationships.

Parenthood has given me the daily opportunity to embody the spiritual teachings I had studied for so many years. As I finish this book and reflect on my journey through motherhood, I find myself gently crying with gratitude. I thank my daughter daily, for her radiant essence is guiding me into the Heart of God, Goddess, All That Is.

I urge you to take on parenthood as a Path to Eternal Love.

Creative Exercise:
A Plan for Holistic Parenting

1. What does holistic parenting mean to you? Write about this in your journal.
2. With your partner make a detailed list of the ways you'll take care of your physical health once your baby has been born. How do you want to fulfill your dietary, exercise, and other physical health care needs? How will you see to your financial needs?
3. With your partner make a detailed list of the ways you'll take care of your emotional health once your baby has been born. How do you want to fulfill your emotional need for self-understanding and self-love, and to gather support from others?
4. With your partner make a detailed list of the ways you'll take care of your mental health once your baby has been born. Clarify your personal beliefs about being a parent. What principles will you apply in raising your child?
5. With your partner make a detailed list of the ways you'll take care of your spiritual health once your baby has been born. How do you see parenting your child as an essential part of your spiritual practice?
6. If you could wish something for your child's whole health, what would that be? For your own whole health? For your partner's whole health? For your new family's whole health?

Appendix A

The PreSeeding Birth Program: A Holistic Model

The following guidelines of the PreSeeding Birth Program are designed to inspire you to create your own custom-designed preconception and prenatal health care plan. These suggestions offer a holistic perspective that recognizes equally the importance of the physical, emotional, mental, and spiritual health of your baby, you, and your partner. In preparing your whole health so that you can be a healthy parent, you will learn to integrate the ideas and behavior that will offer your child the greatest opportunity to unfold his full potential.

For your child to express and embody her innate vitality, authenticity, radiance, and love from the beginning of life, you will need to consistently nurture the conditions for these qualities and others to flourish. As you consciously nourish the seeds of the incarnating soul's physical, emotional, mental, and spiritual bodies before conception and throughout the pregnancy, your baby will blossom into a beautiful and bountiful human being. Enjoy the process of cultivating your true self and those of your family members.

The holistic approach to preconception and prenatal health care includes equal care for:

- **Physical Health:** Maintaining and nurturing your physical well-being and that of all family members, as well as optimizing your lifestyle choices, including environmental influences and financial planning.

- **Emotional Health:** Ease in experiencing and appropriately expressing the full spectrum of emotions, from love to anger.
- **Mental Health:** How you use your thoughts and beliefs to perceive yourself, your family members, and all aspects of life.
- **Spiritual Health:** Understanding and expressing your spiritual nature, religious beliefs, virtuous qualities, values, and ideals.

It includes equal care for:
- **Your Health**
- **Your Partner's Health**
- **Your Future Child's Health**
- **Healthy Dynamics of the Family System**

Equal concern for:
- **Your History:** Understand how your past can affect your relationship with your child and partner, and your identity as a parent.
- **Your Present Lifestyle Choices:** Determine if your lifestyle supports your custom-designed prebirth and postbirth health goals.
- **Your Future Needs and Preferences:** Specify how your future goals affect your prebirth preparation and planning.

Equal concern for defining the unique health care requirements for each of the three phases *before* birth:
- **Preconception Preparation**
- **Prenatal Development**
- **Birth Preparation**

Equal concern for what is *not* healthy:
- Anything that is harmful to yourself or your partner, child, or family.
- Addictions—food, drugs, alcohol, money, sex.
- Any form of abuse—physical, psychological, sexual.
- Dysfunctional relationship patterns between partners, as well as between a parent and child.

Create Your Own Holistic Prebirth Health Plan

Physical Health Care

Explore body health, finances, genetics, medical support, environment, sexuality, home and work concerns, diet, supplements, exercise, alternative medicine, and education. See chapter 3 for details.

1. Diagnose general, reproductive, and genetic health risks.
2. Balance and nourish your hormones.
3. Test for sexually transmitted diseases.
4. Develop a diet for fertility health.
5. Learn which supplements and herbs can help tonify your reproductive system and your unique physiological needs.
6. Improve sperm and egg health.
7. Prevent unnecessary miscarriages by managing stress and diet.
8. Make lifestyle changes before conception.
9. Before conception, review prescription and recreational drugs for both the man and woman with a doctor.
10. Identify stress patterns.
11. Understand how to predict ovulation and pace ejaculation for conception.
12. Avoid exposure to any viral or bacterial infections that could cause a fever in either partner before conception, and in the woman after conception.
13. Build your immune system before pregnancy.
14. Clarify what type of exercise is appropriate once you are pregnant.
15. Identify occupational and home health hazards that can cause infertility and birth defects—and if necessary, change your home or job at least three months before pregnancy.
16. Specify short- and long-range financial needs and goals. Remember that prebirth and postbirth requirements differ (see appendix C, Financial Investments before and after the Birth, on page 283).
17. If you're concerned about infertility, educate yourself about Assisted Reproductive Technologies and medication in conjunction with natural holistic modalities.

Psychological Health Care

Clarify your feelings in order to heal, develop, and express yourself, including reactive patterns, childhood traumas, and feelings with yourself, your partner, and your child. See chapter 4 for details.

Clarify your thoughts, attitudes, and beliefs that are dysfunctional or unhealthy. Again, chapter 4 has more details.

1. Create healthy communication dynamics with yourself, your partner, and your child.
2. Assess whether your emotional intimacy patterns are healthy.
3. Reveal and heal emotional or verbal abuse between you and your partner or anyone else.
4. Clarify ambivalences and fears about parenthood.
5. Specify the ways you feel confident to be a parent.
6. Affirm the ways you feel psychologically healthy to be a parent.
7. Express your concerns about balancing parenthood, career, relationship, and self-care.
8. Establish emotional support sources.
9. Explore and heal unresolved childhood issues and traumas.
10. Make a list of all psychological patterns and behaviors that you want to begin to heal before becoming pregnant.
11. Heal the emotional issues behind addictive or abusive behavior.
12. Learn how to make a genogram to identify transgenerational family patterns potentially affecting your parenting and your child.
13. Discuss your changing self-identity in becoming a parent.
14. Face your future life changes consciously.
15. Deepen your experience of self-love, self-understanding, and self-care.
16. Keep a journal of your preconception and prenatal journey.
17. Let your goal be doing your best to prepare, rather than aiming for perfection.
18. Remember to consciously affirm the love, joy, wonder, and miracle of preparing for your baby.

Spiritual Health Care

Clarify your virtuous qualities, highest ideals, visions of parenthood, religious values, and spiritual practices that support the expression of your true self and highest potential. See chapter 5 for details.

1. Clarify your visions of parenthood.
2. Surround yourself with and contemplate positive images.
3. Listen to harmonious music.
4. Specify your ideals and principles for parenthood.
5. Explore embodying and expressing virtuous qualities for your child.
6. Consider your child's spiritual education.
7. Develop meaningful meditation and spiritual practices.
8. Perceive parenthood as an art form.
9. Create a sacred altar for your future child.
10. Study metaphysical realities and paradigms relevant to parenthood.
11. Focus on the true nature of your child as a blend of personality and soul.
12. Include the presence of mystery beyond the human forces that are creating your child.
13. Create your own prebirth plan based on your values and wisdom.
14. Enjoy the process of preparing and have fun discovering new aspects of yourself, your partner, your child, and the mysteries of life.

A Step-by-Step Holistic Health Worksheet

My Preconception Preparation Goals

1. Optimizing my *physical* health:
   a.
   b.
   c.
   d.

2. Optimizing my child's *physical* health:
   a.
   b.
   c.
   d.

3. Supporting my partner's *physical* health:
   a.
   b.
   c.
   d.

4. Optimizing my *psychological* health:
   a.
   b.
   c.
   d.

5. Optimizing my child's *psychological* health:
   a.
   b.
   c.
   d.

6. Supporting my partner's *psychological* health:
   a.
   b.
   c.
   d.

7. Optimizing my *spiritual* health:
   a.
   b.
   c.
   d.

8. Optimizing my child's *spiritual* health:
   a.
   b.
   c.
   d.

9. Supporting my partner's *spiritual* health
   a.
   b.
   c.
   d.

My First-Trimester Health Care Goals

1. Optimizing my *physical* health:
   a.
   b.
   c.
   d.

2. Optimizing my child's *physical* health:
   a.
   b.
   c.
   d.

3. Supporting my partner's *physical* health:
   a.
   b.
   c.
   d.

4. Optimizing my *psychological* health:
   a.
   b.
   c.
   d.

5. Optimizing my child's *psychological* health:
   a.
   b.
   c.
   d.

6. Supporting my partner's *psychological* health:
   a.
   b.
   c.
   d.

7. Optimizing my *spiritual* health:
   a.
   b.
   c.
   d.

8. Optimizing my child's *spiritual* health:
   a.
   b.
   c.
   d.

9. Supporting my partner's *spiritual* health:
   a.
   b.
   c.
   d.

My Second-Trimester Health Care Goals

1. Optimizing my *physical* health:
   a.
   b.
   c.
   d.

2. Optimizing my child's *physical* health:
   a.
   b.
   c.
   d.

3. Supporting my partner's *physical* health:
   a.
   b.
   c.
   d.

4. Optimizing my *psychological* health:
   a.
   b.
   c.
   d.

5. Optimizing my child's *psychological* health:
   a.
   b.
   c.
   d.

6. Supporting my partner's *psychological* health:
   a.
   b.
   c.
   d.

7. Optimizing my *spiritual* health:
   a.
   b.
   c.
   d.

8. Optimizing my child's *spiritual* health:
   a.
   b.
   c.
   d.

9. Supporting my partner's *spiritual* health:
   a.
   b.
   c.
   d.

My Third-Trimester Health Care Goals

1. Optimizing my *physical* health:
   a.
   b.
   c.
   d.

2. Optimizing my child's *physical* health:
   a.
   b.
   c.
   d.

3. Supporting my partner's *physical* health:
   a.
   b.
   c.
   d.

4. Optimizing my *psychological* health:
   a.
   b.
   c.
   d.

5. Optimizing my child's *psychological* health:
   a.
   b.
   c.
   d.

6. Supporting my partner's *psychological* health:
   a.
   b.
   c.
   d.

7. Optimizing my *spiritual* health:
   a.
   b.
   c.
   d.

8. Optimizing my child's *spiritual* health:
   a.
   b.
   c.
   d.

9. Supporting my partner's *spiritual* health:
   a.
   b.
   c.
   d.

Preparing for the Birth

1. Optimizing my physical, psychological, and spiritual health during the birth:
   a.
   b.
   c.
   d.

2. Optimizing my child's physical, psychological, and spiritual health during the birth:
   a.
   b.

c.

d.

3. Supporting my partner's physical, psychological, and spiritual health during the birth:

    a.

    b.

    c.

    d.

4. What kind of support do I need?

    a.

    b.

    c.

    d.

5. What sources do I need to include to educate myself and prepare for the birth?

    a.

    b.

    c.

    d.

6. What is my birth wish list? (See an example in appendix B.)

My Postnatal Health Care Goals

1. Optimizing my *physical* health:

    a.

    b.

    c.

    d.

2. Optimizing my child's *physical* health:

    a.

    b.

    c.

    d.

3. Supporting my partner's *physical* health:

    a.

    b.

    c.

    d.

4. Optimizing my *psychological* health:
   a.
   b.
   c.
   d.

5. Optimizing my child's *psychological* health:
   a.
   b.
   c.
   d.

6. Supporting my partner's *psychological* health:
   a.
   b.
   c.
   d.

7. Optimizing my *spiritual* health:
   a.
   b.
   c.
   d.

8. Optimizing my child's *spiritual* health:
   a.
   b.
   c.
   d.

9. Supporting my partner's *spiritual* health:
   a.
   b.
   c.
   d.

10. What are my long-term goals and vision for sustaining a holistic health care reality for my family?
    a.
    b.
    c.
    d.

11. What specific soul qualities can enhance my preparation for parenthood? (See the Embodying Spiritual Virtues on page 161).

    a.
    b.
    c.
    d.

12. What specific soul qualities can enhance my relationship with myself and with my partner?

    a.
    b.
    c.
    d.

13. What are the benefits of perceiving and parenting my child as an incarnating soul with innate wisdom, talents, karma, abilities, and virtues previously developed in past incarnations?

    a.
    b.
    c.
    d.

14. What other concerns, challenges, ideals, principles, visions, beliefs, values, or paradigms do I want to include in my preconception and prenatal health plan?

    a.
    b.
    c.
    d.

Appendix B

Birth Wish List

The experience of giving birth is full of mystery as spiritual forces pour into you and the incarnating soul. All the uncontrollable forces of nature, your body, and your psyche ensure that even the best-planned birth will be full of surprises. Many pregnancy books advocate writing a birth plan to inform those attending the birth of your preferences. Most births, however, do not go according to plan, so I recommend calling these directions a birth wish list.

While you do not yet know how your body will respond to the birthing energies or how your baby will respond to his birth journey through your body, you can still use the wish list to organize your thoughts on paper and declare your desires for the birth. This is a good way to align your doctor, midwife, and all birth attendants with your philosophy, special needs, and fears.

Now is the time to inform yourself, whether you choose a home or hospital birth. If you decide on a home birth, be thoroughly aware of the midwife's style, procedures, and philosophy, making sure they are compatible with your personality. If you do not feel relaxed and safe with your midwife or doctor, it will be more challenging to trust this professional to assist you during the birth.

If you are preparing for a hospital birth, know that this is *your* birth experience. Take charge of it by educating yourself about all of the hospital's standard medical protocols. Question the routine use of any drug or procedure that does not support you in trusting your body to give birth naturally. Monitors, episiotomies, forceps, vacuum extractions, cesareans, anesthesia, and sedatives are often not medically necessary and can definitely have short- and long-term consequences for your baby's physical, psychological, and subtle energy bodies. Although it is true that the vast majority of women submit to the standard protocols of hospitals, do not be fooled into believing that these practices are necessarily appropriate for you and your baby.

If, after routine research, you choose a medicated and technological birth, you can still personalize your birth wish list by specifying the kind of attention and care you need. In your list write a detailed description of your concerns about interventions.

Even in the hospital you may have a degree of control over your birth environment when it comes to light, sound, and privacy. Request that there be no time limits or constraints placed on your labor as long as your baby and you are enduring labor well. Make yourself responsible for using self-help alternatives such as massage, relaxation, breathing, emotional support, aromatherapy, chanting, toning, homeopathy, herbal remedies, and acupressure. Specify your preferences for delivery and for your first contact with your baby. State how you want to care for your newborn, including your choices about breast-feeding, immunizations, circumcision, supplemental feedings, full rooming-in, and so forth.

You must allow your birth wish list to be flexible, since unexpected medical complications may necessitate intervention. Specify, however, that in such an event you and your partner expect to be educated about both risks and benefits of any medical procedure that you did not plan to experience. Then if there are complications, be willing to yield your wishes and cooperate in whatever way will support the healthy labor and delivery of the baby, as well as the health of the mother.

State your wishes in a simple, clear, direct, and positive way. Review your list with all people involved with your birth, and make sure any hospital staff on duty have access to a copy of the list in your chart. Express your wishes in the spirit of partnership with your birth attendants, yet always reinforce that *you* are the parents, and this is *your* body and *your* baby.

The following is a sample of a comprehensive birth wish list for a couple who wish to be supported in experiencing a natural birth without drugs, technology, or any unnecessary intervention. In the spirit of creating a "wish list" rather than a fixed plan, they also acknowledge their openness to interventions if medically necessary, or in the event that they consciously choose to alter their original desires. You may choose to use this list as a basic outline, adding or subtracting your own wishes.

Birth Wish List

We would like all attending midwives, nurses, and doctors (obstetrical and pediatric) to be supportive of our requests and desires and committed to giving us the birth experience we choose unless there is a medical reason to proceed differently. If medical intervention is necessary, we require to be educated about our options. Thank you for your cooperation and kind attention during this special time of our lives.

Prefer Limited Intervention

- Strong preference for no drugs. If drugs are recommended or medically necessary, we want to be supported in a clear understanding of the implication and effects on mother and child; it is also important for us to be made aware of the least-detrimental options. The mother prefers pain relief through massage, relaxation techniques, homeopathy, breathwork, emotional support, herbs, and freedom of movement, provided by husband and labor assistant.
- If the mother should request drugs for coping with labor pain, she wants caregivers to estimate how close she is to delivery or the next phase of labor.
- Strong preference not to have the mother's waters broken unless it is medically necessary. In this event we want to be consulted.
- No monitors (internal or external) unless determined medically necessary. The mother does not want her physical mobility restricted. Prefer listening to heart tones and FHR monitored with fetoscope rather than ultrasound devices.
- Episiotomy only if medically necessary. Mother wishes to be consulted and presented with her options. Prefer perineal massage with oil and hot compresses performed by labor assistant or nurse to avoid tearing.
- Vaginal exams only when medically necessary and upon consent, and as few as possible to avoid premature rupture of membranes.
- No use of forceps or vacuum extraction unless medically necessary. We want to be consulted about choices and implica-

tions of each procedure. Most likely prefer suction rather than forceps if this assistance to help the baby be born is needed for health reasons.

- Use of tub or shower as desired (open to medical evaluation once membranes have ruptured).
- Cesarean birth only if medically necessary, and the father will remain at all times with the baby immediately after the baby is born. The father or mother wishes to be able to hold the baby if the baby is not in distress, and the mother wishes to breast-feed as soon as possible.

During Labor

- The mother wises to be supported and encouraged to work with her baby and gravity. She wants to be kept active when appropriate, including any position that will assist with the delivery. She requests freedom of choice of position when pushing.
- The mother requests that the labor coach or labor and delivery nurse model proper breathing when necessary and encourage her to stay focused and express the sounds that will keep her body and energy open and flowing. Since it is not her tendency to express her emotions, she requests encouragement to express fear, pain, and joy.
- If it appears that labor is slowing, the mother wants to be encouraged to express her fears and concerns about what is going on.
- The mother requests gentle reminders to tune in to the baby during labor and delivery. The mother wishes the use of verbal and visual metaphors to help her stay focused on and welcome the baby. Remind and encourage her to relax, and to touch and speak to the baby.
- Maintain a quiet room. Dim lights and soft music are requested during the first stage of labor.
- No interns or residents observing the birth so that a quiet and intimate atmosphere can be maintained.
- No routine IV drip. If necessary, please use a heparin lock.

After Delivery

- Immediate skin-to skin contact with the mother.
- Allow time for bonding. The baby is to be kept with the mother

after birth for breast-feeding. No separation from the mother unless absolutely medically necessary, in which case the father will go with the baby.

- Breast-feeding immediately to assist in the natural delivery of the placenta—no pulling on the cord or routine Pitocin. Pitocin administered only if medically necessary.
- Only breast-feeding. No bottles, pacifiers, artificial nipples, glucose, water, or formula without our permission.
- Delay administration of eyedrops and any unnecessary bathing, measuring, testing, or routine exams.
- The baby is to stay in the mother's room unless urgent medical care is required; no nursery visits unless medically necessary. Perform all routine exams and procedures with us present. Bath given by us if we choose.
- The cord is to be cut by the father, and not until pulsing stops, unless the baby needs emergency medical assistance.
- No circumcision.
- No vaccinations in the hospital.
- Low lights and sound during bonding.
- The father or mother shall be present during all medically necessary testing procedures.

- Support us in maintaining a sacred quiet time with our new family after the birth. We ask all unnecessary medical staff to please leave the room as soon as possible.

Thank you for your support and sensitivity to our desires. We are aware that if there is a true medical need to deviate from these requests for the health of the baby or mother, we will swiftly align with the need of the moment.

Appendix C

Financial Investments
before and after the Birth

Let's take a more detailed look at the financial impact your decision to have a baby will have on your life. First, how much can you afford to invest in optimizing your preconception health? Preconception health care options can include nutritional and genetic counseling, medical exams, acupuncture and herbs to tone the reproductive system, nutritional supplements and vitamins, psychological counseling, chiropractic treatments, exercise, as well as any other form of health care that you feel inspired to undertake to be as healthy as possible *before you conceive* your child.

How much prebirth treatment is covered by your insurance, and how much will you have to pay for yourself? Since it is extremely difficult to obtain medical coverage once you have conceived, securing an insurance plan that covers your prebirth and postnatal health needs should be part of your preconception planning. A general health exam is essential for both partners to assess the quality of your blood, the balance of your hormones, and any diseases that may cause health challenges for you or your future child. Some of the alternative health insurance companies will cover home births and alternative medicine such as acupuncture and herbs.

If you want to strengthen and tone your general and reproductive health before and after conception, then acupuncture, herbal supplements, fitness programs, and chiropractic or homeopathic treatments can be included in your prebirth financial plan. Find the appropriate health practitioners and get an estimate of the treatment's cost. If your insurance will not reimburse you for these extras, clarify how much money you can allocate for your health care out of your personal funds.

Because they had miscarried three times, Peg and Sam wanted to do everything possible to be healthy themselves before their next attempt to conceive. Their attention to their health became even more important during their pregnancy when they discovered that they had conceived twin girls! Peg recalls:

> I knew I was vulnerable to the possibility of miscarriage because of my very stressful work schedule. I also had irregular ovulation times because of my poor diet and irregular sleep patterns. My acupuncturist put me on a six-month program of weekly treatments and daily herbs to balance my hormones, tone my uterus, and regulate my menstrual cycle. Due to his use of recreational drugs and fast foods, Jim had a low sperm count that was corrected with specific herbs and a major dietary change. We went to psychological counseling to evaluate how to reduce the stress between us and our professional commitments.
>
> After our six-month health program, we immediately conceived our daughters. I remained on the diet and supplements that supported my body in "holding" the pregnancy. I felt healthier during my pregnancy with twins than I had my entire life. It cost us much less to invest in natural medicine than the many thousands of dollars we might possibly have paid for infertility tests and technological assistance. I encourage everyone I know to invest in preconception health care. Get healthy before you conceive so your body can say yes to all of the incredible demands of being pregnant, and you have the time *and energy* to nurture and enjoy your unborn child miraculously growing within you.

Prenatal Health Care Investments

Once you have chosen your prenatal doctor or midwife, take the time to investigate the costs for all the specific services you will need. For some, the fees may be a consideration even in their choice of caregiver. Clarify with your health care providers, the hospital, and your insurance company their policies and payment arrangements. If you have insurance, remember to include your deductible or copayment as an actual cost to you. Ask your insurance representative to specify exactly what your policy does and does not cover. Your total obstetric care includes the hospital fees, the fee of your prenatal visits, the delivery itself, laboratory services, and prenatal testing. In the absence of complications a home birth can be a less expensive option than a hospital birth. Once you have established the total cost of these basic services, you can decide how much you want to invest in additional prenatal health care.

Some additional health care options to consider are:

- Prenatal exercise classes.
- Pregnancy massage.
- Chiropractic adjustments when you feel continual stress on any part of your back or body (a common result of pregnancy weight gain).
- Prenatal supplements prescribed by a qualified health practitioner. Consider a high-quality prenatal vitamin—which you can actually take before you conceive. Fortifying herbs prescribed by a licensed acupuncturist or herbalist can be extremely beneficial, but somewhat costly.

Treating yourself to a weekly massage or chiropractic adjustment when you are pregnant will not be an indulgence, especially if you are working every day. After all, your body will be working hard to grow your baby, and it will need constant support and nourishment. Pregnancy is a time to nurture yourself, because every time you give to yourself, you give to your unborn child. You both deserve to be healthy!

Without insurance coverage laboratory services and prenatal tests can be very expensive. You should minimally plan to have a complete prenatal laboratory work-up in the beginning of your pregnancy. Other lab tests may be needed during your pregnancy as well; ask your primary care provider which tests are essential, which are optional but recommended, and how much each test will cost. Subtracting the insurance reimbursement will give you the actual cost that you can use in your planning. For example, Matilda and Stewart were on a very strict budget and had not planned for amniocentesis. The procedure cost $1,200 and since their insurance deductible of $500 had not been met, their total cost was $740: $500 plus a 20 percent copayment.

It is wise to be prepared for prenatal tests even if you think you do not want them. Unexpected medical questions may arise, for which you will be glad you allocated some emergency funds. It is important to allow for some unknown costs even if you have insurance, and especially if you do not have coverage. Leave some room in your budget for things that you may not have considered during your preconception exploration.

One prenatal cost that is certainly never covered, even by the most comprehensive insurance plans, is the mother's wardrobe. Many women enjoy buying new clothes for their pregnancy, while others choose hand-me-downs or their partners' large-size shirts. Go to a maternity store and price items you may want. Several complete ensembles can really add up, but at the very least you should plan to invest in several new bras. Remember that you will be pregnant for more than one season, and consider buying clothes you can use after your child's birth as well.

Pregnancy is a special time to give to yourself those things that enhance your health and remind you that you are becoming a mother. Plan a budget that allows you to celebrate the life unfolding within you!

The Birth

The birth of your child is one of life's greatest joys, and although the cost of the birth can be very high, the gift of a precious new life is worth every penny you will ever have to spend. Because nature has a will of its own, the experience of giving birth is filled with unpredictable decisions—financial and otherwise. However, you will be more prepared for the unusual concerns that may arise once you are familiar with those costs that are predictable.

The cost of a hospital birth depends on the medical and technological procedures used. Fees for the doctor, the hospital room, and any specialists such as an anesthesiologist can be significant. Depending on your insurance coverage, the necessary medications, technology, and medical procedures will cost you money. A cesarean delivery costs many thousands of dollars more than a natural birth, in or out of the hospital. A home birth is the least expensive, the midwife's fee is your only consequential expense. Not all insurance policies will cover midwives, however, even though their cesarean rate is significantly lower. With a home birth you must be psychologically and financially prepared to go to the hospital if there is a medical need.

As part of your preconception financial planning, it is useful to call your obstetrician or midwife, local hospital, and other potential resources to assist you in understanding the standard fees for labor and delivery. Know the payment policies as well. Remember to plan for hidden costs if you are on a limited budget.

An additional fee that you may incur is the cost of a labor coach. Good labor support can greatly contribute to a positive birth experience. I highly recommend this investment because it can prevent any number of medical and technological procedures during the birth. Women often resort to medication or monitors because they are not prepared to handle the pain of birth. A labor assistant can guide you through the phases of labor and choices that will arise along the way—and her fee may be less expensive than the cost of drugs.

The pediatrician who is present to give your baby a checkup immediately after birth is another person to be paid. Call a local pediatrician to find out the fee, and check with your insurance company about how much is covered. The pediatrician will begin a relationship with your newborn at the birth. If there are complications, naturally this doctor's fees will include more than a regular checkup. Then well-baby checkups will begin at two weeks after the birth; these are often recommended monthly for the next three months, and bimonthly the rest of the first year. Thereafter, consult your doctor as to how often wellness checkups are advised. Of course, you can count on the seasonal viruses and bacteria that can send you to the pediatrician unexpectedly.

If you plan on immunizing or circumcising, these will be additional fees for you or your insurance company to pay. Both immunization and circumcision are optional, and I recommend that you become educated about the pros and cons of exposing a vulnerable newborn to these invasive medical procedures.

If you plan on nursing, purchase your nursing supplies in advance, including a breast pump and a few quality nursing bras. Some women invest in special nursing clothes—which are very useful and comfortable but can often be quite costly. A visit to your local maternity store will help you assess your potential purchases.

A cost rarely planned for, but almost always incurred, is film and developing. Plan on buying *lots* of film. As a new parent, you will want to take loads of pictures of your adorable new baby. Your child's delightful presence and developmental milestones will most likely keep you clicking away.

Postnatal Purchases

Future expenses will depend on your personal choices, but there are ways to save money in the beginning of your newborn's life. You might like for your child to sleep in your bed rather than a crib; hand-me-down clothes (or "heirlooms") save the cost of store-bought ones for the first few months; and breast-feeding costs less than using formula. Still, it must be faced: a child in your life means continual unexpected costs.

The basic layette includes the clothing and accessories that make up a baby's first wardrobe, and the average cost will be several hundred dollars even for the minimum. Any major department store or children's store can give you a layette list to organize your plans for the true basic needs of your newborn, or you can ask other parents what they needed. Some items that are certain to appear on this list are undershirts, socks or booties, sleepwear, hats or caps, sweaters, blankets, and a bunting or snowsuit for those born during cold weather. You will find it a rewarding use of your time to explore these suggestions as a part of your preconception or prenatal planning.

Diapers! You cannot have a baby without them. Whether you use a diaper service or disposable diapers, the average cost is ten to fifteen dollars a week (yes, that is forty to sixty dollars a month!) the first year. Most kids spend two or three years in diapers, sometimes longer. In three years' time, you will shell out about two thousand dollars just to diaper your precious one. Washing cloth diapers at home, which incurs the cost of diapers, detergent, water, electricity, and the depreciated cost of appliances, is significantly cheaper, although time consuming. Unfortunately, diaper costs are one of those very basic necessities that every new parent just has to accept. But believe me, once your child is born, you will gladly pay the money for those items that are indispensable—even if they are disposable!

Formula feeding is a significant weekly expense. In fact, for most parents formula is the most costly food item the first year. Bottles and sterilizing equipment must be bought before the child is born. Once solid feeding begins, usually at around six months of age, the food can be bought or homemade with the use of a food grinder or blender. The cost of your child's food will grow as her developmental needs change.

The decision to breast-feed can be cost-effective as well as having significant physical and emotional benefits for your child. You should plan on renting or buying a breast pump, which you will need after the first month if you want the option of other people being able to feed your baby breast milk. Dotty personally discovered the difference in cost between breast-feeding and using formula:

> Jim and I didn't realize that breast-feeding our first child for over a year saved us about one thousand dollars in formula. Our second child could not breast-feed because of my medical condition, and it was a large unexpected expense we had not planned on.

Unless you choose to have your child sleep in the family bed for an indefinite period of time, a bassinet or cradle is common for the first months of the child's life; plan on your child graduating to a crib by the fourth month. Crib mattresses, a comforter, a bumper, blankets, and linens are additional costs. Baby changing tables, a dresser or chest for clothes, an adult rocking chair, as well as an infant carrier are frequent purchases for new parents. In most states an infant or convertible car seat is mandatory when your child travels with you. A carriage or stroller is essential once you want to be in the world with your little one and is often used for several years, so it is worth investing in a sturdy one. Once your child is eating solids and can sit up, at around six months, a high chair will complete your list of basic baby furniture.

Non-necessities that make life easier can wait until after your child is born and you decide what conveniences make sense for your lifestyle. Some possibilities are diaper hampers and disposable wastebaskets, lamps, nursery monitors, diaper bags, vaporizers, rocking chairs, toy hampers, portable cribs, baby bouncers, playpens, soft infant carriers, and a frame backpack. There will also be a seemingly infinite number of inexpensive items such as bath and feeding supplies, as well as many nursery accessories. But be careful. Those little things do add up.

Childproofing your home is very important as soon as your child becomes mobile, often around six to eight months. Covering electrical outlets and wires, as well as placing childproof safety gates in dangerous areas, are among the best investments you can make to keep your child safe and give yourself peace of mind as he explores the world. Window, cabinet, drawer, and door locks are also commonly used. The cost of childproofing your home can run hundreds of dollars, depending on the size of the house or apartment, the number of household items that will be affected, and whether you do the installation yourself or hire someone.

It will be up to you how much you spend in the future on toys and books based upon your child's developmental needs and your finances. Rattles, stuffed toys, activity centers, and swings are common items to request as baby presents from doting family and friends. Many new parents keep their investments simple and offer their plastic Tupperware and other safe household utensils for their child's delight. Once your child begins to crawl and toddle, there will be a need for additional clothes and toys. As the years go by you will have to continually evaluate how much you spend in many areas of your child's growing needs.

Another major expense to consider before conceiving a child is child care costs, especially if both parents need to work or either parent needs personal time away from parenting responsibilities. A child care facility is usually cheaper than a private caregiver in the home. In most major cities parents pay an average of five to eight dollars an hour for day care, and six to twelve dollars an hour for a person in the home. If you plan on returning to work for a forty-hour week, your child care costs can range from two hundred to five hundred dollars a week. Thus, some full-time professional parents can pay ten thousand to twenty-five thousand dollars a year in child care costs. Plan when you will return to work and how many hours of child care you need per week. Then use an estimated fee to calculate your expenses.

Child care costs include baby-sitting if you want to leave your child for activities that may or may not be work related. An evening at the movies and dinner can cost you twenty to fifty dollars just in baby-sitting fees. It is worth paying for experienced child care. Of course, having supportive family or friends to watch your child can cut the cost of a relaxing date. Make sure your child is happy and safe with whomever she is entrusted to, even if it is for a short time. Always ask for references and request that the caregiver be certified in CPR (a three-hour course offered by the American Red Cross).

Be sure to choose a child care provider who models your values and principles and honors your style of parenting. Your child's birthright is to feel safe and be consistently loved. Invest in dependable, creative, and compassionate child care providers because your child's sense of self will be profoundly affected, either positively or negatively, by these individuals.

An additional source of financial challenge for many new parents is the prospect of planning for the educational needs of one or more children. The cost of a basic college education in the next several decades is staggering. An estimate of several hundred thousand dollars for a four-year state school (tuition, room, and board) is considered conservative. A good financial investor can help you sort through the projected fees and learn how to begin establishing a strategy of clearly defined goals and priorities for your child's education.

Some parents know that they want to have the funds available to pay for a private preschool and the entire thirteen years of their child's education even before college investments. Such costs can be very demanding, averaging from several thousand to more than ten thousand dollars a year. Consider Charlene's experience:

> When we had Brad, we knew he was a slow learner before he was a toddler. We did not want him to get lost in the impersonal relationships of our large public school classrooms. We knew if we did not immerse him in an intimate situation with a small teacher-to-student ratio, Brad would never stand a chance to develop his full potential. We spent more on his preschool education than I did for my college tuition twenty years ago! But it was worth it because now he is thriving and loves to learn. We had not planned for his learning disabilities before he was born so we had to take out some education loans. Imagine that—for preschool! In our preconception planning we never considered that we would be investing so much in a little kid's education, and who knows?—maybe our next child will be exceptionally gifted and need a special school to develop his unique talents. No one told us to plan on this.

Determine whether you want a systematic program to invest in your child's immediate and future needs. Saving money for your child's life requires a lot of intuition, risk taking, goal assessment, and practical thinking. It may be as simple as focusing on the financial need of the month or as complex as developing a broad-based financial strategy that includes large-scale goals such as saving money for a new home or renting a larger home with room for future children. The following creative exercise will help you clarify your own potential costs of having a child. Every child deserves to live in a healthy home with a feeling of physical and psychological security. What factors represent that for you? When you understand the practical costs of having your baby before he is conceived, you can plan accordingly to make necessary resources available. Then, when your child is born, you will be able to fully welcome and enjoy his magical presence in your life.

Creative Exercise:
Your Financial Fitness Plan

Use your creative imagination, intuition, and practical sense to estimate the following potential expenses. You can call the necessary people to get realistic estimates—yet remember that unexpected costs will arise. Even if you are not able to gather completely accurate figures, review the list so that you will become familiar with what fees you may have to, or choose to, pay. Which will be a onetime expense and which will be monthly? Remember to include your current living expenses to examine the total cost of having a baby and its impact on all of your finances.

I encourage you to have each partner independently use the following questions to clarify financial commitments for your future child. Then compare your answers and create your combined financial goals.

What to Expect for Preconception Health Care

1. Doctor visits $_____
2. Preconception medical tests $_____
3. Acupuncture $_____
4. Herbs $_____
5. Chiropractic $_____
6. Counseling $_____
7. Exercise classes $_____
8. Nutritional supplements $_____
9. Health insurance $_____
10. Additional items (specify) $_____
11. Allowance for unknown expenses $_____

   Total estimated preconception costs = $_____

What to Expect for Prenatal Health Care

1. Doctor visits $_____
2. Prenatal tests $_____
3. Prenatal lab services $_____
4. Acupuncture $_____
5. Herbs $_____
6. Chiropractic $_____
7. Counseling $_____
8. Exercise classes $_____

9. Nutritional supplements $_____
10. Health insurance $_____
11. Prenatal massage $_____
12. Pregnancy clothes $_____
13. Layette items for the baby (list items) $_____
14. Furniture for the nursery (list items) $_____
15. Bedding items for the baby $_____
16. Nursery needs and accessories $_____
17. Childbirth classes $_____
18. Additional items (specify) $_____
19. Allowance for unknown expenses $_____

   Total estimated prenatal costs = $_____

What to Expect for the Birth

Remember to calculate the initial cost of the service, minus your insurance reimbursement, to determine the actual cost to you.

1. Labor and delivery (doctor or midwife fee) $_____
2. Anesthesia services $_____
3. Pediatric services $_____
4. Circumcision (optional) $_____
5. Hospital charges (room and board, labor and delivery room, nursery, regular or intensive care; laboratory, medications, supplies, nursing care, and so on) $_____
6. Home birth supplies (ask your midwife what is needed) $_____
7. Labor coach $_____
8. Lactation consultation (if breast-feeding) $_____
9. Formula and supplies (if not breast-feeding) $_____
10. Additional items (specify) $_____
11. Allowance for unknown expenses $_____

   Total estimated prenatal costs = $_____

What to Expect Postnatally

1. Breast-feeding pump and supplies $_____
2. Diapers (and wraps if using cloth) $_____
3. Additional furniture $_____
4. Additional baby clothes $_____
5. Additional nursery accessories $_____

6. Toys $_____
7. Bath supplies $_____
8. Well-baby care/pediatrician $_____
9. Additional items (specify) $_____
10. Allowance for unknown expenses $_____

Total estimated postnatal costs = $_____

What to Expect after the First Year

1. Childproofing $_____
2. Child care $_____
3. Additional baby clothes $_____
4. Additional nursery accessories $_____
5. Developmental toys $_____
6. Well-baby care/pediatrician $_____
7. Diapers $_____
8. Additional items (specify) $_____
9. Health Insurance $_____
10. Allowance for unknown expenses $_____

Total estimated costs = $_____

What to Expect Long Term Thereafter:

1. Education:
   Extracurricular activities (dance, music, sports lessons) $_____
   Preschool $_____
   Early education $_____
   High school $_____
   College $_____
2. Child care for work and entertainment needs $_____
3. Additional clothes $_____
4. Food $_____
5. Toys, books, audio and video games $_____
6. Well-child care $_____
7. Insurance for the child $_____
8. Additional items (specify) $_____
9. Allowance for unknown expenses $_____

Total estimated costs = $_____

Creating Your Goals

With your partner review your separate answers, then consider the following questions as you together create a way to reach your goals. Be specific with your answers.

Be assured that these are just plans. You can provide a child with a good life even if you don't have a lot of money. In your new life with your child, there will be lots of surprises, financial and otherwise. Although these financial exercises can be used to guide you in ways that will give you greater financial clarity, the greatest security you can give your child is your abundant love and faith in a happy, healthy future together.

1. Now that you have reviewed the expenses of having a child, what have you discovered?
2. How do you feel about learning what it can cost you to have your child?
3. What are your financial goals in preparing for parenthood?
4. How can you implement a plan for achieving your goals?
5. Do you want to make a current inventory of your major assets?
6. Do you have any benefit programs?
7. Do you need to review existing financial arrangements?
8. Do you need a comprehensive financial analysis? Do you need a financial professional to assist you?
9. How do you feel about your savings habits and current investments?
10. How do your current debts and liabilities affect your confidence in providing for your child?
11. What is your household income, and how much of it is used to pay your monthly expenses before including a child? How much is left over to invest in the child?
12. What do you need to do to be financially ready to conceive a child? How much time do you need to create this reality?

Appendix D

From Soul to Cell:
The Process of Reincarnation

*The body is the soul, it is the soul's replication in flesh and blood,
the simultaneous impact of . . . its prior incarnations.*

Corrine Heline

Perhaps a soul will choose you as its future parents, and you will be
graced to give birth to a baby. But how will the soul experience incarnation into a human form that will become your future child? Is there a
detailed plan for how the soul develops its human self? According to
ageless wisdom teachings—the "golden thread" connecting the mystical
teachings of East and West—once the soul chooses to reincarnate, not
only does the physical body go through a very complex process of
growth, but so do the etheric, emotional, and mental bodies.

Though even the most advanced human development texts struggle
to fully comprehend this process, there is yet a general consensus of who
we are and how we are made. The descent of a soul into a human being
combines natural and spiritual laws, material and invisible structures,
objective facts and subjective realities. I have found the Theosophical
Society texts to most clearly describe the process of reincarnation.

Based on Theosophy's inclusive and universal presentations about
reincarnation, I am offering my distilled interpretation of the writings
that share beliefs about the nature of a soul's return to human embodiment. I have attempted to describe this complex phenomena in a simple
way that will inspire you to compassionately and wisely use the information to more deeply embrace your future child as an evolving soul with
very specific developmental needs. The following offers a streamlined

understanding of the multidimensional reality underlying the rebirth process of your future child.

Past Seeds Blossom into New Life

According to Theosophy, during each incarnation the new personality body is built of the exact quality as the one left behind at the death of the previous incarnation. This same notion is suggested by Rabbi Berg, a contemporary Kabbalist. He states that "every soul, returning after death, must find a place in which conditions will be similar to those just left behind."[1] For most souls, being reborn is for the purpose of unfolding and expressing through a human embodiment our latent divine potentials. For advanced souls, it also may be for the purpose of serving humanity to support the fruition of the divine plan on earth.

The personality form is created by the soul to anchor itself in the three worlds of human experience: physical existence, emotional experience, and mental endeavor and understanding. Each of these worlds embodies different qualities of life energy. The parts of life that the soul deems important for a specific phase of its evolution will receive more power in a given lifetime. Thus some people may have a greater orientation toward their physical development, while others may emphasize their emotional, mental, or spiritual aspects in a particular life cycle. It can be beneficial to deepen your understanding about the specific developmental sequence of your child's physical, emotional, and mental bodies, which begin forming before physical conception.

Theosophy holds that our body, emotions, mind, and intuition (the gateway to our soul) are all innate aspects of our inner nature. Death is described as a recurring incident in an endless life—each lifetime creating the opportunity for the incarnating soul to experience a fuller and more radiant existence. Rebirth is an aspect of the cyclical law seen everywhere in nature, alternating between periods of activity and times of rest and assimilation.

To better comprehend what happens when a soul begins the rebirth process, it is useful to understand what the soul experiences at the end of a human life cycle. When a human being dies, it casts off its material self, the human personality, by shedding the physical body, disintegrating the emotional and mental bodies, and withdrawing that portion of itself that was put forth at the beginning of the life cycle before physical conception—the soul aspect. No longer seeking growth and evolution in the physical, emotional, and mental realms, the soul returns to its own plane of consciousness, the causal plane (in a stage called *devachan* in Sanskrit, a vivid dreamlike state), bringing with it the memory of all of the experiences through which the personality has passed on earth. Then a gestatory period begins during which all of the life experiences of the past incarnation are reviewed and translated into various corresponding powers and gifts. These are added to those already developed in previous cycles.

When this integration is over, the soul begins to thirst for new experiences, for it will desire to reincarnate over and over again until every possible latent divine power has been unfolded and every human lesson has been learned. It will desire to be nourished again by the senses of a human personality. As it prepares to reincarnate, the soul begins to turn its attention outward to the lower three worlds—the physical, emotional, and mental.

How a Soul Incarnates to Become Your Child

In order for a soul to become your infant, there are specific steps it will go through. Motivated by an impulse to be born, the soul sends forth a part of itself into the dense world of matter, and based on the conditions of its past lives (especially the most recent), it begins to gather the materials of its subtle bodies—the etheric, emotional, and mental vehicles—to create its new personality for the present incarnation. While this complex process is underway, it awaits the appropriate opportunity to create a physical body for birth.

During each incarnation, the soul projects down into the three lower worlds a pulsating ethereal cable of energy called the silver cord (also known in Sanskrit as the *Sutratma*, the Life Thread, or life line), which connects all of the personality bodies to the soul consciousness. The silver cord is a dual current of life and consciousness threads. The life thread is anchored in the heart; the consciousness thread, in the head. The body can live without the consciousness thread (as in cases of senility, coma, fainting, and so on) but will die if the life thread leaves the heart. This lifeline is like the main energy circuit of the physical body, and without its current the body cannot remain "on."

The silver cord bears three focal points of energy, which Hindu and Theosophical texts refer to esoterically as the mental permanent atom, the astral permanent atom, and the physical-etheric permanent atom. These permanent atoms are not really "atoms" per se, but rather energetic points that absorb experiences and condense them into an extremely concentrated vibrational essence. They hold together the substance that the soul needs to create its human form. The vibration of each permanent atom determines the character of the body it functions through, and the experiences of each lifetime modify these vibrations. The mental permanent atom is split in two parts. One part remains with the soul within its sphere of influence; the other is called the mental unit and functions within the mental body. In the Bible these permanent-seed-atoms are called "Books of Life."[2]

All consciousness, memory, and faculty are stored in these permanent atoms. And these three seeds of consciousness hold the blueprint for what will be your child's human personality (see The Soul Consciousness Prior to Incarnating, page 301). All three permanent atoms are essential mechanisms of incarnation, for they are the force centers around which the personality bodies are built.

These tiny concentrated reels of energy contain all of an individual's past thoughts and deeds and are not dissipated at death along with the rest of the personality material. When the soul is between incarnations, and not functioning in the physical, mental, and emotional worlds, its permanent atoms of these realms are dormant. When it again focuses on reincarnation, "it draws to itself and activates its permanent atoms in each world, using them as the seeds from which the full bodies are constructed. The permanent atom functions like the seed molecule of a crystalline substance in solution—the solution will crystallize around it. So the unique vibrations of each permanent or seed atoms give a characteristic stamp to the bodies built up around them. These atoms, then, are the link between lives, the carriers of influence from one life to the next."[3]

After our physical death, each of our subtle bodies also dies in succession. As each body dies, its permanent atom is retracted back into the soul in its realm. Once there, a kind of cocoon forms around the permanent atom and it goes into a suspended animation, during which the soul will harvest from it all of its virtuous qualities. You can think of these as the distillations of all the experiences of a human life that have been condensed into vibrational essence by the permanent atoms. The soul adds these qualities to itself, rounding out its character and growing spiritually.

After the soul absorbs this wealth of experience, it seems to say, "I want to learn more! Let's create another human personality." In some cases this impulse on the part of the soul is strengthened by a group or planetary need that, in essence, calls the soul back. For example, a future family system on earth may need this soul for its growth, or this soul may be needed in a future vocational role to serve humanity. The soul's excitement begins to awaken the permanent atoms from their peaceful rest with the soul on the causal plane. Based on the soul's next lessons, its karma, and its present as well as its future purpose, the permanent atoms are vivified and energized for their long journey into creating the human personality. It is a miraculous pilgrimage the soul goes through in order to become your child.

Multidimensional Conception

Many medical texts and pregnancy books depict the ordered sequence of gestation and growth once physical conception has occurred. Yet rarely do these resources illustrate that the etheric, emotional, and mental bodies have sequential growth as well.

The teachings defined in Theosophy texts generally describe four conceptions that occur as soon as a soul begins its process into incarnation. In the subtle realms the mental body is conceived first, then the emotional, then the etheric. The physical body is the last to be conceived. Each of these four bodies goes through a precise order of developmental phases as it stabilizes and matures.

By the time it begins creating its physical body, a soul coming into the world actually has gone through a profound personal evolution. It has begun the formation of the etheric body in the etheric realm, the emotional body in the emotional realm, and the mental body in the mental realm. As with the physical body, all of the personality bodies will continue to grow both in utero and postnatally. We can begin to appreciate the genuine sophistication of what appears to be a helpless newborn at birth: In fact many lifetimes are held within this beautiful new form. To call a baby "new life" is less accurate than to refer to it as "old life in a new form." The diagrams on pages 310–305 can assist you in understanding the complex journey unfolding for your future child.

When a soul is ready to make its appearance in the material world to further its knowledge and power, it projects its three permanent atoms along the silver cord. Each of the permanent atoms sends out a unique vibrational code, often referred to in Theosophical texts as the "word." This inaudible sound is a magnetic frequency that attracts the life

THE SOUL CONSCIOUSNESS PRIOR TO INCARNATING

I. SOURCE/SPIRIT/GOD

This is the One Consciousness that permeates all life.

II. THE SOUL REALM

At the end of a life cycle the soul harvests the virtuous qualities gained through that incarnation and absorbs them into its being. After fully absorbing the fruits of one incarnation, the soul desires another human experience, which reawakens and vivifies the permanent atoms from their rest. The soul pours its energies into the permanent atoms so that it can send them into their own realms to grow a body for the human personality vehicle. The first to awaken and grow is the mental body, followed by the emotional body and then the physical-etheric body. During the nine months of pregnancy, the four bodies continue to grow and align, beginning a lifetime process of integration and balancing.

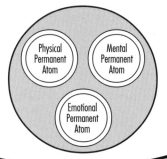

There is no activity in the lower three realms (mental, emotional, physical-etheric) until the soul chooses to reincarnate and sends its consciousness into them through the permanent atoms.
The physical and etheric bodies share the same physical permanent atom.

III. THE MENTAL REALM

The first body to begin forming the new human personality as
the soul begins to reincarnate.

IV. THE EMOTIONAL REALM

The second body to begin forming as the new human personality forms.

V. THE PHYSICAL-ETHERIC REALMS

The last personality bodies to begin forming.

THE SOUL PREPARING TO CREATE A NEW PERSONALITY

I. SOURCE/SPIRIT/GOD

This is the One Consciousness that permeates all life.

II. THE SOUL REALM

Physical Permanent Atom

Mental Permanent Atom

Emotional Permanent Atom

The soul consciousness is still focused only in the soul realm, preparing to incarnate and create a new human form with new mental, emotional, and physical-etheric bodies.

III. THE MENTAL REALM

There is no mental body formed yet.

IV. THE EMOTIONAL REALM

There is no emotional body formed yet.

V. THE PHYSICAL-ETHERIC REALMS

There is no physical or etheric body formed yet.

THE FORMATION OF THE MENTAL BODY

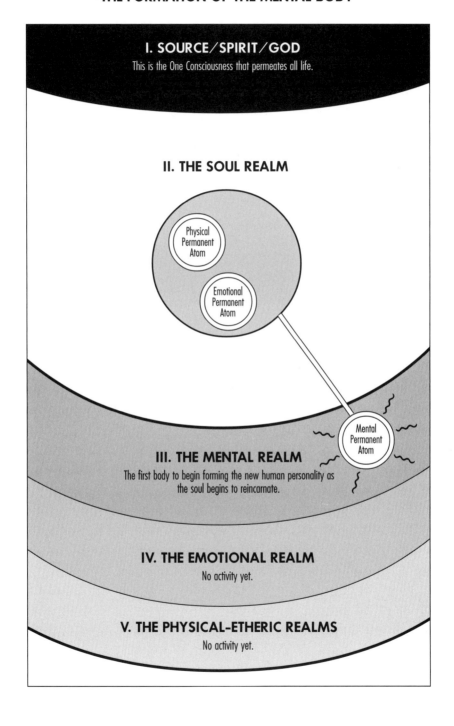

I. SOURCE/SPIRIT/GOD
This is the One Consciousness that permeates all life.

II. THE SOUL REALM

Physical Permanent Atom

Emotional Permanent Atom

Mental Permanent Atom

III. THE MENTAL REALM
The first body to begin forming the new human personality as the soul begins to reincarnate.

IV. THE EMOTIONAL REALM
No activity yet.

V. THE PHYSICAL-ETHERIC REALMS
No activity yet.

THE FORMATION OF THE EMOTIONAL BODY

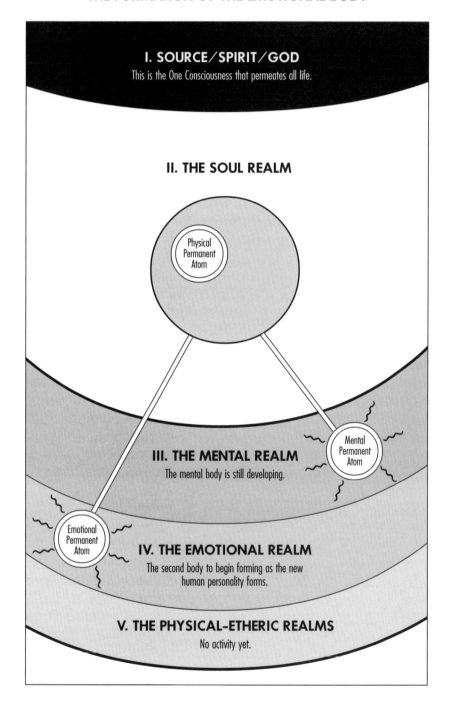

I. SOURCE/SPIRIT/GOD
This is the One Consciousness that permeates all life.

II. THE SOUL REALM

Physical
Permanent
Atom

Mental
Permanent
Atom

III. THE MENTAL REALM
The mental body is still developing.

Emotional
Permanent
Atom

IV. THE EMOTIONAL REALM
The second body to begin forming as the new
human personality forms.

V. THE PHYSICAL-ETHERIC REALMS
No activity yet.

THE DEVELOPMENT OF THE PHYSICAL AND ETHERIC BODIES

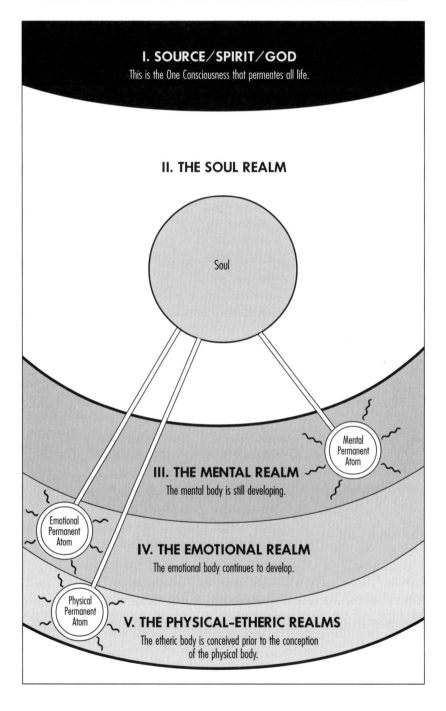

I. SOURCE/SPIRIT/GOD
This is the One Consciousness that permeates all life.

II. THE SOUL REALM

Soul

Mental
Permanent
Atom

III. THE MENTAL REALM
The mental body is still developing.

Emotional
Permanent
Atom

IV. THE EMOTIONAL REALM
The emotional body continues to develop.

Physical
Permanent
Atom

V. THE PHYSICAL-ETHERIC REALMS
The etheric body is conceived prior to the conception
of the physical body.

substance that matches it. Under the soul's influence, each permanent atom becomes, in effect, a magnet drawing to itself the material appropriate to its specific vibration that will create the body of its particular realm.

Once the sperm has fertilized the egg, the creative sound actually sets up a kind of vortex into which surrounding matter is drawn; the etheric, emotional, and mental bodies each are gradually shaped into an ovoid of energy that surrounds the human embryo.

Throughout the prenatal life, this magnetic vibration is gathered around the permanent atoms and organizes the consciousness of each of the personality bodies according to karmic divine design. As the clairvoyant Geoffrey Hodson states, "Resonance and magnetic properties ensure this."

Karma does modify the formation of these bodies. This controlling factor of karma is carried over from previous incarnations. Karmic deficiencies—which can appear as disease in the physical body and personality aberrations in the emotional and mental bodies—are in the projected blueprint carried in each of the permanent atoms. They also carry the seeds of past negative tendencies, which will be offered to the personality consciousness of this incarnation as opportunities to learn from and transform.[4]

The Formation of the Mental Body

See The Formation of the Mental Body on page 303. For humans, the mental unit is always the first of the personality aspects to mature, and it is conceived before the physical-etheric and emotional bodies. When ripened by the desire of the soul to return to human form, the mental unit is projected outward from the causal (soul) plane into the subtle matter of the mental realm. Once residing in this realm, the mental unit vibrates with the general qualities it has condensed into itself from the previous life, as well as qualities modified by its karmic needs. The specific resonant frequency of "the word," an essence of consciousness, affects the matter of the mental realm, attracting mental matter of a similar nature to itself. The soul begins to assemble the mental body of the child-to-be—the mental personality through which it will think during its next lifetime.

The Formation of the Emotional Body

See The Formation of the Emotional Body on page 304. The emotional permanent atom is next to ripen and develops its emotional body through a process similar to that of the mental permanent atom. It also vibrates within its own unique spectrum of frequencies, but it does so in the emotional realm. As it attracts similar emotional matter to itself, it is forming the emotional body of the soul's personality vehicle. The mental and emotional bodies continue to grow in their specific gestational sequence.

The Formation of the Physical-Etheric Body

See The Development of the Physical and Etheric Bodies on page 305. Finally, the physical permanent atom is sent by the soul to the etheric realm. This permanent atom actually creates two personality bodies—the etheric body and the physical body. In most models of esoteric anatomy the physical and etheric are considered one body, often referred to as the physical-etheric body. This is because of the esoteric relationship between the etheric and physical realms. The etheric realm is often perceived as the juncture between matter and energy. It is a subtle energy field that represents a refined order of matter that surrounds the physical body. With its subtle magnetism, it constructs the personality blueprint of this incarnation by receiving soul impressions, as well as influences from the mental and emotional bodies that are embodying into physical matter. This etheric body creates the physical body from organic matter by forming a vehicle through which the soul may influence bioelectric fields and living systems. The etheric body serves as a battery for the physical body's health and vitality and includes the meridians, acupuncture points, and chakras.

Once the mental and emotional permanent atoms have been established in their own realms, then "the soul sends a thread of itself through the silver cord passing through the mental and emotional realm, and into the newly forming etheric body in the etheric realm. The soul establishes organizational codings in the etheric body, which attracts more bioelectric energy of increasing levels of complexity into its growing field. This eventually creates a stable and dynamically fluid electromagnetic field that will determine the precise blueprint for the physical body of the incoming soul."[5]

Out of these four conceptions—the mental, emotional, etheric, and physical—a human being is formed inside the mother's womb. According to Theosophy, this miraculous sequence from "soul to cell" has happened to every soul that is eventually born as a little baby. In my preconception journal, I wrote about my sense of these phenomena several months before my daughter was conceived:

> About two months ago I sensed my own mental body was con- sumed with the idea of having a baby. I intuitively knew that the mental body of the Soul was being conceived on the mental plane for I could feel it drawing on the substance of my own thoughts, yet not on my emotions. Concepts and ideas of its existence were stimulated, and an inner sense to focus my thoughts on the good- ness of life was suggested. This week I felt a new emotional presence activated in my own emotional body, which makes me wonder whether the emotional body of the Soul is being conceived. I could feel my love for this Soul consume me, as if it were already born and in my life. Whether any of this is truly happening is unclear, yet I feel my heart opening to a Soul who I sense is descending steadily from the heavens to become my baby. I wonder how I will sense the conception of its physical-etheric body.

Once conception has occurred, the personality bodies continue to develop in a sequential way throughout the prenatal journey. Inspired by the Theosophical perspective, I have created a Multidimensional Trimes- ter Chart of the Human Personality (see page 310), which illustrates the way the physical-etheric, emotional, and mental bodies develop and inte- grate each trimester of the pregnancy. Unlike the Holistic Trimester Chart of the Human Personality (see page 198), this version includes the impact of the permanent atoms on the prenate's growing personality.

During the first trimester, the growth of the physical-etheric body predominates while the emotional and mental bodies, although already conceived in their own emotional and mental realm through the perma- nent atom conceptions, are still only mildly influencing the physical life of the young fetus.

During the second trimester, the emotional body joins with the developing prenate, integrating and responding to the physical-etheric and emotional body influences from the mother. The child in utero is able to directly experience more complex emotions. The emotional per- manent atom is now absorbed into the human personality vehicle, while the mental permanent atom in the mental realm is building the mental body but has only a limited influence on the young human personality.

By the third trimester, the mental body of the growing child is actively establishing itself as the mental permanent atom is absorbed into the human personality. The developing child is more responsive to thoughts, and the emotional body continues to mature in its ability to experience feelings in the womb. The physical body is growing to "full term." The individual personality of the incarnating soul is unifying as the physical-etheric, emotional, and mental bodies now interact together. By the end of the third trimester, with all personality bodies established yet still slowly unfolding in consciousness, it is time for the soul to be born and fully embody its new human form—body, heart, mind, and spirit.

Use Your Imagination to Assist the Soul's Growth

When you physically conceive your child, she has already been developing the majority of her human personality on other planes of consciousness. What you may have thought of as a chance event of a sperm finding an egg is merely the final step of the soul's multiple conception journey.

If you embrace this perspective as a possibility, you will discover ways to intentionally optimize the whole health of your future child. The emotional and mental stability of the chosen parents can undermine or enhance the reincarnation process for the soul. Before physical conception, the soul will use your thoughts and feelings to develop its emotional and mental bodies. The soul will greatly benefit if you strive to sustain a vibrant state of psychological and spiritual well-being each day.

Now is the time to refine your relationship with your own physical, emotional, and mental bodies so you can become receptive enough to perceive the needs of an incoming soul. By using your imagination, you can open to receiving intuitive impressions about the activity of the soul as it begins its preparation in the subtle realms of its existence to become your child. Djwhal Khul uses the term *mystical perception* to describe a quality available to every human being if it is developed. Mystical perception "includes the mystical vision of the soul, Spirit, God, the universe. It also is the power to contact, understand, and appreciate the meaning of the subjective world. It is the power to love and experience that which is other than self. It is the capacity to grasp and intuit ideas. It is the ability to sense the unknown. It is the power to sense, register and record the good, the beautiful and the true. It is the urge to discover, and to penetrate to the secrets of God and of nature."[6]

MULTIDIMENSIONAL TRIMESTER CHART OF THE HUMAN PERSONALITY:
Blueprint of Creation and Alignment of the Physical-Etheric, Emotional, and Mental Bodies

SOUL REALM

This is where the soul consciousness resides, and where the permanent atoms are stored each incarnation before they are projected down into the physical-etheric, emotional, and mental realms to create the next human personality.

All permanent atoms are now absorbed into human personality vehicle.

MENTAL REALM	Mental Permanent Atom Mental body conceived but not actively integrating with etheric or physical body.	Mental Permanent Atom Mental permanent atom still attracting mental substance to further develop mental body.	Mental Body more responsive to thoughts now as mental permanent atom is absorbed
EMOTIONAL (ASTRAL) REALM	Silver thread sending consciousness and life force from soul to human form to keep it alive. Emotional Permanent Atom Emotional body conceived in emotional realm, not yet fully active with physical-etheric, but mildly influencing.	Emotional Body responds with more feelings as emotional permanent atom is absorbed	Emotional Body continues to mature in its ability to respond to and experience feelings in the womb
PHYSICAL-ETHERIC REALMS	Etheric Body Physical Body conceived and growing	Etheric Body Physical Body "quickening"	Etheric Body Physical Body matures to full term
First Trimester: Cellular memory begins at conception.		**Second Trimester:** Emotional body integrating and responding to physical-etheric body and emotional influences from mother.	**Third Trimester:** Physical-etheric, emotional, and mental bodies are interacting, unifying individual personality of incarnating soul.

You can use your mystical perception and your understanding of the developmental stages of reincarnation to perceive, or at least imagine, an image or feeling of the etheric, emotional, mental, and spiritual bodies of your incoming child. Also, you can practice developing an intuitive dialogue between the incarnating soul and yourself. In meditation you can ask the soul to impress upon your awareness specific things you can do from the human side to assist in the formation of each of its four personality bodies, before and after they are conceived.

For example, when communing with my daughter's soul, I would first go into a deep state of stillness and contemplate the mystical sense of the incarnating soul's presence. Then I would ask her soul, "Is there anything I can do today to prepare for your arrival?" and allow some moments to receive an intuitive response. Sometimes the guidance would be specific, such as, "Please meditate more on inner peace," or, "Eat less protein and increase calcium." At other times it was simply an undeniable certainty that all was going along well without my detailed awareness. I stayed conscious of tuning into all aspects of her being, sometimes focusing on one personality body or another if my intuition guided me to do so. Some days I would imagine her seven chakras as brilliant spheres of radiating light—the light purifying anything that was not itself.

Kyla applied her understanding of reincarnation theory in a practical way:

> I had heard about the theory of the permanent atoms, and even though I was not sure I really grasped it all, it did inspire me—right from the time of conception—to think of our tiny child as a very old soul who had worked diligently to establish its life inside my body. I wanted to give those permanent atoms—whatever they were—my total respect, like I would any and all parts of my child. I was very conscious about eating healthy, thinking uplifting thoughts, and praying regularly. I experimented with meditating on the essence of each of the personality bodies. It felt as if I was nourishing the four permanent atoms like four seeds that were about to unfold into four beautiful flowers—together becoming my baby.

Kyla's experience illustrates that even if the reincarnation process seems abstract or complex, you can use the ideas metaphorically in your preparation process.

Creative Exercise:
Co-Creating with the Soul

1. During your preconception health care preparation, how can you practically use the theme of your future child experiencing four conceptions?
    - The conception of the mental body.
    - The conception of the emotional body.
    - The conception of the etheric body (including the chakras and acupuncture meridians).
    - The conception of the physical body.
2. What do you want to do to assist the formation of an incoming soul's mental body? The soul's emotional body? Its etheric body? Its physical body?
3. How do you feel about considering your future "new" baby as an "old" soul?
4. How can you use your mystical perception to assist the personality development of a soul who has chosen you to be its parents?
5. Imagine and draw a picture (using colors) of your future child's soul before it begins the journey of being reborn. Then draw a picture of the multidimensional conceptions as you would like them to be experienced by the soul.

Appendix E

The Implications of Abortion in a Prebirth Health Care Model

As a holistic counselor and metaphysician, my belief is that the consciousness of the incarnating soul exists *prior* to physical conception—thus the soul exists *without* a physical form. Therefore, if abortion is the chosen outcome of a conception, I feel that the physical body is shed while the soul remains alive, sometimes maintaining its focus on the etheric, astral, or mental plane for its next incarnation, or returning to the soul realm before reincarnating. Thus, as I understand it, *the true life stream animating the physical body does not die* when abortion occurs.

Nevertheless, it is also my understanding and belief that there are karmic consequences to all actions. It is up to the man and woman who have conceived a baby to determine the positive or negative effects of releasing the body of their child. Some souls may prefer to be released from the earth plane back to the spiritual realms before being born. Perhaps many of these souls become miscarriages, a natural way to release themselves. On the other hand, karmically, some souls may need the experience of a fully embodied human incarnation despite being born into adverse conditions.

If you have developed the intuitive ability through meditation to commune with your own soul, or that of your child, you can request inner guidance as to whether or not to sustain a pregnancy. In making a decision, I recommend that you follow your own principles, spiritual beliefs, inner truth, and heartfelt sense. The information in this book is not intended to support indiscriminately pro-choice or pro-life positions; my intention is rather to awaken you to the reality of the *eternal life* of the soul.

In addition to biochemical and human laws, there are cosmic and universal laws. This writing is an attempt to offer a holistic perspective that honors the laws of evolution and life.

Appendix F

Resources

Contacting the Author

For information about Dr. Luminare-Rosen's calendar of workshop events, training programs, and additional products being developed, please contact The Center for Creative Parenting. Individual consultations (by phone or in person) with Dr. Luminare-Rosen are available.

Carista Luminare-Rosen, Ph.D.
The Center for Creative Parenting
P.O. Box 2024
Petaluma, CA 94952
(707) 781-3438
E-mail: carista@aol.com
Web site: www.creativeparenting.com

Audiotapes

The following tapes can be ordered by writing to the address above. Each tape is $12 plus $2 shipping and handling in the United States, $5 overseas. Please make checks payable to The Center for Creative Parenting.

- *Preparing for Your Baby: An Interactive Prebirth Program for Couples*

One side of this tape is for the female partner, and the other is for the male partner. Your relationship to yourself, your partner, your childhood, and your future child are explored as you answer the questions out loud. Together you and your partner can discuss the issues that the tape awakens in you.

- *Commune with Your Future Child: Preconception and Prenatal Bonding*

This tape includes a relaxation technique so that you can open your intuition and commune with the soul of your child-to-be. Discover how to receive impressions from the incarnating soul to prepare and care for your child's physical, emotional, mental, and spiritual health before she is conceived and/or born.

Other Resources and Organizations

Most of these organizations have Web sites, but because site addresses often change rapidly, we have not included them here. A search engine can point you to the most current information.

American Gentle Birthing Association
1804 Southwest Oak Knoll Court
Lake Oswego, OR 97034
(503) 636-7823
Multidisciplinary group dedicated to gentle birthing.

American Holistic Medical Association
4101 Lake Boone Trail
Raleigh, NC 27607
(919) 787-5181
Information for the public, physicians, and other health care practioners on holistic medical options.

American Psychological Association
750 First Street NW
Washington, DC 20002
(202) 336-5500
The largest scientific and professional organization representing the field of psychology in the United States. Its membership includes researchers, educators, clinicians, consultants, and students.

American Society for Past-Life Research and Therapy
P.O. Box 20151
Riverside, CA 92516
(714) 780-1030
Promotes research and education in the field of regression or past-life therapy.

American Society for Reproductive Health
1290 Montgomery Highway
Birmingham, AL 35216-2809
(205) 978-5000
Offers information and supports reproductive health care services nationwide.

The Anthroposophic Press
R.R. 4, Box 94A1
Hudson, NY 12534
Offering numerous books on the Waldorf Steiner approach to education, health care, parenting. Holistic approaches to honoring the body, mind, and soul of the child before and after birth.

The Association for Prenatal and Perinatal Psychology and Health (APPPAH)
P.O. Box 994
Geyserville, CA 95441
(707) 857-4041

An educational organization dedicated to a comprehensive exploration of the physical, emotional, mental, and spiritual development and health of the unborn and newborn child. The association holds a biennial international conference and publishes a quarterly journal.

The Theosophical Publishing House (Quest Books)
306 West Geneva Road
Wheaton, IL 60187
(630) 665-0130

Publishes classical and contemporary works on Theosophy and allied subjects, including transpersonal psychology, meditation, new science, deep ecology, holistic health and healing, spirituality, and comparative religion.

Center for Sexual Abuse Counseling
214 Market Street, No. 14
Brighton, MA 02135
(617) 782-7664

Resources for adults who were sexually abused as children.

Christiane Northrup, M.D.
Health Wisdom for Women
Phillips Publishing, Inc.
P.O. Box 60042
7811 Montrose Road
Potomac, MD 20859-0042
(800) 221-8561

Dr. Northrup offers a monthly newsletter discussing safe, effective, and natural solutions to women's health problems.

Emerson Training Seminars
4940 Bodego Avenue
Petaluma, CA 94952
(707) 763-7024

Publications, videotapes, training, workshops about treating prenatal and birth trauma in babies. For parents and professionals.

Hoffman Institute
223 San Anselmo Avenue, Suite 4
San Anselmo, CA 94960
(415) 485-5220

Offering intensive programs to heal childhood pain and traumas affecting adult wellness.

International Childbirth Education Association
P.O. Box 20084
Minneapolis, MN 55420-0048

Offers information about family-centered maternity care.

La Leche League International

9616 Minneapolis Avenue
Franklin Park, IL 60131

Local chapters throughout the United States and Canada offering breast-feeding information and support groups.

Lucis Publishing Company

113 University Place, 11th Floor
New York, NY 10003

Publishes and distributes the Alice Bailey writings.

Midwives Alliance of North America (MANA)

P.O. Box 175
Newton, KS 67114
(888) 923-6262

An organization of North American midwives and their advocates, MANA's central mission is to promote midwifery as a quality health care option. Provides information on the legal status of midwifery in various states.

Mind-Body Health Sciences, Inc.

393 Dixon Road
Boulder, CO 80302
(303) 440-8460

Dr. Joan Borysenko's organization, which offers audiotapes and other products on mind-body health.

Mind/Body Medical Institute

Deaconess Hospital
1 Deaconess Road
Boston, MA 02215

Information on Alice Domar, M.D., author of Healing Mind,
Healthy Woman: Using the Mind Body Connection to Manage Stress
and Take Control of Your Life.

Mothering Magazine

P.O. Box 1690
Sante Fe, NM 87504
(505) 984-8116, main office
(800) 984-8116, for subscriptions

A quarterly magazine offering thoroughly researched alternative parenting information.

National Association of Parents and Professionals
for Safe Alternatives in Childbirth (NAPSAC)

P.O. Box 646
Marble Hill, MO 63764

Promotes safe alternatives in childbirth with an emphasis on home births and opposing unnecessary medical interventions. Publishes books and newsletters.

National Organization of Circumcision
Information Resources Centers (NOCIRC)
P.O. Box 2512
San Anselmo, CA 94979
(415) 488-9883

Information, newsletter, book orders, conferences to address the harm caused by circumcision.

National Women's Health Network
514 10th Street NW, Suite 400
Washington, DC 20004

Offers a Women's Health Information Clearinghouse, which provides unbiased health information for women.

New Atlantean Press
P.O. Box 9638
Santa Fe, NM 87504
(505) 983-1856

Extensive resource catalog and books about the dangers of childhood immunizations. Alternative parenting books available.

Niravi Payne, M.S.
Whole Person Fertility Program
100 Remsen Street
Brooklyn, NY 11201

The Whole Person Fertility Program offers a mind-body approach to fertility health.

Resolve, Inc.
1310 Broadway
Somerville, MA 02144-1731
(617) 623-0744

A national organization offering cutting-edge information and conferences for those struggling with infertility issues.

Single Mothers by Choice
P.O. Box 1642
Grace Square Station
New York, NY 10028
(212) 988-0993

Information for single mothers seeking support.

The Theosophical Society in America
P.O. Box 270
Wheaton, IL 60189-0270
(630) 668-1571

A nonsectarian worldwide organization devoted to promoting human solidarity, cultural understanding, and self-development. The Theosophical Society seeks to reconcile the religions, philosophies, and sciences of East and West.

Notes

Chapter Two

1. Richard Grossinger, *Embryogenesis: From Cosmos to Creature—The Origins of Human Biology* (Berkeley: North Atlantic Books, 1986), 5.

2. William Blake, *The Marriage of Heaven and Hell,* edited by Alfred Kazin (New York: Viking Press, 1946), 250.

3. Piero Ferrucci, *What We May Be* (New York: Putnam, 1982), 67.

4. Ina Crawford, *A Guide to the Mysteries* (London: The Lucis Press, 1990), 184.

5. Virginia MacIvor and Sandra LaForest, *Vibrations* (York Beach, Maine: Samuel Weiser, Inc., 1990), 95.

6. Ina Crawford, *A Guide to the Mysteries,* 175.

7. Ibid., 200.

8. John Algeo, *Reincarnation Explored* (Wheaton, Ill.: The Theosophical Society Publishing House, 1987), 133.

9. Ibid., 28.

10. "Theosophy Northwest," on World Wide Web at www.theosophy-nw.org/theosnw/reincar/re-elo.html, 27 September 1999.

11. Ibid.

12. Rabbi Berg, *Wheels of a Soul* (New York: The Kabbalah Learning Centre, 1995) 30–32, 49–50, 54.

13. Joseph Head and S. L. Cranston, *Reincarnation: An East-West Anthology* (Wheaton: Ill.: The Theosophical Publishing House, 1990), vii.

14. Ibid., 232.

15. Ibid., 299.

16. Ibid., 308.

17. "Theosophical Society in America," on World Wide Web at www.theosophical.org/intro.html, 27 September 1999.

18. Manly P. Hall, *Man: The Grand Symbol of the Mysteries* (Los Angeles: The Philosophical Research Society, Inc., 1972), 20.

19. Joseph Head and S. L. Cranston, *Reincarnation: An East-West Anthology,* 270.

Chapter Three

1. Richard Marrs, M.D., Lisa Friedman Bloch, and Kathy Kirtland Silverman, *Fertility Book* (New York: Delacorte Press, 1997), 13.

2. Alice D. Domar, M.D., and Henry Dreher, *Healing Mind, Healthy Woman* (New York: Henry Holt Company, 1996), 267.

3. John R. Sussman, M.D. and B. Blake Levitt, *Before You Conceive* (New York: Bantam Books, 1989), 150.

4. Bruce H. Lipton, "Maternal Emotions and Human Development," *The Golden Thread* 2 (1): 21–22 (1997).

5. Alice D. Domar, M.D., and Henry Dreher, *Healing Mind, Healthy Woman*, 234.

6. Norra Tannenhaus, *Pre-Conceptions* (Chicago: Contemporary Books, Inc., 1988), 11.

7. Karen Bradstreet, *Overcoming Infertility Naturally* (Pleasant Grove, Utah: Woodland Books, 1995), 40.

8. John R. Sussman, M.D., and B. Blake Levitt, *Before You Conceive*, 28.

9. Ibid., 31–37.

10. Winifred Conkling, *Getting Pregnant Naturally* (New York: Avon Books, 1999), 164.

11. John R. Sussman, M.D., and B. Blake Levitt, *Before You Conceive*, 113; and Karen Bradstreet, *Overcoming Infertility Naturally*, 44.

12. Karen Bradstreet, *Overcoming Infertility Naturally*, 43–44.

13. Richard Marrs, M.D., Lisa Friedman Bloch, and Kathy Kirtland Silverman, *Fertility Book*, 17.

14. Ibid., 20.

15. John R. Sussman, M.D., and B. Blake Levitt, *Before You Conceive*, 22.

16. Karen Bradstreet, *Overcoming Infertility Naturally*, 43–44.

17. John R. Sussman, M.D., and B. Blake Levitt, *Before You Conceive*, 101.

18. Winifred Conkling, *Getting Pregnant Naturally*, 59.

19. John R. Sussman, M.D., and B. Blake Levitt, *Before You Conceive*, 41.

20. Karen Bradstreet, *Overcoming Infertility Naturally*, 58.

21. Niravi B. Payne and Brenda Lane Richardson, *The Whole Person Fertility Program* (New York: Three Rivers Press, 1997), 58.

22. Alice D. Domar, M.D., and Henry Dreher, *Healing Mind, Healthy Woman*, 4.

23. Niravi B. Payne and Brenda Lane Richardson, *The Whole Person Fertility Program*, 74.

24. Christiane Northrup, M.D., *Women's Bodies, Women's Wisdom* (New York: Bantam Books, 1998), 418.

25. Niravi B. Payne and Brenda Lane Richardson, *The Whole Person Fertility Program*, 6.

26. Christiane Northrup, M.D., *Women's Bodies, Women's Wisdom*, 418.

27. Honora Lee Wolfe, *Healthy Pregnancy, Healthy Birth* (Boulder, Colo.: Blue Poppy Press, 1994), 3.

28. Mantak Chia and Maneewan Chia, *Awakening Healing Light of the Tao* (Huntington, N.Y.: Healing Tao Books, 1993), 31.

29. Bob Flaws, *Path of Pregnancy* (Brookline, Mass.: Paradigm Publications, 1983), 165.

30. Leslie Ann Oldershaw, "Infertility According to Chinese Medicine" (El Cerrito, Calif.: self-published, 1998), 1–2.

31. Ibid.

32. Bick Jane Tang, "Infertility: Traditional Chinese Herbal and Acupuncture Treatment of Female and Male Infertility" (Mill Valley, Calif.: self-published, 1991), 40–41.

33. Leslie Ann Oldershaw, "Infertility According to Chinese Medicine," 3.

34. Honora Lee Wolfe, *Healthy Pregnancy, Healthy Birth*, 8–9.

35. Mantak Chia and Maneewan Chia, *Awakening Healing Light of the Tao*, 57.

36. Honora Lee Wolfe, *Healthy Pregnancy, Healthy Birth*, 9.

37. Bick Jane Tang, "Infertility: Traditional Chinese Herbal and Acupuncture Treatment of Female and Male Infertility," 11.

38. "Can Toxins Affect Your Children?," *Bostonia* (Jan/Feb, 1990): 12.

39. John R. Sussman, M.D., and B. Blake Levitt, *Before You Conceive*, 119.

40. Winifred Conkling, *Getting Pregnant Naturally*, 165–66.

41. John R. Sussman, M.D., and B. Blake Levitt, *Before You Conceive*, 83–85.

42. Ibid., 17.

43. Karen F. Schmidt, "The Dark Legacy of Fatherhood," *U.S. News and World Report* (Dec. 1993): 94–96.

44. Ibid., 96.

45. John R. Sussman, M.D., and B. Blake Levitt, *Before You Conceive*, 28–29.

46. Ibid., 28.

47. Ibid., 55.

48. Ibid., 31–37.

Chapter Four

1. Thomas Verny, M.D., and John Kelly, *The Secret Life of the Unborn Child* (New York: Summit Books, 1981), 20.

2. Ibid., 30.

3. John Bradshaw, *Reclaiming and Championing Your Inner Child* (New York: Bantam Books, 1993), 39.

4. Patricia Evans, *The Verbally Abusive Relationship: How to Recognize It and How to Respond* (Holbrook, Mass.: Bob Adams, Inc., 1992), 138.

5. June G. Bletzer, *Encyclopedic Psychic Dictionary* (Norfolk, Va.: The Donning Company, 1986), 649.

6. Thomas Verny, M.D., and John Kelly, *The Secret Life of the Unborn Child*, 85.

7. Marshall H. Klaus, M.D., John H. Kennell, M.D., and Phyllis H. Klaus, *Bonding* (New York: Addison-Wesley, 1995), 7.

Chapter Five

1. Deepak Chopra, *The Seven Spiritual Laws for Parents* (New York: Harmony Books, 1997), 46.

2. Gary Zukav, *The Seat of the Soul* (New York: Simon & Schuster, 1990), 41.

3. Rabbi Berg, *Wheels of a Soul*, 82, 123.

4. Alice Bailey, *Serving Humanity* (London: Lucis Trust, 1987), 253.

5. Karen Schultz, *A Theosophical Guide for Parents* (Ojai, Calif.: Parents Theosophical Research Group, 1984), 50.

6. Alice Bailey, *Esoteric Psychology II* (London: Lucis Publishing, 1988), 547.

7. Karen Schultz, *A Theosophical Guide for Parents*, 50.

8. Alice Bailey, *The Rays and Initiations* (London: Lucis Publishing, 1992), 337.

9. Alice Bailey, *Serving Humanity*, 55.

10. Marshall H. Klaus, M.D., John H. Kennell, M.D., and Phyllis H. Klaus, *Bonding*, xviii.

11. Corinne Heline, *Occult Anatomy and the Bible* (LaCanada, Calif.: New Age Press, 1937), 66.

12. Ibid., 63.

Chapter Six

1. Steven Raymond, "Cellular Consciousness and Conception: An Interview with Dr. Graham Farrant," *Pre- and Peri-Natal Psychology News* II (2) (Summer 1988): 4.

2. Ibid., 20.

3. Lisa Alpine, "When Are We Born?" *The Common Ground* 80 (Summer 1994): 156–57.

4. Ibid., 158.

5. Elizabeth Noble, *Primal Connections* (New York: Simon & Schuster, 1993), 144.

6. Ibid., 18.

7. Ibid., 159.

8. Geoffrey Hodson, *The Miracle of Birth*, 45.

9. Karen Schultz, *A Theosophical Guide for Parents*, 53.

10. David Chamberlain, *Updating Parents on the Sentient Prenate* (San Diego: self-published, 1994), 4.

11. Corrine Heline, *Occult Anatomy and the Bible*, 107.

12. Montessori International, ed., *The Science of Motherhood for the New Age* (1986), 40.

13. Ibid., 86.

14. Ibid.

15. Judith G. Bletzer, *Encyclopedic Psychic Dictionary*, 103–04.

16. Ibid., 5.

17. Luminare and Mini, Multidimensional Model of Preconception and Prenatal Care (PPPANA presentation).

18. Montessori International, ed., *The Science of Motherhood for the New Age,* 88.

19. Rabbi Berg, *Wheels of a Soul,* 78.

20. Montessori International, ed., *The Science of Motherhood for the New Age,* 88.

21. Ibid., 88.

22. Rabbi Berg, *Wheels of a Soul,* 134–35.

23. Allen J. Wilcox, Clarice R. Weinberg, and Donna D. Baird, "Timing of Sexual Intercourse in Relation to Ovulation," *New England Journal of Medicine* 333, no. 23 (December 7, 1995).

24. Honora Lee Wolfe, *Healthy Pregnancy, Healthy Birth,* 19.

25. Dosthora Mudalihamy Warnasuriya, *Sri Lanken Science for Conceiving Gifted Children* (Los Angeles: Divine Body Care, 1987), 31.

26. Corrine Heline, *Occult Anatomy and the Bible,* 68.

Chapter Seven

1. Thomas Verny, M.D., and John Kelly, *The Secret Life of the Unborn Child,* 62.

2. Ibid.

3. Karen Schultz, *A Theosophical Guide for Parents,* 51.

4. Manly P. Hall, *Man: The Grand Symbol of the Mysteries,* 109.

5. Richard Grossinger, *Embryogenesis,* 10.

6. Corrine Heline, *Occult Anatomy and the Bible,* 105.

7. Ibid., 102.

8. Richard Grossinger, *Embryogenesis,* 293.

9. Ibid.

10. Karen Schultz, *A Theosophical Guide for Parents,* 47–48.

11. Ibid., 57.

12. David Chamberlain, *The Mind of Your Newborn Baby* (Berkeley, Calif.: North Atlantic Books, 1998), 5–8.

13. Thomas Verny, M.D., and John Kelly, *The Secret Life of the Unborn Child,* 39.

14. David Chamberlain, *The Mind of Your Newborn Baby,* 11.

15. Ibid., 25.

Chapter Eight

1. David Chamberlain, Ph.D., *The Mind of Your Newborn Baby,* 105–120.

2. For information about William Emerson Training Seminars and Products, call (707) 763-7024; for Castellino Prenatal and Birth Therapy, call (805) 687-2867.

3. Marshall H. Klaus, M.D., John H. Kennell, M.D., and Phyllis H. Klaus, *Bonding,* 37–38.

4. Barbara Harper, R. N., *Gentle Birth Choices* (Rochester, Vt.: Healing Arts Press, 1994), 56.

5. Marshall H. Klaus, M.D., John H. Kennell, M.D., and Phyllis H. Klaus, *Bonding*, 38.

6. For an extensive catalog of books about the dangers of immunizations, contact New Atlantean Press at (505) 983-9638.

7. Michel Odent, M.D., *Birth Reborn* (Medford, N.J.: Birth Works Press, 1994).

8. Marshall H. Klaus, M.D., John H. Kennell, M.D., and Phyllis H. Klaus, *Bonding*, 188–197.

9. Murshida Vera Justin Corda, *Cradle of Heaven* (Lebanon Springs, N.Y.: Omega Press, 1987), 149.

10. Joan Salter, *The Incarnating Child*, 72–85.

11. Thomas J. Ritter, M.D., *Say No to Circumcision!* (Aptos, Calif.: Hourglass Book Publishing, 1992), last-page insert.

12. Ibid., 24.

13. Ibid., back cover.

14. Honora Lee Wolfe, *Healthy Pregnancy, Healthy Birth*, 77.

Chapter Nine

1. Marshall H. Klaus, M.D., John H. Kennell, M.D., and Phyllis H. Klaus, *Bonding*, 188–209.

2. Myla Kabat-Zinn and Jon Kabat-Zinn, *Everyday Blessings: The Inner Work of Mindful Parenting* (New York: Hyperion, 1997), 23.

Appendix D

1. Rabbi Berg, *Wheels of a Soul*, 70.

2. Judith G. Bletzer, *Encyclopedic Psychic Dictionary*, 462.

3. John Algeo, *Reincarnation Explored* (Wheaton, Ill.: The Theosophical Society Publishing House, 1987), 120.

4. See Geoffrey Hodson, *The Miracle of Birth* (Wheaton, Ill.: The Theosophical Society Publishing House, 1981), 84–87.

5. Carista Luminare and John Mini, "An Introduction to a Multidimensional Model of Preconception and Prenatal Health Care" (paper presented at the Fifth International Pre- and Perinatal Psychology Association of North America [PPPANA] Conference, Atlanta, 1991).

6. Alice Bailey, *Serving Humanity*, 29–30.

Recommended Reading

Self-Healing and Relationship Healing

Beattie, Melody. *Codependent No More*. San Francisco, Calif.: HarperCollins, 1987.

Bloomfield, Harold. *Making Peace with Your Parents*. New York: Random House, 1983.

Bradshaw, John. *Bradshaw On: The Family*. Deerfield Beach, Fla.: Health Communications, Inc., 1988.

————. *Homecoming: Reclaiming and Championing Your Inner Child*. New York: Bantam Books, 1993.

Chia, Mantak, and Maneewan Chia. *Healing Love through the Tao: Cultivating Female Sexual Energy*. Huntington, N.Y.: Healing Tao Books, 1986.

————. *Transform Stress into Vitality*. Huntington, N.Y.: Healing Tao Books, 1985.

Chopra, Deepak, M.D. *Ageless Body, Timeless Mind*. New York: Harmony Books, 1993.

Evans, Patricia. *The Verbally Abusive Relationship: How to Recognize It and How to Respond*. Holbrook, Mass.: Bob Adams, Inc., 1992.

Forward, Susan, and Craig Buck. *Toxic Parents*. New York: Bantam Books, 1989.

Gabriel, Michael. *Voices from the Womb*. Lower Lake, Calif.: Aslan Publishing, 1992.

Hay, Louise L. *You Can Heal Your Life*. Farmingdale, N.Y.: Coleman Publishing, 1984.

Hendrix, Harville. *Getting the Love You Want*. New York: Harper and Row, 1988.

Leonard, Linda Schierse. *The Wounded Woman: Healing the Father-Daughter Relationship*. Boston: Shambhala, 1992.

Maslin, Bonnie. *The Angry Marriage: Overcoming the Rage, Reclaiming the Love*. New York: Hyperion, 1994.

Noble, Elizabeth. *Primal Connections: How Our Experiences from Conception to Birth Influence Our Emotions, Behavior, and Health*. New York: Simon & Schuster, 1993.

Osherson, Samuel. *Finding Our Fathers: How a Man's Life Is Shaped by His Relationship with His Father*. New York: Fawcett Columbine, 1986.

Preconception and Prenatal Preparation and Health

Arms, Suzanne. *Immaculate Deception II: Myth, Magic, and Birth*. Berkeley, Calif.: Celestial Arts, 1994.

Baker, Jeannine Parvati, Frederick Baker, and Tamara Slayton. *Conscious Conception*. Monroe, Utah: Freestone Publishing Co., 1986.

Chamberlain, David. *The Mind of Your Newborn Baby*. Berkeley, Calif.: North Atlantic Books, 1998.

———. *Updating Parents on the Sentient Prenate*. San Diego, Calif.: self-published, 1994.

Conkling, Winifred. *Getting Pregnant Naturally*. New York: Avon Books, Inc., 1999.

Domar, Alice D., and Henry Dreher. *Healing Mind, Healthy Woman: Using the Mind-Body Connection to Manage Stress and Take Control of Your Life*. New York: Henry Holt and Company, 1996.

Edwards, Margot. *A Stairstep Approach to Fertility*. Freedom, Calif.: The Crossing Press, 1989.

Harper, Barbara. *Gentle Birth Choices*. Rochester, Vt.: Healing Arts Press, 1994.

Huxley, Laura Archera, and Piero Ferruci. *The Child of Your Dreams*. Rochester, Vt.: Healing Arts Press, 1992.

Nilsson, Lennart. *A Child Is Born*. New York: Dell Publishing Co., Inc., 1977.

Northrup, Christiane, M.D. *Women's Bodies, Women's Wisdom: Creating Physical and Emotional Health and Healing*. New York: Bantam Books, 1994.

Payne, Niravi B., and Brenda Lee Richardson. *The Whole Person Fertility Program: A Revolutionary Mind-Body Process to Help You Conceive*. New York: Three Rivers Press, 1998.

Peterson, Gayle. *An Easier Childbirth: A Mother's Guide for Birthing Normally*. Berkeley, Calif.: Shadow and Light Publications, 1993.

Queenan, John T., M.D., and Kimberly K. Leslie, M.D. *Preconceptions: Preparation for Pregnancy*. Boston: Little, Brown and Co., 1989.

Rich, Laurie A. *When Pregnancy Isn't Perfect: A Layperson's Guide to Complications in Pregnancy*. New York: Penguin USA, 1993.

Salter, Joan. *The Incarnating Child*. Glouchester, U.K.: Hawthorn Press, 1987.

Schwartz, Leni. *The World of the Unborn: Nurturing Your Unborn Child Before Birth*. Boston: Sigo Press, 1991.

Sussman, John R., and B. Blake Levitt. *Before You Conceive*. New York: Bantam Books, 1989.

Tannenhaus, Norra. *Pre-Conceptions: What You Can Do Before Pregnancy to Help You Have a Healthy Baby*. Chicago: Contemporary Books, 1988.

Verny, Thomas, and John Kelly. *The Secret Life of the Unborn Child*. New York: Summit Books, 1981.

Verny, Thomas, and Pamela Weintraub. *Nurturing the Unborn Child*. New York: Delacorte Press, 1991.

Weed, Susun S. *The Wisewoman Herbal for the Childbearing Year*. Woodstock, N.Y.:

Ash Tree Publishing, 1986.

Wolfe, Honora Lee. *How to Have a Healthy Pregnancy, Healthy Birth with Traditional Chinese Medicine*. Boulder, Colo.: Blue Poppy Press, n.d.

Metaphysical Perspectives and the Soul

Aivanhov, Omraam Mikhael. *Education Begins Before Birth*. Frejus Cedex, France: Editions Prosveta, 1982.

Bailey, Alice. *Education in the New Age*. New York: Lucis Publishing, 1981.

———. *Esoteric Psychology (I)*. New York: Lucis Publishing, 1984.

———. *The Light of the Soul*. New York: Lucis Publishing, 1989.

———. *Rays and Initiations*. New York: Lucis Publishing, 1992.

———. *Serving Humanity*. New York: Lucis Publishing, 1987.

Berg, Rabbi. *Wheels of a Soul*. New York: Kabbalah Learning Centre, 1995.

Besant, Annie. *The Necessity for Reincarnation*. Wheaton, Ill.: The Theosophical Publishing House, 1984.

Chia, Mantak, and Maneewan Chia. *Awakening Healing Light of the Tao*. Huntington, N.Y.: Healing Tao Books, 1993.

Crawford, Ina. *A Guide to the Mysteries*. London: The Lucis Press, 1990.

Fairfield, Gail. *Choice-Centered Astrology: The Basics*. Smithville, Ind.: Ramp Creek Publishing, 1990.

Grossinger, Richard. *Embryogenesis: From Cosmos to Creature—The Origins of Human Biology*. Berkeley, Calif.: North Atlantic Books, 1986.

Hall, Manly P. *Man: The Grand Symbol of the Mysteries*. Los Angeles: The Philosophical Research Society, Inc., 1972.

Hallet, Elisabeth. *Soul Trek: Meeting Our Children on the Way to Birth*. Hamilton, Mont.: Light Hearts Publishing, 1995.

Hardy, Jean. *A Psychology with a Soul*. New York: Viking Penguin, 1987.

Head, Joseph, and S. L. Cranston. *Reincarnation: An East-West Anthology*. Wheaton, Ill.: The Theosophical Publishing House, 1990.

Hodson, Geoffrey. *The Miracle of Birth: A Clairvoyant Study of the Human Embryo*. Wheaton, Ill.: The Theosophical Society Publishing House, 1981.

———. *Reincarnation: Fact or Fallacy?* Wheaton, Ill.: The Theosophical Society Publishing House, 1979.

Holmes, Ernest. *Living the Science of Mind*. Marina del Ray, Calif.: Devorss and Company, 1992.

Oken, Alan. *Soul-Centered Astrology*. New York: Bantam Books, 1990.

Schultz, Karen. *A Theosophical Guide for Parents*. Ojai, Calif.: Parents Theosophical Research Group, 1984.

Sonsino, Rifat, and Daniel B. Syme. *What Happens After I Die? Jewish Views of Life*

After Death. New York: UAHC Press, 1990.

Walsch, Neale Donald. *Conversations with God: An Uncommon Dialogue: Book 1*. New York: G. P. Putnam's Sons, 1996.

Whitton, Joel L., M.D., and Joel Fisher. *Life Between Life*. New York: Warner Books, Inc., 1986.

Zukav, Gary. *The Seat of the Soul*. New York: Simon & Schuster, 1990.

Birth and Early Parenting

Arms, Suzanne. *Adoption: A Handful of Hope*. Berkeley, Calif.: Celestial Arts, 1990.

Arms, Suzanne, Mary Renfrew, and Cloe Fisher. *Bestfeeding: Getting Breastfeeding Right for You*. Berkeley, Calif.: Celestial Arts, 1990.

Kitzinger, Sheila. *The Complete Book of Pregnancy and Childbirth*. Rev. ed. New York: Knopf, 1996.

Klaus, Marshall H., M.D., John H. Kennell, M.D., and Phyllis H. Klaus. *Bonding*. New York: Addison-Wesley, 1995.

Ritter, Thomas J., M.D. *Say No to Circumcision!* Aptos, Calif.: Hourglass Book Publishing, 1992.

Spiritual Parenting

Alexander, Shoshana. *In Praise of Single Parents: Mothers and Fathers Embracing the Challenge*. New York: Houghton Mifflin Company, 1994.

Berends, Polly Berrien. *Whole Child/Whole Parent*. New York: Harper and Row Publishers, 1983.

Chopra, Deepak, M.D. *The Seven Spiritual Laws for Parents: Guiding Your Children to Success and Fulfillment*. New York: Harmony Books, 1997.Glas, Norbert. *Conception, Birth and Early Childhood*. Spring Valley, N.Y.: Anthroposophic Press, Inc., 1983.

Gray, John. *Children Are from Heaven*. New York: HarperCollins, 1999.

Kabat-Zinn, Jon, and Myla Kabat-Zinn. *Everyday Blessings: The Inner Work of Mindful Parenting*. New York: Hyperion, 1997.

Infertility Education

Cooper, Susan Lewis, and Ellen Sarasohn Glazer. *Choosing Assisted Reproduction: Social, Emotional and Ethical Considerations*. Indianapolis, Ind.: Perspectives Press, 1998.

Indichova, Julia. *Inconceivable: Winning the Fertility Game*. New York: Adell Press, 1997.

Marrs, Richard, M.D., Lisa Friedman Bloch, and Kathy Kirtland Silverman. *Fertility Book*. New York: Delacorte Press, 1997.

Wesson, Nicky. *Enhancing Fertility Naturally*. Rochester, Vt.: Healing Arts Press, 1999.

Index

Page numbers followed by an *f* indicate information that is found in figures or illustrations.

Carista Luminare-Rosen, Ph.D., is a counselor in private practice, who specializes in holistic approaches to preconception and prenatal health care. For more than two decades, she has studied the essential elements that a new life needs for optimal development from the earliest moments of life. Her work has evolved into a synthesis of eastern and western philosophy, psychology, and health care that includes a thorough understanding of personality and soul development.

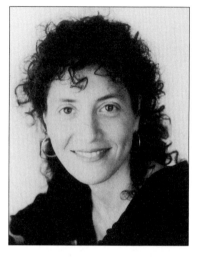

The founder and codirector of The Center for Creative Parenting in Marin County, California, Dr. Luminare-Rosen is a pioneer in the field of preconception education. She teaches classes and workshops throughout the world and lectures frequently at conferences, hospitals, and universities. Her holistic model of early preparation for parenthood has guided and encouraged thousands of women and couples.

She lives in California with her husband, Jared, and daughter, Kylea, with whom she continues to explore many of the themes offered in her work.